Colonial Madness

Colonial MADNESS

Psychiatry in French North Africa

Richard C. Keller

The University of Chicago Press
Chicago and London

Richard Keller is assistant professor of medical history and the history of science at the University of Wisconsin–Madison.

The University of Chicago Press, Chicago 60637
The University of Chicago Press, Ltd., London
© 2007 by The University of Chicago
All rights reserved. Published 2007
Printed in the United States of America

16 15 14 13 12 11 10 09 08 07   1 2 3 4 5

ISBN-13: 978-0-226-42972-4 (cloth)
ISBN-10: 0-226-42972-5 (cloth)
ISBN-13: 978-0-226-42973-1 (paper)
ISBN-10: 0-226-42973-3 (paper)

Library of Congress Cataloging-in-Publication Data

Keller, Richard C. (Richard Calvin), 1924–
    Colonial madness : psychiatry in French North Africa / Richard C. Keller.
       p. cm.
    Includes bibliographical references (p.   ) and index.
    ISBN-13: 978-0-226-42972-4 (cloth : alk. paper)
    ISBN-10: 0-226-42972-5 (cloth : alk. paper)
    ISBN-13: 978-0-226-42973-1 (pbk. : alk. paper)
    ISBN-10: 0-226-42973-3 (pbk. : alk. paper) 1. Psychiatry—Africa, North—History. 2. France—Colonies—Africa, North—History. 3. Psychoanalysis and colonialism—Africa, North—History. I. Title.
    RC451.A42K45 2007
    616.89'00961—dc22

                                                        2006026923

Contents

Acknowledgments

This book would have been impossible to write without the generous support of a number of organizations. The project began in the course of a fellowship from the Council for European Studies and a Fulbright award for study in France, which made much of the research possible. A Bernadotte E. Schmitt grant from the American Historical Association, a travel award from the American Institute for Maghrib Studies, and funds from the Department of History and the Center for Historical Analysis at Rutgers allowed me to conduct research in Tunisia. At the University of Wisconsin–Madison, funding from the Center for European Studies, the Office of International Studies and Programs, the International Institute, the Graduate School, and the School of Medicine and Public Health, along with a travel award from the Society for French Historical Studies, enabled me to conduct critical follow-up research in Paris, Nantes, and Aix-en-Provence. Special thanks go to the Department of Medical History and Bioethics, whose generous support has made this book possible in many ways.

I owe a great debt to Pierre Collombert and Elizabeth Marmot at the Franco-American Commission for Educational and Cultural Exchange in Paris, who facilitated my research in innumerable ways. Georgiana Colvile and Francine Muel-Dreyfus supported this project and provided useful guidance upon my arrival in Paris. Elisabeth Roudinesco invited me to her home (as well as her Freud seminar at the Université de Paris VII) on many occasions, opened doors to several collections, and introduced me to a number of scholars and psychoanalysts who shared my concerns. Françoise Vergès also offered encouragement and insight. At the Bibliothèque Médicale Henri-Ey at the Centre Hospitalier Sainte-Anne, I thank Alexandrie Argouse, Anastasie Melendo, and Nadine Rodary, who time and time again patiently pointed me in the right direction. I am indebted to the personnel at the Bibliothèque Interuniversitaire de Médecine, the Archives de l'Assistance Publique, the Archives Nationales, the Musée de l'Homme, the Bibliothèque Nationale de France, the Ministère des Affaires Etrangères in Paris, the Centre d'Archives d'Outre-Mer in Aix-en-Provence, the Centre d'Archives Diplomatiques in Nantes, and the Institut de Médecine Tropicale in Marseilles. In the United States, Micaela Sullivan-Fowler at the University of Wisconsin's Ebling Health Sciences Library has helped me track down crucial last-minute references, while Jack Eckert graciously allowed me access to Harvard's Countway Library during a fleeting trip to Cambridge.

Without the assistance of Jeanne Mrad and Riadh Saadaoui at the Centre d'Etudes Maghrébines à Tunis my research in Tunisia might have been fruitless. I also thank the personnel at the Archives Nationales de Tunisie, the Institut de Recherche sur le Maghreb Contemporain, the Institut de Belles Lettres Arabes, the Institut Supérieur d'Histoire du Mouvement National, and the Bibliothèque de l'Hôpital Razi-La Manouba, with special thanks to Habib Belaid, Mohamed Ben Achour, Hattem el-Hattab, Mohamed Larbi Ladab, and Fadhel Mrad. Annoir Tebsi graciously allowed me to tour the grounds at Razi-La Manouba and to read in the hospital's library. Meriem el-Gaid offered a helpful introduction to research in Tunis and shared her research on contemporary Tunisian psychology and psychiatry with me. Hamza Es-Saddam and Ridha Mabrouk exposed me to their knowledge of Tunisian medical history, while Lilia Labidi helped me to conceptualize some of this project's fundamental problems. I also thank Essedik Jeddi, who welcomed me into his home and presented me with a number of documents, as did Cherifa Ammar. Finally, Newine Eschadely generously allowed me access to crucial papers in her collection.

Conferences, seminars, and colloquia provided fertile venues for presenting drafts of several chapters. I thank participants at meetings of the Society for French Historical Studies, the American Historical Association, the American Association for the History of Medicine, the History of Science Society, and the Western Society for French History, and especially Alice Bullard, Alice Conklin, Michael Osborne, Torbjorn Wandel, and Gary Wilder for their comments on this project. Thanks also to audiences at the Clinical Ethnography Workshop at the University of Chicago, the History of Science Workshop at the University of Pennsylvania, Johns Hopkins University's History of Medicine Colloquium, and the Wellcome Unit for the History of Medicine at Oxford for their deep insight, and to

David Barnes, Nathaniel Comfort, Mark Harrison, Tanya Luhrmann, Sloan Mahone, Harry Marks, Randall Packard, and Megan Vaughan in particular. Kilala Ngalamulume and Paula Viterbo were gracious enough to invite me to present at their Health and Medicine in Africa Workshop at Bryn Mawr in April 2005, where my fellow panelists, and especially Jonathan Sadowsky, generously shared their ideas. Thanks also to the participants in the Globalizing the Unconscious Research Circle at the University of Wisconsin–Madison, where Warwick Anderson, Alice Bullard, John Cash, Joy Damousi, Didier Fassin, Christiane Hartnack, Deborah Jensen, Shruti Kapila, Ranjana Khanna, Lucienne Loh, Hans Pols, and Mariano Plotkin offered insightful readings of my work in an intense yet critical forum.

The Rutgers Center for Historical Analysis provided an environment conducive for early writing. Thanks to the center's members and staff for their assistance and contributions, and to Omer Bartov, Michael Burleigh, Eric Davis, Matt Matsuda, and Lynn Shanko in particular. An Andrew W. Mellon postdoctoral fellowship at Washington University allowed me to initiate the revisions process; many thanks to John Bowen, Derek Hirst, Walt Schalick, and Steve Zwicker for their support and criticism. Over the years since this project began, I have also benefited greatly from exchanging ideas with a number of colleagues and friends, including Fethi Benslama, Ben Brower, Brady Brower, Lauren Clay, J. P. Daughton, Malick Ghachem, Leor Halevi, Rick Jobs, Tamara Matheson, Roxanne Panchasi, Jared Poley, Todd Shepard, and Luise White, among others. This book benefited in particular from impassioned conversations with Lara Moore before her tragic and untimely death in 2003.

This project began as a dissertation at Rutgers University, where I had the privilege of working with an outstanding thesis committee that offered boundless encouragement, keen insight, and valuable comments. Michael Adas has become a trusted friend as well as a mentor, having guided me through the literature on colonialism and helped me to situate this project within the existing scholarship. John Gillis always kept me focused on wider themes in European history that touch on the scope of the thesis and provided especially useful comments on key chapters. Joan Scott tirelessly read chapters and offered pointed criticism as the project unfolded, and her seminars gave me a crucial grounding in the history of psychoanalysis before beginning work on psychiatry. Richard Serrano directed me to a number of sources on the twentieth-century Maghreb that I might have otherwise missed and provided useful comments on early drafts.

The University of Wisconsin–Madison has offered a perfect environment for completing this project. Graduate students and colleagues have provided encouragement, stimulation, and inspiration since my arrival in 2002. My colleagues in the Department of Medical History and Bioethics, and in particular, Warwick Anderson, Tom Broman, Judy Houck, Judy Leavitt, Gregg Mitman, and Ronald Numbers, have offered unflagging support, as have Jean Von Allmen, Lorraine Rondon, and Sharon Russ. Thanks also to my colleagues in History of Science, the African Studies Program, and the Robert F. and Jean Holtz Center for Science and Technology Studies, and especially to Joan Fujimura, Cindy Haq, Linda Hogle, Florence Hsia, Lynn Nyhart, Eric Schatzberg, Mike Shank, and Richard Staley. Graduate students such as Mitch Aso, Libbie Freed, Camilo Quintero, and Andrew Ruis, among others, have kept me on my toes. Thanks also to Bridget Collins and Kristen Hamilton for invaluable research assistance. Katie Gilbert, Sage Goellner, Aliko Songolo, and Soraya Tlatli generously read early drafts of chapter 5 and refrained from rolling their eyes at a historian's ham-fisted attempts to read literature.

In Bonnie Smith and Ronald Numbers I have had mentors of whom most scholars can only dream. From the very inception of the project, Bonnie provided inspiration, encouragement, and criticism, in addition to unfailing support at every step from dissertation to finished volume. She offered a constantly sympathetic ear, exciting new perspectives, and sharp insight into the project as it developed, and has always been ready to take an emergency phone call from Paris or Madison. This book would never have seen the light of day without her help, and I thank her for her guidance and look forward to her future support. Since our first meeting, Ron Numbers has been a tireless ally. He has always been willing to read a chapter—usually on very short notice—and his sage advice has never missed the mark. He has proven a daunting, yet always encouraging model to follow, and my thanks for his support are profound.

At the University of Chicago Press, Catherine Rice has been a staunch advocate for this project from the start. I have treasured her guidance, and especially her patience with a first-time author. Pete Beatty has cleared up a number of technical questions with great efficiency. Many thanks also to three anonymous referees who conducted very close readings of the manuscript and offered critical advice on improving the final product, to Barbara Norton for her expert copyediting, and to Rosina Busse for seeing the book through production. I of course accept all responsibility for any of the book's failings, especially where I have stubbornly held out against their counsel.

Friends and family provided a measure of sanity and kept me from losing myself completely in this project, while offering toleration and understanding as I immersed myself in research and writing. Many thanks to

Roberta Keller, Rod Keller, and Bruce Cramer, who each helped in their own ways. Thanks also to Jerry Keller, Gean and Bill Lyster, Joanne and Sean Williams, Autumn Marler, Lucy and Ben Cramer, Dianne Cramer, Helene Cramer, and especially Sarah Cramer, who is greatly missed. Jack Cramer has always known when to show up with a bottle of good wine. A special thanks must go out to my son, Max Keller, who arrived in tandem with the book contract and whose smile has often been enough to get me through the day after a sleepless night.

Words will never express clearly enough the immeasurable thanks and the debts that I owe to my wife, Brooke, for all she has done for me, but I will nevertheless try. Brooke has lived with this project every day, and how I might have coped with the difficulties of writing the book without her is unimaginable. Her support has been a constant presence through the highs and lows of research and writing, and I value it almost as much as I value her love. It is with love, then, that I dedicate this book to her.

For Brooke, with love, thanks, and boundless affection

Introduction
Madness and Colonization

Novelists, travelers, and physicians in the mid-nineteenth century conjured a North Africa that was a space of savage violence and lurid sexuality, but also a space of insanity. For many authors who passed through the region during a period of expanding European contact and influence, it was the madness of the Muslim world that constituted its fundamental difference from the West. "Egypt is bursting with hospitals," Maxime du Camp tells us, and it appeared only natural that in Cairo, one of the "largest" of them was "intended for madmen, whom one hears shrieking and moaning behind the thick walls of their padded cells."[1] Alphonse de Lamartine went a step further, proposing that madness offered a sympathetic means of understanding Muslims. The mannerisms of Lady Stanhope, his "Circe of the Desert," evoked "a studied, voluntary madness"; this form of her "génie" helped her to communicate with the "Arab populations living near the mountains" and elicited their "powerful admiration."[2] For his part, Gustave Flaubert suggested the corrupting power of prolonged exposure to this world of unreason. His ruminations on the tensions between reason and insanity in *La première éducation sentimentale* proclaim that the confinements of bourgeois society prompt his protagonist, Jules, to "create the *djinns*" that take him "into madness and into savagery."[3]

It is significant that Flaubert uses the Arabic *djinn*, rather than the roughly equivalent "spirit," as the vector of madness. Lamartine employs the French "génie"—a double entendre signifying "brilliance" and in this context "genie"—but the term conveys the same sense as Flaubert's *djinn*. Both locate

1

the source of madness in an Oriental empire of unreason, a place where surely the "largest" hospitals would house the insane. The authors exploit the central tropes of the Orientalist canon as their characters move into a fantastic space—a physical movement for Lamartine's Lady Stanhope, a figurative one for Flaubert's Jules.[4] Their displacement into another world strips them of Europe's cultural restrictions, giving free rein to indulgent reveries and dark emotional outbursts. Yet while this menacing presence of insanity threatens reason, the Orient is for these authors an experimental space, a blank slate for the inscription of European will. In their treatment of the psychological realm these works operate at two levels. Lamartine, Flaubert, and du Camp produce an Orient and its inhabitants as an absence of reason. But at another level this dehumanized space is a permissive one, one allowing European subjects to experiment while freed from the norms of bourgeois conduct.

A century later, a new literature placed the subject of North African madness in a different light. During the decolonization struggles of the 1950s and 1960s, and in their immediate aftermath, an emerging group of North African writers saw insanity as a consequence of the traumas of colonial rule and the transition to a development state. In autobiographical fiction and in his anticolonial treatises, the Tunisian author Albert Memmi argued that colonialism generated neurosis: the ambivalence of the civilizing mission, which preached the assimilation of France's colonial subjects yet erected insuperable barriers in their paths, wrought powerful emotional tensions by placing the colonized in an impossible position between tradition and modernity. The Algerian novelist and playwright Kateb Yacine employed a more extreme poetics of madness and violence. His works chronicled the anguish of the colonial world through the figure of the insane mother who watches her sons die in the service of revolution, a recurrent character in his works; her flights into madness constitute her primary form of resistance against colonialism's social and political order. For the Algerian author Rachid Boudjedra as well, the insane characters in his novels *La répudiation* and *L'insolation* reflect the chaotic tensions and internecine violence of a postcolonial society in a state of breakdown and disorder.

These two literatures of Islam and insanity—from the Orientalist traditions of the nineteenth century to an emergent postcolonial literature—bracket this story. *Colonial Madness* traces the path between these competing representations by focusing on those who developed the language of North African insanity most extensively. Near the turn of the twentieth century, French psychiatrists who toured and practiced in the colonies seized control of discussions about normality and pathology in Algeria, Tunisia, and Morocco. As the French settlement of North Africa increased—prompted by the loss of Alsace and Lorraine in the Franco-Prussian war and facilitated by the establishment of a Tunisian protectorate in 1881—psychiatrists carved out a new role for themselves as they sought to extend their discipline's authority into new terrains. In the 1880s they began a protracted period of lobbying for the establishment of colonial asylums as a key component of France's imperial project in North Africa. By the interwar period, as new psychiatric hospitals began to open in Algeria, Tunisia, and Morocco, Antoine Porot—the architect of most of North Africa's mental assistance programs—had begun psychiatric instruction at the Algiers Faculty of Medicine. Over the next two decades Porot produced a number of protégés, who contributed to the development of the "Algiers School" of French psychiatry. Members of the school published extensively and quickly became the French empire's leading authorities on the intersection of race and psychopathology by virtue of their daily contact with indigenous patients in colonial hospitals. Far from marginal, these practitioners' contributions to psychiatric research shifted the direction of the French psychiatric discipline between the First World War and the Algerian struggle for independence.

This book focuses primarily on the story of these doctors and their patients. It explores the genealogy and development of the idea of the Muslim world as a space of madness from the beginnings of colonial expansion to the present. Yet it also aims at a wider cultural history of the ways in which the theories, practices, and institutions of French psychiatry in colonial North Africa inscribed the idea of Muslim insanity in a medical language. In so doing it explores that discipline's principal themes—the notion of an inherent mental, intellectual, and behavioral rift marked by the Mediterranean, and the idea of the colonies as an experimental space freed from the limitations of metropolitan society and reason—and their resonance not only in a medical literature, but also, by the postcolonial era, in fiction, memoir, and film. It relates the ideas and practices of the colonial realm to more general developments in the psychiatric profession, and suggests how shifts in the fortunes and attitudes of empire and mental medicine contributed to the discipline's rise and, ultimately, to its decline.

The intersection of psychiatry and colonialism evokes for many the life and work of Frantz Fanon. A central figure in the emergence of the field of postcolonial studies, Fanon was born in Martinique and trained as a psychiatrist in France before moving to Algeria in the early 1950s, where he quickly sided with the insurgency during the decolonization struggle. For Fanon, Algeria was less a space of madness than it was a site of unbearable violence. His patients suffered not from a predisposition to mental breakdown, but instead from their subjection to the unspeakable brutalities of colonial domination. Fanon found science and medicine to be among the most insidious tools of imperial conquest. It was "a good thing," he asserted in 1959, "that a technically advanced country benefits from its knowledge and the discoveries of its scientists." But the colonial situation perverted this order. In the words of Hubert Lyautey, the French field marshal whose battalions conquered Morocco in 1912, medicine was less a healing art than it was "the only excuse for colonialism." Medical knowledge in Fanon's eyes became another source of colonial power, a technology of exploitation. It became a means of extracting intelligence from the colonized population and offered a venue for lording authority over the colonized patient.[5] Among the medical specializations, psychiatry presented the worst of these violations. Fanon's anticolonial manifesto *The Wretched of the Earth* concludes with a searing indictment of psychiatry as a critical weapon in the colonialist's arsenal. Psychiatry, Fanon argued, constituted a form of scientific violence directed against the colonized by seizing the North African in an inescapable language of inferiority and immutability. Beginning in the interwar period, psychiatrists in Algiers, in Blida, in Oran drew on their clinical material to model North African Muslims as "born slackers, born liars, born robbers, and born criminals."[6]

Psychiatrists in the Maghreb contributed significantly to the dehumanizing logic of colonial rule. Yet the history of the discipline is more complicated than Fanon suggests. By placing Fanon's attack on colonial psychiatry in a wider history of psychiatric theories, institutions, and practices, this book investigates the ways in which psychiatric ideas informed the colonial encounter. Psychiatry brought a new degree of sophistication to colonial racism. This was especially the case in Algeria, where a large settler population depended upon a rigid racial hierarchy as a means of defending its social and political status. Yet colonial psychiatry was more than a system for the defense of settler prejudices. At different periods, and from different perspectives, the field was less a weapon in the arsenal of colonial racism than it was a tool for the emancipation of the colonized, an innovative branch of social and medical science, an uncomprehending therapeutic system, a discipline in crisis, and a mechanism for negotiating the meaning of difference for republican citizenship.

. . .

Perhaps more than its rivals, France emphasized its colonial expansion as part of a larger project. The famous "civilizing mission" that undergirded French imperialism in the late nineteenth and early twentieth centuries incorporated a progressivist vision that sought the development of its colonies in every sense. Central to the project was the particularly French concept of *mise en valeur*. Often taken as synonymous with economic development, *mise en valeur* emerged as an important colonial ideology in the late nineteenth century. As historians Michael Osborne and Alice Conklin, among others, have noted, the concept marked a shift from the acquisition of new territories to the "rational" and "progressive" improvement of France's existing colonies. In its most basic sense, *mise en valeur* applied to the economic development of the colonies; hence its connotation of conferring value upon a decadent space. Its initial applications in West Africa, for example, unfolded as the construction of railroads and efforts to improve public health: such endeavors would foster communication and the movement of goods while assuring the best yield from the colonies' human capital. By the interwar period, *mise en valeur* had become a dominant component of France's civilizing mission in its colonies. The practical dimensions of the concept mostly remained limited to efforts to maintain a healthy labor force and to instill (often through forcible means) a work ethic in colonized populations as the backbone of rational colonial exploitation—especially important in a period of economic depression.[7]

Yet for many "progressivists" in colonial politics, the rhetorical uses of *mise en valeur* went far beyond the rationalization of labor. *Mise en valeur* meant the modernization of so-called primitive or barbaric worlds and their inhabitants through the construction of new cities, the education of colonial subjects, the recuperation of infertile soil, and the establishment of new institutions that sought to "civilize" colonial space and colonized peoples according to the ideals of republican virtue. As much recent scholarship has suggested, colonialism was a central element in the formation of the idea of modern citizenship itself. The colonial "primitive" represented a potential citizen in its most abstract form. The demands on settlers in the colonies both to set an example for the colonized and to defend European respectability were thus a driving factor in the making of modern citizenship rather than its result.[8] Psychiatry, along with other biomedical sciences, contributed profoundly to these diverse strains of *mise en valeur*. With their aim to produce physically and mentally sound subjects, epidemiologists, microbiologists, vaccinologists, and psychiatrists played significant roles in the integration of a healthy labor force with the demands of an increasingly globalized colonial market system. Yet they also contributed to debates over the potential citizenship—indeed, the civilization—of colonial subjects in a broader sense.

The role of science and medicine in these projects has generated intense interest among historians, literary critics, and anthropologists. For decades, scholars characterized colonial scientific development as following an established pattern of gradual diffusion as knowledge and innovation moved outward from Europe to the margins of empire.[9] By these accounts, activity at the periphery consisted of simple data gathering and specimen collection, dependent upon and derivative from the center, where prestigious institutions, associations, and organizations confirmed findings and generated conclusions. By the same token, the only legitimate scientific pathway from colony to colony passed through metropolitan sites such as London, Paris, and Amsterdam, hubs for the dissemination of imperial knowledge. Yet scholars from a range of disciplines now see a more complex interaction unfolding under imperialism. As Bruno Latour has noted for the case of Pasteurian biology, to cite one example, the entrepreneurial spirit of many settler scientists, the uses of science and technology in the ideological defense of domination, and the lack of professional scrutiny in many colonial settings created unique opportunities for experimentation and innovation.[10] According to much of this work, overseas territories served as vast laboratories for testing and perfecting a range of medical, scientific, and social projects before their implementation in European settings.[11] Global expansion was by this logic a constitutive factor in the development of modern science rather than its mere by-product.

In the history of psychiatry, however, the notion of productive cores and stultified peripheries has proven resilient. Such arguments appear to hold for the British case: with some notable exceptions, isolated physicians in Nigeria, in East Africa, and even in India with little or no psychiatric training offered, at best, custodial care for the insane and produced little durable research in the process.[12] In the French case—at least before the twentieth century—psychiatry was also largely a metropolitan affair. Whether one dates the origins of French psychiatry to Louis XIV's creation of the Hôpital Général in 1656, to Philippe Pinel's legendary (if apocryphal) liberation of the insane at Bicêtre during the Revolution, or to the law of 1838 that regulated the internment of lunatics, change radiates outward from a Parisian hub.[13]

When one considers the development of French psychiatry in the twentieth century, a different trajectory appears. Pioneers in the United States and in several European locations outside of France developed most of the discipline's novel concepts between 1900 and 1950. But these ideas crossed the Mediterranean to the French colonies in Algeria, Tunisia, and Morocco more easily than they crossed France's European borders. In the twentieth century, colonial psychiatrists honed their discipline's cutting edge by implementing these technologies at least contemporaneously with—and in many cases far earlier than—their metropolitan colleagues. Antoine Porot and his students saw the colonies as a medical void, an ideal experimental location for reinvigorating their discipline. They understood themselves as medical pioneers: rejecting alienism's entrenched traditions, they sought to replace the lunatic asylum of the nineteenth century with the psychiatric hospital of the twentieth, an innovative institution that would break down barriers between hospital and community. The mental assistance networks of French North Africa were therefore the first in the French dominion to develop comprehensive mental hygiene programs and to utilize "open" services to facilitate outreach into indigenous communities. They were also among the first to employ radical new somatic therapies for the treatment of mental illness. While scandal plagued outdated metropolitan institutions during the Second World War, colonial psychiatrists blazed a path toward a new code of mental health care by developing and implementing new ideas in hospitalization and legislation.

Yet colonial psychiatry has an ambivalent and troubling history. New facilities may have improved many patients' mental and physical conditions. But these patients also constituted a data set for wide-ranging forms of experimentation and the development of new knowledge. Much of this work undermined the benevolent image of colonial medicine's civilizing mission. The most novel element that colonial psychiatrists brought to their field was the development of an empirically based sub-specialty within the psychiatric discipline for the study of the relationship between race and mind. Psychiatrists inherited the assumptions of their literary predecessors as well as those of the settler communities in which they practiced, but in addition to granting a scientific veneer to existing prejudices, as these doctors developed into influential authorities on indigenous psychology, they shaped ideas about North African Muslims. Far from neutral, knowledge about North African Muslims' "primitive mentalities" and "criminal impulsiveness" often precluded their membership in the human community. Although based on observations of North African mental patients, French psychiatric knowledge claimed universal relevance, so that at their most inflammatory, psychiatrists proposed that the consciousness of the "normal" North African Muslim represented "a mixture of insanities in varying doses."[14] Most important, this knowledge consistently sought and found practical outlets: the new discipline of ethnopsychiatry informed educational and professional discrimination against Muslims, shaped discourse about immigration into France, and provided the essential background for the French army's psychological warfare programs during the Algerian struggle for independence.

This book explores the history of psychiatry in the French empire and the resistance it generated among patients and the general public by emphasizing this ambivalence. By exploring colonial psychiatrists' obsession with innovation and development, as well as the effects of the knowledge it produced, the book exposes the paradox of how a responsive, nuanced medical circle that positioned itself at the cutting edge of mental science could be at the same time a violent, uncomprehending, racist organism. This is in some ways a problematic endeavor. As several critics have noted, a focus on the colonies as a crucible for innovation and experimentation includes a troubling dimension: reading the colonies as a laboratory perpetuates the conceptualization of overseas territories as a space devoid of indigenous human agency by ignoring the resistance of the colonized.[15] Yet framing the question in this way provides both an opportunity to investigate the manner in which French colonial institutions produced a colonized subject who lacked the essential qualities of humanity and a means of revealing the precise contexts in which the colonized contested the violence of these assumptions.

The history of French colonialism—especially in settler colonies such as Algeria—is one of silence and denial: silence about the violent legacy of the colonial past and denial of the subjectivity of the colonized. As one French Algerian settler writes in her memoirs, "We knew hardly anything about the natives, and when someone asked, 'Was there anyone at the fair?' we sometimes heard the response, 'No, no one. Only Arabs.'" Of Arabs' miserable poverty, "we said, 'They're used to it. They don't *feel* like we do. They don't have the same needs as we do. . . . They are incapable. They refuse civilization.'"[16] Studies of colonial literature have drawn attention to this phenomenon. Emily Apter's work on Albert Camus, for example, highlights the "nullification of Arab characters" in his works: Algerian Arabs are either absent or appear only as underdeveloped set decoration.[17] But although scholars have noted the dehumanizing aspects of colonial history, they are only beginning to study how the processes of colonial dehumanization worked. As the psychoanalyst Fethi Benslama has argued, the most effective means to examine colonialism's negation of the humanity of the colonized is "through a meticulous investigative work which discerns the moments, the peoples, the acts" responsible for this process.[18]

Postcolonial literary critics have been at the forefront of this endeavor, drawing heavily on psychoanalytic concepts to explore the affective elements of the colonial predicament. Often reading Fanon's work on race and identity, violence and dehumanization, and the psychical suffering of the colonial subject through Freudian and Lacanian filters, scholars such as Homi Bhabha and Anne McClintock have identified sexuality, ambivalence, misrecognition, and the fetish as key concepts in the operation of colonial discourses of power.[19] Many of these questions pertain to the Maghreb as well, where a rigidly patriarchal social structure has prompted many critics to interrogate the Oedipal dimensions of social relations.[20] Yet during the colonial period, psychoanalysis was virtually absent in the Maghreb; indeed, Fanon himself was only marginally inspired by psychoanalysis, demonstrating far closer affinities to Hegel, Sartre, and phenomenology than to Freud.[21] More important, in the first half of the twentieth century, psychoanalysis and more orthodox strains of psychiatry were founded on different assumptions about the nature and origins of mental illness and the status of the patient. Most psychiatrists assumed a biological origin of madness, whether in the form of a cerebral lesion, a hereditary defect in the nervous system, or a racially determined organization of the brain structure. By contrast, psychoanalysis assumes the psychogenic rather than the organic origins of mental illness. These disciplinary paradigms entail crucial assumptions about the patient. For all its problems, psychoanalysis considers the patient as a subject—albeit one ruled by drives—who participates in the curing process. This theory therefore presupposes a certain degree of sophistication in the patient, which is inherent to the production of the psychological conflicts at the origin of neurosis and necessary to the patient's capacity to participate in the cure. Early-twentieth-century psychiatrists, by contrast, tended to view the patient as an object suffering from organic disorders, and their suppositions stigmatized the patient by proposing that a lesser degree of mental complexity lay at the root of mental illness. Psychiatry thus corresponded much more closely to a colonial order that constantly reiterated natives' biological inferiority, their simplemindedness, and their incapacity to adapt to modern civilization.

Almost unique among medical specializations, psychiatry draws at once on biological, physiological, behavioral, and social dimensions of the subject. For these reasons it has been a critical field in shaping ideas about race. Discussions about race have historically seized on any number of locations of potential difference, and especially the body. Disciplines such as physical anthropology and biology have therefore been central to these debates.[22] But the mind has also been a battleground in the struggle to understand race and difference. Psychiatry offers both obtuse and subtle forms of commentary about the phenomena that guide social knowledge about race, ethnicity, and difference. As a biological and medical science, it touches on the anatomy of the brain and the chemical pathways of thought and consciousness. As a social and behavioral science, it touches on intelligence and educability, but also criminality, recidivism, and the possibility of rehabilitation. Above all, psychiatry offers a medical language for framing the normal and pathological subject according to social and biological criteria, and therefore speaks of the capacity for adaptation of the psyche to a new mental environment—a critical point of contention in debates over French policies of assimilation, modernization, and civilization in the colonies.

This debate went through a range of permutations in North Africa in the nineteenth and twentieth centuries. Many Europeans in the colonies considered Muslim difference and the challenges of assimilation to be functions of psychology. As Gabriel Alapetite, resident-general of the Tunisian protectorate from 1907 to 1918, wrote upon retirement, "Long experience with Oriental Muslims only allows the European to understand one precise fact about their mentality: that their brain does not reason like ours."[23] Colonial psychiatrists argued that what settlers had long understood as an incapacity for logic revealed the Muslim's incapacity for civilization—and indeed, the Muslim's threat to the civilized order. Yet in the context of colonial psychiatric practice patients represented a destabilizing presence. The psychiatric encounter between French doctors and North African patients produced a key environment for resistance against colonial authority. In contrast with the insistent repetition that Edward Said presents in *Orientalism*, through which Western thought from Homer to *Harper's* has constituted a savage "Orient" as the obverse of Western rationalism, colonial psychiatrists' contact with real patients in changing historical contexts forced their rhetoric to evolve according to developments in psychiatric practice and along with crucial shifts in French colonial administration.

...

Colonial Madness examines the complexities of this question in the Maghreb, the region of northwest Africa that includes Algeria, Tunisia, and Morocco. But it is important to note the major distinctions that mark the national histories of the region. French expansion into the Maghreb followed a number of different spatial, temporal, and political trajectories. After conquering the city of Algiers in 1830, the French army engaged in a nearly two-decade struggle that ended in the effective pacification of Algeria and the proclamation of the territory as three French departments in 1848. By the late nineteenth century, in conjunction with the establishment of the Tunisian protectorate in 1881, Europeans began settling Algeria in significant numbers. France's strategic expansion into Morocco unfolded just a few decades later, with initial military incursions followed by the establishment of a protectorate in 1912. None of the territories was a colony per se. Algeria was a constituent component of the French interior, its European population enjoying full benefits of citizenship. By contrast, French residents-general administered Tunisia and Morocco as protectorates under the rubric of France's Ministry of Foreign Affairs, while indigenous authorities technically ruled their own populations. Even Tunisia and Morocco present startling differences considering their ostensibly parallel administrations. The French ruled Tunisia much like any other colony. Settlers, while smaller in number than in Algeria, held significant political authority through mechanisms such as the Tunisian High Council (Grand Conseil de la Tunisie, hereafter GCT), whereas Marshal Hubert Lyautey, Morocco's conqueror and first resident-general, ruled the protectorate with convincing authority. Although his policies ostensibly sought to preserve local interests and customs, his programs never precluded direct manifestations of French influence in Morocco.

Despite these important differences, geographical proximity and frequent contact among administrations ensured that French rule in the Maghreb shared certain characteristics. De facto segregation ruled, giving very few colonized subjects a political voice, and the sorts of large-scale projects that aimed to inculcate European culture in Muslims—including schools, museums, and hospitals—bore strong likenesses to one another. Medical projects, in particular, were integral to French efforts in all three domains. Colonial practice of course helped the careers of Nobel Prize winners such as Alphonse Laveran and Charles Nicolle, who capitalized on the prevalence of local infectious diseases to contribute to bacteriology and parasitology. But science and medicine were also instruments of colonial power that contributed to the advancement of France's so-called civilizing mission through what many scientists and colonial administrators labeled the "pacific penetration" of new regions. From the moment of the conquest of Algiers, natural historians, physical anthropologists, social scientists, and physicians developed far-reaching demographic, zoological, and biological knowledge about climate, race, and disease that frequently enhanced colonial power and marginalized indigenous populations.[24]

Throughout the Maghreb, clinical medicine and public health served as important initial sites of confrontation between colonialists and indigenous populations. The conquest of Algeria, for example, was construed in both medical and military terms: the French army's expedition in 1830 included nearly three hundred pharmacists, physicians, and surgeons, many of whom saw diagnosis and treatment as a contest over civilization as well as one over health and disease.[25] In Tunisia, medical "colonialism" preceded the establishment of the protectorate: European interventions in Tunis's typhus and cholera epidemics of the 1860s provided an entrée for French assertions of political control over the region.[26] The relationship was even more direct in Morocco. In 1907, a mob in Marrakech murdered

a French physician rumored to be working as a spy; reparations for the attack offered a pretext for invading the territory, a move the French had long
sought as a means of protecting Algeria's borders.[27]

Colonial medicine was only rarely consistent across space and time.
Whereas in the mid-nineteenth century, physicians worried about the
potential dangers of the Algerian climate for the European constitution,
within a few decades the ostensibly salubrious effects of sun and heat signaled the Maghreb as an ideal site for tuberculosis convalescence. By the
turn of the twentieth century, Biskra in Algeria was the logical setting
for the consumptive antihero of André Gide's *The Immoralist* to seek his
recovery. Medical and ethnographic knowledge about local populations
also varied widely. In Algeria, for example, physical anthropologists, physicians, and social scientists insisted upon a marked distinction between
the personalities, behaviors, and physiognomies of Arab and Berber populations for much of the nineteenth century. Yet with increasing colonial
settlement, the importance of these differences was gradually supplanted
by the more politically relevant boundaries between Europeans and Muslims. Likewise, colonial administrators and physicians insisted on marking
significant differences between the personalities of "typical" Algerians,
Moroccans, and Tunisians: where nineteenth-century physicians saw Algerians as tending toward violent criminality, for example, Tunisians were
often understood to be a more tranquil population.[28]

Yet any consideration of psychiatry in French North Africa benefits
from examining the region as a unit. Despite major ethnic and cultural
differences in the region, French psychiatrists in the early twentieth century treated the Maghreb as a piece. Psychiatric development unfolded simultaneously in Algeria, Tunisia, and Morocco: reformers in each context
spoke in unison, the same individuals conceptualized the major psychiatric
institutions in each country according to similar models, and the hospitals
began treating patients within several years of each other. Psychiatrists
in the Maghreb were in constant contact with one another and published
regularly in the same journals. Finally, and most important, while many
authorities recognized significant differences in populations both within
administrative regions and across national contexts, psychiatrists emphasized the shared characteristics of North African personalities. Although
psychiatrists occasionally discussed problems specific to Algerians, Moroccans, or Tunisians, by and large they saw hereditary biology and religious culture as contributing to a homogeneity of personality in North Africa unmatched in Europe, and used terms such as "Algerian," "Muslim,"
and "indigenous North African" interchangeably. As one author argued in
1913, "Observing the Arabo-Berber soul amounts to attempting to deter-

mine the product of the force and cohesion of many wide-ranging ethnic elements forged through heredity and education in a clearly shaped and rigid crucible: ISLAM."[29]

As an extension of this phenomenon, this book focuses on French psychiatry's intersection with indigenous populations in the Maghreb. French psychiatric hospitals in North Africa confined many European patients: in some cases they constituted roughly half of the patient population. Yet between the First and Second World Wars, psychiatrists dedicated their research almost exclusively to the study of normal and pathological psychology in the indigenous population. In the nineteenth century the reverse was true: physicians and psychiatrists worried constantly about Europeans' psychological capacity to live in the colonies. Even in the early twentieth century, European doctors argued that hot climates transformed the brain: one physician wrote in 1902, "As the thermometer rises physical and psychological strength diminishes," while another proposed that "the nervous system and the brain are hypersensitive to" the "abnormal conditions of temperature and light" that characterized colonial terrains.[30] Yet by the 1910s, medical theorists argued that the chief threat to European sanity in the colonies lay in tropical illnesses such as sleeping sickness or the victim's hereditary predisposition to madness, and that sound moral and physical hygiene could ward off the psychological effects of excessive heat. At the same time, the scientific vogue for the study of "primitivism" in the interwar period encouraged researchers throughout the empire to explore "indigenous mentalities." Thus, although colonial psychiatrists cared for Europeans and North African Muslims in roughly equal numbers, their research in the twentieth century focused almost exclusively on natives as they attempted to establish a psychiatric hierarchy of races.

...

Psychiatry accordingly offers a privileged site for the study of the relationship between knowledge and power under colonialism. This conjunction has encouraged a wave of critical studies of colonial psychiatry, most of which have taken the uses and abuses of psychiatry in the British Empire as their focus. Waltraud Ernst, for example, has signaled the ways in which colonial asylums functioned as key symbols of European civilization in colonial India, serving as markers of European medical superiority and sources for the propagation of the idea of benevolent rule.[31] For sub-Saharan Africa, Meghan Vaughan and Jonathan Sadowsky have produced fascinating studies of British efforts to define a specifically "African" insanity in Nyasaland, Rhodesia, Nigeria, and British East Africa.[32] Scholarship on psychiatry in French North Africa remains much more limited.

Aside from biographies and critical studies of Fanon (discussed in chapter 5), studies of French colonial psychiatry have been the work of practitioners rather than historians. The Algerian-born psychiatrist Jean-Michel Bégué, for example, has produced a remarkable thesis on the development of a racial ethnopsychiatry in Algeria between 1830 and the Second World War, and the psychiatrist Robert Berthelier has reiterated much of Bégué's work and extended its periodization to the postcolonial era.[33] Yet because of an exclusive focus on medical sources, their research remains limited: neither author explores the institutional, political, and social contexts for the development of knowledge about the "North African mind," for example, or the cultural dimensions of psychiatric practice in the Maghreb.

Colonial Madness tells a more complex story about psychiatry in the Maghreb by situating the field in a wide historical context. One way of examining this complexity is by focusing on the idea of *development* in colonial psychiatry. From the field's beginnings in the late nineteenth century through the present, development and its many possibilities have been a significant focus of psychiatry in the French empire. From the project of modernizing the colonies via the development of colonial space to the advent of the postcolonial development state, psychiatrists have insisted on their essential role in mediating change and facilitating progress.

Development and its potential applications in the colonial world—of the subject, of institutions, of knowledge—are central to this book. The first two chapters explore the question of psychiatric reform and colonial possibilities in the early twentieth century. Chapter 1 is the most rigorously comparative component of the book, exploring the condition of the mentally ill and reform efforts in Tunisia, Morocco, and Algeria respectively. The establishment of the Tunisian protectorate in 1881 and increasing European settlement in the Maghreb drew the attention of French doctors, students, politicians, tourists, and concerned citizens to the plight of the indigenous insane. For French psychiatrists, abusive treatment of the mentally ill in the North African colonies prompted a humanitarian call to arms. Images of fettered patients languishing in the *maristans,* or hospices for the mentally ill, called to mind the condition of the European insane before the reforms of the eighteenth century led by Philippe Pinel. Citing Pinel's legacy, French psychiatrists sought to modernize the care of the mentally ill in Algeria, Tunisia, and Morocco in the name of scientific progress. Their efforts, however, drew attention to the central paradox of asylum-based psychiatry. Reformers' propositions to deliver these patients from their chains aimed at confining the insane in institutional settings, limiting this liberation to the boundaries of the asylum. As with many of

France's colonial projects, psychiatry promised the Maghreb a form of emancipation that entailed submission to a European order.

Yet as chapter 2 illustrates, psychiatry in metropolitan France had itself reached a state of crisis. The asylum-based model of care through confinement that had marked the profession's development in the nineteenth century had largely failed as a therapeutic solution. Given the undesirability of merely transplanting a failed technology for the management of insanity to a new environment, the intense scrutiny of the problems that plagued the North African *maristans* also prompted a reassessment of the foundational principles of modern psychiatry. By focusing on the struggle to build a psychiatric infrastructure in Algeria in the 1920s, the chapter explores an emphasis on innovation that guided colonial psychiatry through the twentieth century. Psychiatrists such as Porot imagined North Africa as a blank slate, unencumbered by the mistakes of psychiatry's history in Europe. It was therefore fertile terrain for the implementation of a new model for the management of mental illness, one that fulfilled Pinel's legacy by "elevating the madman to the dignity of the patient." Where reformers in France had failed to remake the asylum in the same period, they succeeded in the colonies, marking North Africa as a site of innovation. Yet the debates that surrounded these innovations—which included the establishment of "open" psychiatric services in general hospitals and an emphasis on mental prophylaxis and acute care, as opposed to the custodial treatment of chronic patients—also entailed a debate over France's colonial obligations to its subjects. For those who saw colonialism solely as a system of economic exploitation, social commitments were an unnecessary distraction. But for those who saw imperialism as a project for the renewal of colonial space, *mise en valeur* necessitated investment in the colonial population and its welfare. The debate thus pitted the material economies of exploitation against moral economies of care in a moment that witnessed a reconsideration of the nature of the colonial project itself.

The next two chapters explore the operation of psychiatric institutions and the production of knowledge within their walls. Chapter 3 explores the everyday realities of life and practice in colonial hospitals. It analyzes the mechanisms of confinement that brought European and Muslim patients into psychiatric care and highlights the differences in their experiences of treatment. It also details the pragmatic effects of colonial psychiatrists' efforts to place themselves on the cutting edge of their field. Focusing on the period from the early 1930s to the mid-1950s, it explores a moment of prodigious experimentation in psychiatry that saw the development of a range of radical new technologies for the treatment of chronic patients, including the convulsive therapies and psychosurgery, but also a "softer" form of treatment in the form of social work and mental hygiene. These new treatments promised to bring psychiatry into parity with other medical specializations, but they did so at an often painful cost to the patient populations of the Maghreb. The "softer" treatments advocated by reformers in the 1920s—mental hygiene and social work programs—were implemented to great effect in Algeria's European enclaves, where they drew attention to the possibility of an effective management of society through the focused application of science. But Muslim patients constituted instead a field of experimentation for the testing of more invasive treatments. Chapter 3 explores the stories of these patients as a means of understanding the cultural rifts that opened in the colonial psychiatric clinic, in which the seeking of cures often amounted to a contest over cultural hegemony.

Chapter 4 elaborates the theoretical underpinnings of the knowledge these institutions produced. Beginning from an emblematic case history published in 1939, it traces the development of colonial psychiatric ideas as a practical form of knowledge. The psychiatrists of the Algiers School offered scientific support to settlers' prejudices, but they also changed the terms of discussion about indigenous mentalities. Whereas theorists in the mid-nineteenth century suggested that climate determined the Muslim's psychological difference from Europeans, Porot and his students insisted that the North African native's "primitivism" was overdetermined: Muslims' "bodies, culture, and traditions" prevented them from assimilating into French civilization. This "primitivism" manifested itself in a capacity for violent criminal impulses—especially sexual violence. These ideas enjoyed an extensive circulation. Members of the Algiers School published widely in prestigious medical journals, and by the 1950s they had become France's foremost authorities on ethnopsychological phenomena. More importantly, ideas about Muslim psychological difference had multiple practical outlets. Psychiatrists argued that colonial initiatives such as education were wasteful, because the Muslim was incapable of adapting to civilization, and proposed that these funds be directed to other institutions that could preserve the colonial order, chiefly police forces and psychiatric hospitals. In France, mental health practitioners and criminologists cited works by the Algiers School to support their demand for an end to immigration, which in their view threatened to overwhelm France with criminal lunatics from North Africa. Psychiatric ideas also played a significant role in the interpretation of the origins and course of the Algerian war for independence by contributing to programs for *action psychologique*, or psychological warfare. This was a logical culmination of psychiatrists' emphasis on the utility of their research, which they had deployed as a weapon in the interests of colonial rule since the beginning of the twentieth century.

Both the military form of *action psychologique* and the scientific racism of psychiatry in the service of empire elicited strong reactions from North Africans. Frantz Fanon, the Algiers School's most prominent detractor, was merely one voice in a cacophony of protest against colonial psychiatric racism in the twentieth century. Chapter 5 argues that Fanon must be placed in a wider context of resistance that included not only physicians, but also budding postcolonial theorists such as Albert Memmi and fiction writers such as Kateb Yacine. An analysis of works by Fanon's contemporaries—especially Kateb—reveals the extent to which colonized intellectuals inscribed their experiences of suffering and violence in a medicalized language. Central themes for Fanon, including the psychological effects of colonialism, the violence of the colonial encounter, and the regulatory function of colonial psychiatry, made lasting impressions on North African novelists, political theorists, and physicians who contested the colonial order. Borrowing from recent work in medical anthropology, Chapter 5 charts the development of an intellectual culture of resistance that took aim at medical and psychiatric forms of knowledge while highlighting the experiences that shaped local imaginings of violence and suffering in the twentieth-century Maghreb.

Chapter 6 explores the broad legacy of colonial psychiatry for the relationship between France and North Africa in the postcolonial era. Through an analysis of postcolonial film, literature, and medical writings, it highlights the vestiges of the Algiers School's work in the global present as well as the ongoing resistance it has engendered. At once an intellectual history and a cultural study of the postcolonial period, it speaks to the problems of dislocation, deracination, and development that have shaped political and social debates in France and the Maghreb, particularly those over immigration, the place of multiculturalism in the republic, and the place of the welfare state in the resource-poor postcolony. Chapter 6 details the ways in which psychiatrists have sought to smooth both France's and the Maghreb's transitions to global modernity, but also highlights the ways in which that transition has forced both sides to confront the traumas of decolonization and the violences of the colonial past.

...

This book argues that studies of colonial psychiatry must explore more than the field's contributions to medical racism. Scientific racism was of course central to the colonial psychiatric encounter. But illustrating that colonial psychiatrists were bound by their cultural roots shows only the most apparent aspect of a complex historical problem. As the Moroccan psychoanalyst Jalil Bennani argues, putting historical personalities and disciplines "on trial" is not the only way to elucidate the ways in which race operated as an organizing category in colonial psychiatry.[34] As a location for historical and ethnographic inquiry, colonial psychiatry provides a new lens through which we can interpret the intentions and realities of the civilizing mission. European psychiatry may have brought measurable improvement to the care of the mentally ill, but rather than using technological advances as apologias for psychiatry's darker side, we can look at the ways in which colonial politics used the establishment of medical institutions and assistance networks to perpetuate the illusion of Western munificence. Lay sources offer a means of situating colonial medicine in its social context and reveal the experiences of patients and their families with confinement. If European psychiatrists saw the development of colonial mental institutions as a key location for reinvigorating their field, a study of the day-to-day operations of colonial hospitals can reveal distinctions between the realities of colonial practice and the ideals behind these systems.

Colonial psychiatry represents one instance of scientific collusion with a racist social and political regime. But the field also included a utopian dimension, in which psychiatrists saw the future of mental medicine unfolding before them in their grandiose dreams of revolutionizing the profession. This vision entailed a blindness to the agency of the colonized, one that psychiatric theories about indigenous mentality supported. Only by denying the legitimacy of Arab medicine could psychiatrists conceptualize the North African colonies as a medical void. The chapters that follow address the ways in which the two principal aspects of colonial psychiatry—institutional innovation and the dehumanization of the colonized—were inextricably entwined. Psychiatrists such as Antoine Porot and his students saw North Africa not only as an experimental space for testing new institutional structures, new medical legislation, and new therapies before importing them back to the metropole. They also saw the Maghreb as an ideal space for redefining psychiatry as a discipline with multivalent practical applications. But the insistent presence of the colonized reveals that despite psychiatrists' intentions to deploy a unidirectional exercise of medical power in the colonies, the colonial psychiatric encounter was a site of intense contestation and negotiation of authority.

1

Pinel in the Maghreb
Liberation and Confinement in a Landscape of Sickness

Two photographs illustrate one of the defining paradoxes of French psychiatry in the North African colonies. The first was taken by two French physicians during a 1910 investigation of treatment for the mentally ill in Morocco (figure 1). At the request of the French Ministries of the Interior and Public Education, Solomon Lwoff and Paul Sérieux toured the countryside inspecting the kingdom's *maristans*, a survey undertaken as the French prepared for the establishment of an official protectorate in the region. Depicting a mental patient's thin, childlike legs and feet locked in crude fetters atop an intricate carpet, the image juxtaposes the barbarism and refinement that characterized North African Islam in much of French Orientalist discourse. The doctors indicated that the fetters "are formed from a plate of heavy iron . . . pierced with holes at each end which allow half-spiraled rings to pass through, encircling the ankles. . . . Walking is quite painful and falls are frequent."[1] They also noted other signs of brutality in the *maristans*: the insane were usually provided insufficient shelter and subsisted on food offered by charitable relatives.

The second photograph illustrates a transformation in care for the insane in Morocco under French control (figure 2). This image, published in a 1949 issue of *Maroc médical*, shows the realization of French psychiatric advocates' goals. Depicting an isolation ward in the Berrechid Psychiatric Hospital, founded in 1920, the photo presents a Moroccan orderly in Western medical dress looking into the camera as a nurse stands further down the hall. Locked doors line the corridor like perspective guidelines, suggesting an infinite capacity for confinement. Tiny windows

19

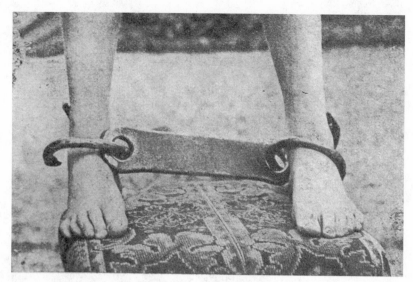

Figure 1.   A Moroccan patient in leg irons. From Solomon Lwoff and Paul Sérieux, "Sur quelques moyens de contrainte appliqués sur les aliénés au Maroc," *Bulletin de la Société clinique de médecine mental* 4 (1911). Reprinted by permission of Bibliothèque nationale de France.

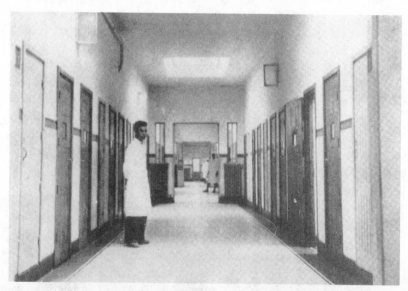

Figure 2.   Isolation ward at the Berrechid Psychiatric Hospital. From C. A. Pierson, "L'assistance psychiatrique au Maroc," *Maroc médical* (April 1949). Reprinted by permission of Bibliothèque nationale de France.

allow physicians to observe confined patients. Mechanical restraint has become unnecessary: architecture and the watchful eyes of a carefully trained staff appear to provide a hygienic, modern alternative to the harsh realities of confinement in the *maristans*.[2]

This chapter follows the sequence of these images in demonstrating how a simultaneous emphasis on liberation and confinement marked the movement to reform mental health care in French North Africa. Like psychiatric reformers in Enlightenment Europe, colonial psychiatrists in the early twentieth century sought to deliver North African lunatics from their chains. Loudly proclaiming the humanitarian motives for these concerns, they proposed significant improvements in conditions for the care of the indigenous mentally ill. Yet the rhetoric of emancipation also conveyed passionate advocacy for the extension of psychiatric influence and authority into the colonies. Colonial psychiatric reformers tempered their call for deliverance by proposing the further confinement of an even larger proportion of the insane in more humane institutions, limiting this liberation of the colonial mad to the boundaries of the asylum. As often as they decried the brutal conditions for the confinement of the Moroccan, Algerian, and Tunisian insane, they also lamented that vast numbers of mentally ill North Africans were left to their own devices in cities and villages, where they posed a significant threat to public safety.

French psychiatric reformers in the Maghreb shared a vision of the North African colonies as a prime terrain for the reenactment of their profession's foundational myth, Philippe Pinel's liberation of the insane in Paris's Bicêtre and Salpêtrière hospitals during the French Revolution (figure 3). As the legend goes, in a fit of utopian fervor, Pinel brought the ideals of liberty, equality, and fraternity to those most marginalized of *citoyens*, replacing the bonds of the insane with the invisible chains of the asylum and its injunction to moral responsibility. Arguing that these chained "beasts" were so unmanageable "only because we have deprived them of air and freedom," Pinel sought to reconfigure the clinical relationship as one between doctor and patient, rather than one between trainer and animal. Historians have since demonstrated that the story is apocryphal.[3] Yet this vision of modern psychiatry as a liberating force had enormous symbolic value and was constantly invoked by French psychiatrists in the course of the nineteenth century. The framing of the nascent psychiatric profession in the language of emancipation highlighted a victory of science and civilization over ignorance and tyranny. Yet as the psychiatrist Jacques Postel has argued, this representation amounted to an "alibi" for the continued subjugation of the insane to medical and state authority for much of the nineteenth century.[4]

The Pinel myth merges seamlessly with a commonplace theme in colonial

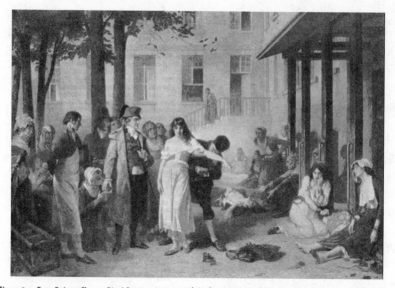

Figure 3.   Tony Robert-Fleury, *Pinel Freeing the Insane* (1887). Bibliothèque Charcot, Hôpital de la Salpêtrière, Paris. Public domain.

literature: the trope of sickness and suffering in exotic landscapes. Missionaries, explorers, travelers, and physicians frequently portrayed the voyage into colonial space as a regressive journey away from civilization into a foreign universe of misery, filth, and infectious disorder. Yet, at least in the case of North Africa, they also connected this decadence to republican ideologies about the "civilizing" project of French imperial expansion. Borrowing from the work of Jean Comaroff and Sander Gilman, I suggest that French colonial physicians' readings of madness in North Africa consistently invoked the theme of the "suffering native": a figure who at once signaled the collapse of an exotic society into a state of morbid decay and heightened a sense of French accomplishment in a recalcitrant zone.[5] Through its emphasis on the humanitarian impulses of medical progress, the Pinel legend echoed a range of other colonial mythologies of regeneration and renewal. It suggested the capacity of psychiatric science to blaze a pathway of enlightenment through a landscape of sickness in order to conquer the tyranny of madness and injustice in a space that colonialists imagined as having rejected modernity centuries earlier. As Françoise Vergès has argued, both the Pinel legend and colonial psychiatry functioned as "screens" that concealed political agendas with medical language.[6] Psychiatric reformers promised the emancipation of North Africa's Muslim population from its own barbaric customs, but, as with the colonial civilizing mission, the deliverance they promised entailed the expense of a transition to European institutionalization.

"The Moral Conquest of the Native": Framing Madness in Tunisia

By the end of the nineteenth century, references to insanity had become a cliché in the accounts of Orientalist writers, artists, and physicians who traveled through North Africa. The North African insane represented an essential component of the Orientalist tableau—a picturesque symbol of the pathological strangeness of a civilization in decline, representing the frisson of moral transgression that these authors found so emblematic of the Muslim world. Yet none so compellingly captures the ambivalence provoked by the insane as Guy de Maupassant in his 1887 description of the Sadiki hospital in Tunis. Curiosity drove him to the hospice—an institution for male lunatics founded in 1663—but upon witnessing the hospital's interior, he "could scarcely dream of what made [him] want to go there":

> All around me, on all four sides of the courtyard, narrow cells with bars
> like cages confined men who rose up when they saw us, and pressed their
> hollow, pallid faces between the iron bars. Then one of them, extending
> his hand and shaking it outside his cage, shouted some insult. The others,
> jumping up suddenly like animals in a zoo, raised their voices, while in the
> upstairs gallery, an Arab with a large beard, his head covered with a thick
> turban, his neck encircled with copper necklaces, let his bracelet-covered
> arm and ringed fingers hang over the balustrade. He smiled at hearing this
> noise. He is a madman, free and calm, who believes he is the king of kings
> and that he reigns peacefully over the furious madmen confined below.[7]

As he surveyed this mad dominion, Maupassant found these "frightening and admirable demented men in their Oriental costumes" to be "more curious . . . by virtue of their strangeness, than our poor European fools." Some of these madmen had only recently arrived; others, like the "king," had been there for over a decade. Some had "a rare beauty" and a "perfect distinction"; others were more disconcerting. Sensing "a breath of unreason penetrating into [his] soul, a contagious and terrifying emanation," Maupassant departed the hospital with mixed emotions, "full of pity, perhaps desire, for some of these hallucinating men."[8]

Maupassant also recounts his "horror" at their state. The madmen he describes are "furious," "frightening," "terrifying"; their actions are "frenetic" and "vigorous," and the ambient sound is "a continuous laughter with a menacing air." Disturbing though their condition may have been, for Maupassant there was no question that they required enforced isolation. In addition to their unpredictability and agitation, these dangerous madmen exhaled their "breath of unreason," a "contagious" force that taunted society with its

inscrutability. Maupassant's fantastic narrative is emblematic of the idiom in
which French reformers spoke of madness in North Africa, manifesting both
fear of and fascination with the indigenous insane: a sentiment underscored
by the implication that only French assistance could improve their lot.

Maupassant wrote at a moment of expanding French authority in the
Maghreb. Algeria had experienced some degree of French direction since at
least the 1830 conquest of Algiers, and certainly since the 1848 proclamation of the territory as three French departments. Yet the displacement of
populations through political upheaval in France, Spain, and Italy in the late
nineteenth century, which unfolded alongside the establishment of the Tunisian protectorate in 1881, contributed to the massive civilian settlement of
Algeria. By the 1890s, French military and civilian expansion into Morocco
appeared imminent.

Despite major differences in the political administration of the Maghrebian
territories, key ideological similarities marked much of colonial rule in the
region. Chief among these was an emphasis on French renewal or regeneration
of a decadent space. Often citing the legacy of Roman imperial expansion
into the region, many French administrators and settlers saw themselves as
renewing Latin influence in North Africa, which had been under assault since
the spread of Islam to the Maghreb in the early medieval period. By the early
twentieth century, this notion had profoundly shaped French colonial sentiment, having attained what Patricia Lorcin has called "the status of foundation myth" in Algeria in particular, where links to a Roman heritage across
the Mediterranean fostered a "spiritual" connection between settlers and
Maghrebian soil.[9] Ideals of renewal worked in the other direction as well: many
of those who touted this link to North Africa's Roman past saw the colonial
project as capable of regenerating not only a "decadent" society and a dead
landscape, but also a lost culture of Latin greatness that had been weakened
through overcivilization in the modern era. The "rebarbarization" of French
culture through settlement in a harsh terrain meant that colonial *mise en valeur*
promised lasting benefits for both the Maghreb and for France.[10]

These dual mythologies of regeneration deeply influenced medical projects
throughout the Maghreb. Across the region, physicians played key roles as
promoters of France's civilizing mission, shoring up in turn the broader mission of French colonial rule. Psychiatrists in particular spoke in unison about
poor provisions for the indigenous and European insane in Algeria, Tunisia,
and Morocco, arguing that traditional means of caring for the insane in the
Maghreb were intolerable blemishes on France's record of North African
administration. Yet they also clearly saw the reform of colonial institutions as
a strategic tool for the regeneration of a profession—and a national psychi-

atric tradition—that they perceived to be in sharp decline at the turn of the twentieth century.

As Jan Goldstein has persuasively argued, the making of a psychiatric profession in France was a process of long duration rather than a circumscribed event.[11] Yet the discipline's most pervasive symbol, the asylum, remained fixed for much of the nineteenth century. Beginning with the medical reforms instituted under the French Revolution and Napoleon, the first half of the nineteenth century witnessed the development and consolidation of most of the key principles and strategies that marked French psychiatric orthodoxy for the next hundred years. Many of the profession's initial practitioners were concerned principally with the organization of an appropriate institutional and therapeutic structure for managing insanity according to rational-positivist principles. Early psychiatrists such as J.-E.-D. Esquirol dedicated significant energy to devising an elaborate administrative structure to guide state policy on the insane. A student of Pinel and an important theorist of insanity, Esquirol played a key role in designing the law of 30 June 1838, which established asylum psychiatry as the sole legal model for the care of the insane.

Beginning with Pinel in the late eighteenth century, alienists imagined the asylum as a revolutionary healing technology. With its rigid classifications of patients both by disorder and by disposition, the asylum placed a premium on the function of confinement for the reordering of the mind. Esquirol was convinced that isolation "acts directly on the brain," with the effect of "repressing the liveliness and mutability of impressions" and "moderating the exaltation of ideas and affectations" in asylum patients.[12] But this emphasis on the asylum as a therapeutic machine necessitated strict professional control to prevent abusive internments and to offer patients the best possible prognosis. Diagnostic science and classification were emphasized because only an accurate picture of the patient's illness could maximize the possibility of a cure through the properly directed influence of the alienist.

Where French institutional psychiatry saw the asylum and its practices (including water treatments, work therapy, sedation, and confinement itself) as a panacea for a range of disorders, North African Muslims coped with mental illness in a number of ways.[13] Many in the Maghreb recognized no distinction between illnesses of the mind and those of the body; the pluralism that obtained in much of North African medicine therefore marked approaches to mental as well as physical disorder. Although the tradition of humorally based Avicennian medicine that had prevailed in the court culture of many medieval Islamic cities remained influential in those circles into the early modern period (and in some sectors to the present), by the late nineteenth and early twentieth centuries this tradition had largely given way to positivist medicine among the ruling elites of Morocco and Tunisia, as well as many Algerians. Among the urban poor and in rural areas, however, the early modern period had witnessed the rise of the *marabouts*, or spiritual healers (from the Arabic *m'rabit*, or "man connected to God") and cults of saints, which constituted a significant challenge to both humoral and positivist medical traditions, and which remain a primary source of healing for many contemporary North African Muslims.[14] The therapeutic strategies embraced by the *marabouts*, especially for milder afflictions, were largely benign. Many patients sought religious forms of healing for illnesses they believed originated in possession by *j'nun*, or invading spirits. The *marabouts* therefore practiced exorcisms, proposed means for reconciling oneself to possession, and offered protection against future possessions. For the chronically or violently ill and for those without the means to seek spiritual forms of healing, treatment was both more limited and more severe. Families often kept their insane relatives locked in the home to protect them from themselves and others. For those who proved uncontrollable in the home, however, and those without family resources, the standard response was confinement in the *maristans*.

The *maristans*, from the Persian *bimaristan* (house for the sick), originated in Baghdad in the ninth century. In the medieval *maristans*, physicians treated the insane at public expense according to orthodox Islamic medical theories, which drew on Galenic ideas about humoral pathology (and Avicennian revisions of them) as the explanatory framework for understanding sickness and health. Practitioners administered water treatments as a means of rectifying bodily equilibrium in addition to soothing patients with music and aromatherapies.[15] The institutions spread through the Islamic world, and by the fifteenth century hospitals had opened in Kairouan, Salé, and Fez. Yet by the late nineteenth century, most of the North African *maristans* had abandoned their therapeutic functions and merely served as decrepit housing for the mentally ill. Patients in this period tended to come from disenfranchised groups and entered the *maristans* after scandalous behavior brought them to police attention. With most patients spending only three or four days in wretched conditions before being sent back to the streets, the hospices' punitive dimensions earned them a notorious reputation.[16]

Beginning in the late nineteenth century—concomitant with the Third Republic's increasingly pronounced rhetoric about the "civilizing" capacity of colonial expansion[17]—French descriptions of the *maristans* seized on this reputation, singling out these institutions as characteristic of the brutality and decline of Muslim civilization. A description of the Sadiki published by the physician Gaston Variot in the *Revue scientifique* in 1881 indicates how doctors and scientists adapted the lurid rhetoric of Orientalist writers as a means of promoting change. After wandering through "many twists and turns in narrow alleys of the Souk," Variot found that the exterior of the hospital looked "not at all different from the other Moorish houses" in the Tunis medina. But Variot was aghast at what he saw inside. On the ground floor, the cells "only receiv[ed] air and light from the door that opened onto the courtyard." At his feet lay "a blind old man sleeping on a damp woven mat, covered up to his waist with a worn woolen blanket. On his doorstep, a clay bowl in which someone had left a pittance for him." Sickly, feverish patients lay in a "sad, wasting state." The upper story was populated by patients held behind iron bars: "They are, for the most part, completely naked in their cells, I should say in their cages. Heavy chains fixed to the wall . . . fettered the most agitated" among them.

The sensational images of the Tunisian insane in Variot's description suggest an analogy to the Pinel myth: an enlightened physician tours a wretched space, moved by the sight of chained, pathetic inmates languishing in their own filth. Perhaps most disturbing to Variot was the absence of professionalism at the hospice. The very appearance of Dr. Kaddour, the hospital's director, stunned him: "his manner had nothing of the medical about it; he wore a large red *chechia* and a *gandourah* like a true Tunisian."[18] The hospice lacked administrative offices or an admissions bureau, and was unprepared to treat any medical or surgical problems, leading Variot to conclude that the Sadiki was "scarcely, strictly speaking, a shelter." This was a common complaint. Psychiatrist Auguste Voisin, who toured the Sadiki in the late 1890s, focused on the absence of bureaucratic procedure as he decried the feeble administration of the hospice: he was horrified to find that "Arab lunatics are admitted and held in the hospital quarters without a certificate, and they are released without a certificate": even those patients "recognized as madmen in the prison . . . are admitted without a certificate of mental alienation."[19]

For French critics, a lack of professionalism lay at the root of the Sadiki's problems. This assertion was at the core of Henry Bouquet's thesis, "Les aliénés en Tunisie" (Lunatics in Tunisia), which appeared a decade after Voisin's observations. The most extensive analysis of the lunacy problem in the protectorate, Bouquet's study of Jewish, Muslim, and European methods for coping with insanity detailed the plight of the entire Tunisian population of the mentally ill. Asserting that France "was the nation of Pinel and Esquirol," Bouquet concluded that formal assistance for the colonial insane was thus "very much the order of the day." Tunisia was a "racial crossroads" where "the most diverse ethnographic origins encounter one another," and the protectorate thus constituted a crucial location for a sophisticated mental assistance network. Because each race had its "own defects, predispositions, and reactions," each of these populations naturally had its own means of managing the insane.[20] None was without major problems. Tunisia's Jewish community attempted to care for the mentally ill through family charity, but many Jews lived in abject poverty, limiting their means to provide adequate care: Bouquet found the "horror" of many of Jewish Tunisians' hovels "impossible to translate."[21] The situation for European settlers was also "deplorable." Tunis's European hospital (the Hôpital Civil Français, or HCF) was ill equipped to handle psychiatric cases. The hospital had no therapeutic capacity, and architects had "*not even foreseen the separation of the sexes!*" Such inattention to detail gave rise to scenes of debauchery, including seduction games and jealous riots among the inmates. Among other incidents, Bouquet described "a vicious epileptic seeking to awaken the ardors of a demented senile man"—only "Providence" had prevented the arrival of an "enfant du miracle" in this "phalanstery."[22]

The only alternative to confinement in this "shameful penal colony" consisted in transporting particularly difficult cases to asylums in France. Yet records show that this proved a cumbersome, protracted, and ineffective solution. As in Algeria, many European settlers in Tunisia were originally from Italy or Malta; yet unlike the Algerian case, where the law of 26 June 1889 had extended French citizenship to all those of European descent born in the colony, non-French Europeans in Tunisia did not share this privilege. Departmental asylums in France therefore often refused admission to such patients, forcing protectorate authorities into extensive negotiations with foreign ministers and shipping companies to secure transportation of these patients back to their nations of origin, their placement in hospitals, and payment of all associated fees. Beyond the expense and bureaucracy, such transfers also offered increased opportunities for dangerous patients to escape custody, as happened with one Spaniard in April 1921.[23] Even for French citizens, transportation across the Mediterranean was carried out in "disastrous conditions": a long passage under a police guard led to long-term confinement away from one's family, with poor prospects for a cure.[24]

Egregious as conditions for Europeans and Jews may have been, Muslims posed the greatest problem to solve. Bouquet argued that Muslims tended to treat violent madmen with the utmost brutality. Confinement in the "penitential system" of the Sadiki and Tékia hospices was an atrocity: "Everything here has a miserable air about it," and "one breathes in a bizarre indefinable odor, a mixture of antiseptic fumes and the foul stench of the incontinent." The tiny cells reminded Bouquet of "dark and musty dungeons," furnished with only straw mats and blankets. One patient was practically "naked, wrapped in a torn and sodden *burnous*." The twenty patients confined here often burst into spontaneous brawls, and "the asylum's neighbors . . . continually gripe about the din and the screams that emerge from here." The Tékia, a facility for Tunisian women founded in 1775, was cleaner than the Sadiki, and its whitewashed walls and well-maintained tile floors provided a "cheerful clarity in this lunatic ward," but the cells resembled "cages," several with chains attached to their walls. The "establishment [was] generally in good order," but the building's architecture and the use of the straitjacket as the sole means of treatment indicated that a "penitential" rather than a medical atmosphere surrounded the Tunisian response to mental illness.[25]

Ironically, Bouquet argued, Tunisians in fact venerated the mad, and only turned to such hostile measures when patients became unmanageable. Yet this epistemological difference in the interpretation of madness precluded the possibility of submitting the insane to medical treatment. Tunisians "consider[ed] the insane not as sick patients, but as the possessed, who should be respected" rather than healed. Moreover, conditions in the *maristans* discouraged Tunisians from bringing deranged family members to authorities' attention, with the consequence that most Arab lunatics were "confined, chained, and hidden away, but at home." For Tunisia's indigenous mad, Bouquet concluded, "it is either too much freedom or confinement that is too severe"—a predicament that demanded French intervention. In the same way "Pinel" had "elevated madmen to the dignity of patients," medical patrimony obliged France to renovate Tunisia's mental health care system. Hospitals that segregated violent and calm patients and that substituted "all means of restraint" with "direct surveillance" offered the only means for improving the lot of Tunisia's mentally ill, a move that mandated French investment in modern facilities for their care.[26]

Although powerful, these critiques remained isolated until taken up by French psychiatry's most powerful professional organization. The Congress of French and Francophone Alienists and Neurologists (Congrès des médecins aliénistes et neurologistes de France et des pays de langue française) first addressed the problem in 1908, when a delegate discussing the plight of the colonial insane argued that "in the country of Pinel, such a state of affairs should not exist."[27] By 1912 the organization took decisive action on the issue, electing to hold its meeting that year in Tunis. As a means of celebrating the inauguration of a neuropsychiatric clinic at the European hospital in Tunis, the Congress made "the grave and important question of assistance for lunatics in our colonies" the meeting's central concern.

Emmanuel Régis, a professor of psychiatry, and Henri Reboul, a physician and the director of public health in Indochina, presented the meeting's plenary report on colonial psychiatric assistance. Arguing that colonial dominion "created not only rights, but also imperative duties," the authors asserted that foremost among these was the "duty of medical assistance" to those in need.[28] The report attracted significant attention from medical and lay audiences alike. Gabriel Alapetite, Tunisia's resident-general, acknowledged the vast progress made by France in the protectorate, which, "scarcely thirty years ago, was several centuries behind in the path to civilization." But noting that the French had "not yet brought sufficient improvement" to the mentally ill, Alapetite indicated that "the moral conquest of the native through medical welfare is a long-term effort" to facilitate French interests in North Africa.[29] Antoine Porot, who founded Tunis's psychiatric clinic for European settlers in 1911, agreed. A product of the Lyon medical faculty, where he trained under the psychiatrist Jean Lépine, Porot had moved to Tunisia in 1907 and practiced general medicine until opening the neuropsychiatric clinic. Porot, who became in the interwar period the French empire's leading proponent of establishing pioneering institutions in the colonies, already found medical work "one of the most powerful means of penetration" in colonial terrains and urged the government to "complete this assistance and extend it to the natives whom France has the duty to protect."[30] Echoing Bouquet, Porot argued that the "penitential" environment of Tunisia's "notoriously insufficient and insufficiently organized" hospices needed to be "completely modified"; most important, it was "necessary to create an insane asylum in Tunisia *as soon as possible*."[31]

Conceding the point, the Tunisian interior ministry began preliminary studies for an asylum. The outbreak of war in 1914 tabled the plans, however, and significant problems continued to beset psychiatric assistance in the protectorate. For example, the Tunisian criminal code of 1913 stipulated that mentally ill criminals be confined "in the interest of public security."[32] Compounding the problem, in 1920 the resident-general promulgated the French law of 1838 in Tunisia, mandating the internment and observation of French lunatics in Tunisia.[33] Yet facilities for confining these cases remained limited. Conditions at the Tékia and Sadiki hospices had declined, if anything, since Bouquet's analysis. Porot's tiny ward at the European hospital, meanwhile, had no secure facilities for violent patients. Tunisian lunatics confined in their homes or wandering through villages represented a constant threat to public order. Finally, even as the newly created Tunisian High Council (Grand Conseil de la Tunisie, or GCT), the protectorate's main fiscal assembly, authorized the construction of the Manouba Hospital for Mental Diseases on the outskirts of Tunis in the early 1920s, conservative members stalled the project.[34] As one official phrased the problem, "To spend four or five million per year to care for madmen when we don't have enough food for our hospitals and clinics [is] the real act of madness."[35]

In the face of this opposition, reform activists redoubled their efforts. Some members of the GCT's Tunisian Section joined the campaign, bringing isolated Tunisian voices to the debate. Mahmoud Cheffnoufi asked in a 1925 report: "What, gentlemen, is more miserable than the state of abandonment in which our insane patients stagnate, packed far too tightly into makeshift premises as poorly adapted as possible to the conditions of modern hygiene? . . . Is this not a situation worthy of moving us, and could we remain insensitive to this lot so deserving of our compassion and pity?" The indigenous population, he argued, had the right to expect better from the administration.[36]

Several of the GCT's French delegates joined Cheffnoufi. One physician-delegate described the Tékia as "a tragedy whose horrors cannot be described."[37] Another called the Tékia a "Hell" and a "garden of supplication." A native confined in the Tékia "is considered as erased from the realm of the living: that's the situation. They inflict treatments on the patients in this hospice that you would not find in Chinese torture." Many Tunisians kept their mentally ill relatives at home "to avoid these tortures," and the delegate accused the government of racist inaction: "Your Commissions have swept away these projects because they only pertain to Muslims!" Even the protectorate's interior director acknowledged that conditions in the Tékia were an atrocity. Designed for forty patients, the Tékia currently interned seventy-five, forcing many patients to share the tiny cells, facilitating the spread of infection: of 120 patients who passed through the Tékia in 1925, nineteen died of tuberculosis.[38]

Resident-general Lucien Saint responded to such criticism by commissioning an independent report on Tunisian health services in early 1926. The report described the Tékia as "a scandal and a defiance of the most basic humanitarian sensibilities," where three and four patients often shared cells designed for one. Several had died from exposure, given their cells' feeble shelter from the weather. Because the asylum had no therapeutic facilities, one was forced "to watch powerlessly the passage to chronicity of mental disorders at the same time as the evolution of tubercular infection." The author found the patients' condition the most powerful evidence for the urgency of reform:

> This one is young and pretty. Dressed in her beautifully colored finery as if for a reception, she was seated behind her iron bars and repeated with a gentle obstinacy, in French: "Bonjour, Monsieur. Tomorrow, I will leave." She said this with a calm stubbornness, without raising her voice, without anger, without gesture, while in the neighboring cell, in a striking contrast, one saw an idiot's face, frighteningly ugly, dazed, with a hanging lip, fixed like a stone. It is profoundly sad, like the spectacle of all human decay! But another courtyard reserves a horrible impression for the visitor!
>
> The door opens. What are these furious barks? Completely naked, squatting, clinging to the heavy bars, slavering, frothing, this unchained demented woman leaned toward the one who approached her and she bayed, she bayed desperately. Suddenly, the raucous scream stopped, her fiery eyes

fixing furiously like those of a defensive guard dog, her spittle hissed and the scream started again, more violently until [her voice] cracked. Next to her, a little thing rolled in a ball threw itself right, then left, like a poor squirrel in a cage, without a sound, then stopped itself in the corner, like a bat. Then this little thing, which was a thinking being, began pounding a pendulous, rhythmic beat, in a jerking movement of her head and shoulders, chanting the scream of this furiously frothing woman. . . . It is terrifying![39]

Whereas the Tékia confined its patients too brutally, the Sadiki was too lax: Potentially rabid patients who had been bitten by mad dogs were sent to the Pasteur Institute for vaccines "in complete freedom, unguarded, across the city," and escapes were frequent. The reporter noted, "How beautiful the sun is when leaving this place! It is urgent to begin construction on the pavilions at La Manouba." He concluded that the "creation of a psychiatric asylum thrusts itself on us" for two reasons: because patients "have the right to medical care, but also because they are dangerous for themselves, for those around them, and finally for public order. It is not only a humanitarian question, but even more it is a question of social security."[40]

In the same year, the nascent asylum's director, Dr. George Perrussel, clarified the issue. The brutality of confinement exacerbated Tunisia's other major problem with the insane: those who wandered the streets or otherwise escaped official attention. The *maristans* "enjoyed so sinister a reputation" that it was unsurprising that "so many lunatics are hidden and sequestered at home for as long as possible."[41] This theory resonated with medical and public officials, whose fears fixated on the vast numbers of *aliénés en liberté*. The "stagnation" of the insane in cages like "wild beasts" posed an affront to humanitarian sensibility, but every unfettered lunatic also constituted an impending threat to public safety. France's administrative responsibilities mandated reform of hospital conditions, then, if only as a means of establishing public order.

This awareness fostered a transition in the language and strategy of colonial psychiatric reform from the mobilization of concern to a mobilization of resources. With the endorsement of key political figures, psychiatrists emphasized the palpable dangers posed by madness in colonial society while insisting on the obligation France had to serve its colonial subjects. Administrators sympathetic to the cause of psychiatric reform sought to quantify the dangers presented by the native insane. In 1921, the residence-general attempted to determine "the numbers of individuals susceptible of forming the population of the envisaged asylum, and their approximate classification."[42] Responses signaled the presence of several hundred freely roaming lunatics who represented a clear danger to public safety. Yet this figure most likely underestimated the population of the untreated insane: as one district officer noted, since Tunisians were "generally reluctant . . . to be separated from their lunatic relatives," he had only reported the number that was unambiguously "recognized as dangerous" in the region.[43] The study outlined a scenario in which local ideas about the nature of mental illness and a failure to recognize the legitimacy of Western medicine conspired to preserve the dreadful status quo. Officials contended that superstition and fear made most Muslim families guard their sick relatives at home, while trepidation about the *maristans* discouraged active reporting of cases. As the district officer mentioned earlier noted, Tunisians scarcely appreciated the "care given in asylums": instead, their "conception of madness makes them prefer the direct or indirect intervention of *marabouts* to that of physicians."[44]

In amassing these statistics, protectorate administrators, psychiatrists, municipal authorities, settlers, and Tunisian Muslims collaboratively framed a pattern that became visible only in its aggregate form. As historians and anthropologists have noted for other contexts, projects such as these contributed to broad endeavors of colonial governance. Establishing dossiers and case files for recognized yet unconfined lunatics in Muslim communities rendered that population visible and knowable for the first time.[45] As with other forms of sanitary policing, censuses of madness sketched the colonial population in all its variances.[46] Yet they also revealed an elaborate calculus of risk and pointed to clear strategies for optimizing safety in colonial space.

The solution therefore lay in constructing a gentler asylum with an immeasurably greater reach. Other problems also pointed toward the construction of the Manouba hospital. Perrussel had been hired to direct the asylum in 1924, but when construction lapsed he spent his time "doing his best to care for patients at the Tékia" and "for all lunatics for whom he is consulted."[47] Yet he needed an asylum to put his years of French institutional training to work, and his public salary had been squandered for the past two years while he served as a little more than a warden. Moreover, the transportation of mentally ill French settlers to metropolitan asylums—along with their guards—entailed inordinate expenses and extensive paperwork for Tunisian officials.[48] Considering these escalating costs, along with the tandem issues of philanthropy and fear surrounding the Tunisian insane, those who had initially resisted funding the hospital relented, dedicating nearly half the public works budget for 1927 to the hospital's construction.[49]

Barbarism and Decay: Hygiene, Persuasion, and Reform in Morocco

In October 1951, a French public health official in Morocco alerted his superiors to what he considered an extraordinary political opportunity. French authorities had recently completed construction on the new Sidi Fredj *maristan* in Fez. This was a hospice designed to care for mental patients according to their own traditions, but in a space that conformed to French hygienic standards. An inauguration ceremony—with the Moroccan sultan presiding— would offer a venue for French authorities to demonstrate publicly "that the Protectorate respects Muslim traditions and revitalizes them, by bringing them into harmony with the needs of hygiene and the teachings of modern science." Moreover, the ceremony provided an opportunity to stage a "demonstration of a political order" that would display the ways in which the French had invested heavily in "a domain that interests Moroccans alone." To facilitate this goal, the official offered to produce a press release on the conditions of Morocco's *maristans* prior to the establishment of the protectorate, detailing "their decay, their decrepitude, even their inhumane character." Such a report "would allow anyone of good faith, who was concerned about this issue, to determine the road taken since that date."[50]

Issued forty years after Lwoff and Sérieux published their survey of Morocco's *maristans*, the report recapitulated their findings. The author signaled the plight of the mentally ill as a metaphor for the larger decline of Moroccan civilization since the medieval period, but simultaneously pointed to the protectorate's efforts to incorporate Moroccan traditions in its institutional reforms. "In the eleventh century," for example, Morocco's Andalusian kings created "a hospital without equal in the world," graced with shade trees and fruit orchards, plentiful running water, marble baths, and rooms whose "luxury surpassed description." Cured patients were even given a stipend to reestablish their lives upon release. Yet with the collapse of the Almohad and Marinid dynasties, Morocco's hospitals fell into "a state of decadence." By the early sixteenth century, the *maristans* had become purely custodial facilities, offering little in the way of treatment to inmates who relied on charity in order to survive. Held in cells "deprived of both air and light," patients were locked away by request of their families and by order of the pasha—a procedure recalling the Bourbon monarchs' use of *lettres de cachet* to confine enemies of the regime or wayward nobles under France's ancien régime. Even in the twentieth century, patients languished in *maristans* such as Sidi Fredj, "chained practically naked, resting on the bare ground amid their own excrement." The "repugnant filth" and "nauseating stench" that emanated from the hospice shocked the senses, and as patients often exceeded available space, "some slept outside, chained to the columns of the courtyard." At Sidi Ben Achir in Salé, starvation compounded such filth: with "*no regular sustenance*" patients "died little by little from deprivations of all kinds, without anyone pitying them or caring for them." One visitor claimed that the "madmen of Sidi Ben Achir" were at "the last stage" of misery.[51]

The report and its context highlight major themes in the struggle to reform the *maristans* across the Maghreb but also point to significant Moroccan particularities. Physicians and politicians employed similar sanitarian and humanitarian rhetoric in Tunisia toward the goal of establishing modern hospitals in a European mode. Yet in Morocco, an ideology of "indirect rule" shaped a complex public health discourse. The explicit use of health care as tool for political persuasion—rather than domination—was more pervasive in Morocco than in France's other North African colonies, informing the development of hybrid institutions unimaginable in the more assimilationist regimes to the east.

Upon the establishment of the protectorate in 1912, French observers found Morocco's health problems to be far more deeply rooted than those of the rest of the Maghreb. Thirty years of occupation in Tunisia—and eighty in Algeria—had provided significant opportunity for authorities to establish programs designed to "modernize" public health infrastructure. Morocco had had no such "advantages," having remained stubbornly resistant even to the Ottoman colonization that had so powerfully influenced Tunisia and Algeria since the seventeenth century. It was thus the region's *timelessness* that most powerfully impressed many French observers, who characterized pre-protectorate Morocco as a space of sickness and death, forsaken by modernity. Morocco was a "vast country, nearly as big as France," but one where "the absence of bodily hygiene, the precariousness of the environment, the ignorance of basic rules of collective hygiene, and periodic famines" marked a state of general "anarchy."[52] In the domain of public health, "everything remained to be done": according to one critic, "in a word," authorities were forced to "*equip* the country in the fashion of a modern nation."[53] Summing up a career beset by such difficulties, the protectorate's public health director, Georges Sicault, characterized the hygienist in Morocco as condemned to performing a "balancing act, with one of his feet planted in the twelfth century, the other in the twentieth."[54]

The situation of Morocco's mentally ill was particularly troubling. *Maristans* operated throughout the protectorate, confining patients in wretched misery, while administrators continued to evacuate French patients to metropolitan asylums, resulting in further bureaucratic complications. Hubert Lyautey's particular approach to the protectorate form in many ways compounded the problem. Powerfully committed to medicine as a tool for colonization, Lyautey threw his influence behind the construction of modern institutions, such as the Berrechid Neuropsychiatric Hospital, which opened in 1920. Yet Lyautey effectively established a system that provided modern facilities for Europeans while leaving Moroccans to fend for themselves in more "traditional" settings. In this way, the program of psychiatric reform bears a powerful resemblance to urban planning initiatives in the protectorate. As Paul Rabinow has characterized the problem, Lyautey sought to invigorate the protectorate without eviscerating tradition through mindless assimilation of Moroccan society into a French state. In theory, these programs had the potential to produce a seamless integration of modern hygienic standards of urban organization with Morocco's "timeless" society and culture. The reality, however, was decidedly less successful. As with the inauguration celebrating the opening of the Sidi Fredj *maristan* in 1951, such programs amounted to little more than a staging of reform: in Rabinow's words, a "theatrical" performance of indirect rule's capacity to shepherd the protectorate toward modern civilization while preserving its exotic essence. Yet also like the inauguration of Sidi Fredj, the protectorate's approach to health reform was explicitly political. As with education and housing, a rhetoric that emphasized both preservation and modernization betrayed a dual standard for the remaking of colonial space, one that provided extensively for Europeans while condemning Moroccans to substandard facilities.[55]

Pre-protectorate accounts of conditions in Morocco's *maristans* emphasized rampant mismanagement that affronted both the humanitarian and the coercive impulses of modern medicine. Lucien Raynaud, the inspector general of public health in Algeria, published a "Study of Hygiene and Medicine in Morocco" in 1902, a decade before the establishment of the protectorate. Raynaud found the Dar-el-Arifa prison in Marrakech to be emblematic of other such facilities in Morocco. A women's institution that dated to the sixteenth century, it "still serve[d] as an asylum for the mad." Inside, the "prostitutes bear chains, and receive beatings." Wrongful internment was common. Husbands incarcerated disobedient wives with horrifying frequency and disastrous consequences: a woman here immediately "became the prey of libertines," and "when she has spent the night in Dar-el-Arifa, there is nothing left to do but divorce her."[56] In Tangiers, another *maristan* was reminiscent of Louis XIV's Hôpital Général: "These rooms are in reality dungeons, locked with padlocks, and aerated only by a small dormer window installed above the door; they confine madmen, the sick, the poor." Twenty patients lived together in three tiny cells, where "the greatest uncleanliness reigns" and "the stench of dirty rags, rotten food thrown in all the corners, and spaces that have never been cleaned or washed follows you long after you have left." Such brutal confinement constituted only part of the problem, as these same prisoners wandered freely through the city in the daytime: "The lodgers are only there at night; during the day they are found in the street or go into the city to beg for alms."[57]

Raynaud and other critics argued that Morocco desperately required enlightened technologies for coping with insanity, as much for public safety as for the care of the sick. Doctors Lwoff and Sérieux, who led the official investigation of Morocco's *maristans* in 1910, concurred: they found that most lunatics "who appear to be inoffensive wander freely," while those who became dangerous were either chained at home or thrown in prisons. Visiting the Sidi Fredj *maristan* at Fez, the doctors appear as anthropologists coming across a lost tribe, witnesses to a barbaric culture of madness. Describing themselves as the first Europeans to enter the hospice, they found "fifteen patients, their iron yokes around their necks, pulling forcefully at their chains so they could come as close as possible to these unfamiliar visitors."[58] Lwoff and Sérieux lamented that despite Muslims' extensive advances in mental medicine during the medieval period, a civilizational decline had preserved only the most uninformed elements of treatment. Most patient care consisted of "benevolent, demonic, or Koranic magic, or magico-medical practices, all having the same goal of expelling demons." And as most of the insane wandered the streets with no supervision, one "cannot exaggerate the role of lunatics in Muslim countries as disturbers of public order." Even in France, unhindered lunatics committed crimes every day; in Morocco, the authors assumed, the problem could only be worse.[59]

Lwoff and Sérieux's papers provided substantial evidence for the 1912 report on colonial mental assistance presented at the Tunis psychiatric congress, where Régis and Reboul concluded that "it is certainly premature to speak here about assistance for lunatics in Morocco."[60] But as in Tunisia, the outbreak of war swept aside all questions of colonial social welfare. Immediately after the war, however, Lwoff and Sérieux picked up their campaign with renewed vigor, asserting that French dominion over Morocco obliged the Republic to dedicate significant resources to the care of the insane. Employing the standard combination of philanthropic pleas and scare tactics, Lwoff and Sérieux sent a copy of their report to the French foreign minister, arguing that "it appears to us as if the time has come to pursue our mission and bring it to a good end." Virtually "everything remained to be done." The immediate construction of an asylum was crucial in order to provide medical care for deserving patients and to protect the innocent public: the presence of "unrecognized lunatics" in every Moroccan city was responsible for "numerous acts of violence (murders, rapes, arson, rebellions)."[61]

Such achievements contributed to the persuasive image of Lyautey's capacity to rule through investment rather than coercive domination as a means of consolidating French authority in Morocco. Yet although some portrayed these achievements as heroic, the reach of these facilities was decidedly limited, as the case of patient M. illustrates. M. had been interned in the Rhône departmental asylum after killing his parents in Lyon in 1919. Yet the asylum discharged him as "completely cured" in the beginning of 1921, and he moved to Tangiers. After committing an unspecified crime, he was placed under medical observation in Morocco. Medical authorities eagerly sought his placement at the Saint Pierre asylum in Marseille, citing a lack of local psychiatric resources. But the placement reveals the protracted negotiations required for the internment of colonial patients: some twenty-five exchanges passed between seven different agencies in France and Morocco, and five years after his internment M.'s Mediterranean passage still had not been paid by any authority.[62]

This new assistance network also served only European patients, accomplishing little for Morocco's indigenous insane—those singled out by Raynaud as well as Lwoff and Sérieux as most in need. As with M., some indigenous patients found themselves interned in metropolitan asylums.[63] But for the majority of Moroccan patients, the *maristans* remained the primary institutional recourse, and efforts to improve them were slow-going. In graphic 1925 testimony about the persistence of abominable conditions at the Sidi Ben Achir *maristan* in Salé, one witness offered a familiar litany of criticisms. Finding "several unfortunate souls deprived of their reason confined in narrow cells, without air or light, and with such low ceilings that even a short man could not stand erect," the observer was incredulous that "such an establishment" could exist "in the twentieth century, within a French protectorate." The site was filthy: patients "bedded down in their own excrement and the bread they were stingily given swam amid fecal matter." Yet it was the "barbaric procedure used for restraining these poor demented souls in their infectious dungeons" that astonished this visitor most:

> Their necks are squeezed into a thick iron ring with a heavy chain . . . solidly fixed to the inner wall of the cell. This chain is so short that the captive is forced to remain crouching in a sort of vertical immobility of the torso that after several hours must become a form of torture. The straitjacket is a child's toy next to this instrument of torture. Loud screams that these unfortunate souls emit seem to be provoked more by the inhibition that their painful position produces than by the ill defects of their mental faculties.

Such treatment reflected a therapeutic paradigm that "preceded the generous efforts and the charitable reforms of Pinel and Esquirol." If the local authorities in Salé "hoped to cure [madness] by the intervention of forces from beyond," this observer argued that "it would be wiser to seek simpler remedies on earth and to coordinate the regime of lunatics in Morocco, admitting all madmen without distinctions of nationality, race, or religion" into asylums.[64]

Lyautey rejected such criticism, arguing that the protectorate had undertaken serious steps toward improving all *maristans*, including Sidi Ben Achir.

He noted that "currently the asylum at Sidi Ben Achir is in a state of cleanliness that is difficult to surpass," and patients' waste and sustenance were "never mixed in a horrible mélange." But Lyautey's response to accusations about mechanical restraint suggests that he understood the chaining of lunatics as a sign of cultural difference rather than brutal mistreatment. He admitted that chains were widely used in Moroccan institutions, but insisted they were "no more barbaric than the straitjacket." The chains allowed patients to move, and medical observers from Paris who had seen Sidi Ben Achir "perfectly understood that even medical institutions should vary according the peoples' mores, customs, and religions." These physicians "never dreamed of protesting against this barbaric procedure." Lyautey conceded that "it is difficult to bring change" to Moroccan traditions, but, he lamented, "Moroccan Islam is not yet ready for the creation of asylums in the medical and scientific sense."[65]

Lyautey thus acknowledged the limitations of reform in the protectorate. But speakers at the Congress of French and Francophone Alienists in Rabat in 1933 were far less ambivalent. Despite significant evidence to the contrary, Morocco's public health director signaled in his opening speech that "for many years, Morocco has no longer evacuated its lunatics to metropolitan establishments." Lyautey's successor Urbain Blanc also saluted French efforts, announcing that prior to conquest the only therapy offered to the mentally ill in Morocco consisted of "playing a little music for them to soothe their sufferings." Lyautey himself sent a letter to the congress president, where he acknowledged the importance of health services to the French mission in Morocco, "not only from the medical and hygienic point of view, but also from the social and political points of view."[66]

While some therefore extolled the protectorate's successes in curtailing abuses in the *maristans*, others drew attention to the regime's incomplete reform of hospitalization practices. Marise Périale, a travel writer with close connections to the Moroccan administration, toured Sidi Ben Achir while researching a book about Salé in 1936 and published her observations in *Paris médical*. The hospice was divided into two sections: one held pilgrims while they visited the saint's tomb, while the other housed the chronically insane. In the pilgrims' section, "one notes a certain comfort": certain residents kept pet cats, and their rooms had a "homey feeling." But Périale's perspective shifted when she passed into the section for the insane. "Brrr! It was dark and damp." Patients lived behind iron bars as if in "cages for wild beasts." And most important, patients were still chained in their cells. Périale noted that the chains reflected an alternative medical epistemology: Moroccans considered them symbols of their illnesses, and donning chains represented a crucial step in an elaborate curing ritual, the acceptance of one's role as patient. Yet she argued that this interpretation "shocks our sensibilities, because we can only see the brutal fact of a human being attached to a chain in a dungeon, a condition worse than that of a criminal in a penal colony." Although many patients therefore actually requested to be chained, Périale found the practice chilling, and she "hastened to get back to the bright light, the invigorating air outside. . . . What a difference! It is night and day."[67]

Like others before her, Périale found the chains that bound patients to be the most powerful indicator of the "medieval framework" of mental health care in Morocco. The chain had a powerful symbolic value for these Moroccan patients as a signifier of their illness and harbinger of their cure. But as testimonies like Périale's indicate, the chain had symbolic value for Europeans as well. A vestige of treatment of the mad before Pinel, it indicated to French witnesses just how far Islamic ideas about insanity remained behind European sciences of the mind. Only the extension of modern institutions into the everyday lives of all Moroccans could bring this population up to date; only the efforts of French civilization could conquer a recalcitrant indigenous culture. In the minds of reformers such as Périale, the protectorate form offered an excuse for inaction rather than a productive way to serve the interests of Moroccans. Psychiatric advocates embraced the Pinel myth as a rallying cry for reform in the protectorate, but the ubiquity of *maristans* alongside modern facilities defined the exceptional nature of the Moroccan protectorate's regime for the insane through the 1950s.

Compassion and Endangerment: Confining the Mad in Algeria

The French conquest of Algiers predated intervention in Moroccan or Tunisian affairs by fifty years. Yet even by the interwar period, the state of mental assistance in Algeria was no further advanced than in the two protectorates. In contrast to Morocco and Tunisia, however, in Algeria reformers took aim at French rather than indigenous treatment of the mentally ill. The fact that authorities had suppressed Algeria's *maristans* by the mid-nineteenth century did little to assuage critics, who censured their compatriots as virulently as Moroccan and Tunisian reformers had attacked indigenous mistreatment of the insane. Pinel's legacy thus came to the forefront in Algeria as well, although the ensuing debates over psychiatric administration unfolded in dramatically different ways.

In the aftermath of conquest, medical expeditions in Algeria focused on the local population's dreadful state of health, exposing conditions similar to those described in Morocco nearly a century later. The natural environment vacillated between the intense heat and sterile landscapes of the Saharan desert and its arid, mountainous borders, and the humid, mosquito-infested marshlands of the coastal regions: a space whose climatic and topographic

characteristics engendered fierce debate about Europeans' prospects for acclimatization and productive colonization.[68] Physicians, ethnologists, and
administrators during the period of military rule—which lasted from 1830
to 1870—often ascribed the diseased state of the nascent colony to a general
collapse of civilization in the Muslim world, laying blame primarily on the
selfishness and fatalism of Algeria's Arab population. As Patricia Lorcin and
Yvonne Turin have noted, French medical officials found that pervasive filth,
crowded cities, and the close atmospheres of Muslims' homes compounded
the epidemics of smallpox and cholera that laid waste to Algerian Arabs.
Combined with the diabolical tyranny of Algeria's rulers and the "deprav-
ity" of its populations, these epidemics and the foul hygienic practices that
facilitated their spread provided medical evidence for the decline of Islamic
civilization, at least to French observers.[69]

Limited calls for provision for the insane in Algeria began as early as the
mid-nineteenth century. The passage of the law of 30 June 1838—which mandated the construction of a public asylum in each French department—and
the division of Algeria into three French departments in 1848 raised the question for the colony's military authorities, but a still-minuscule French settler
population postponed any serious action for decades. Sustained consideration
of the plight of the European and indigenous insane only took hold with the
passage of the Crémieux decree during the early Third Republic—which offered French citizenship to Europeans and Jews in Algeria—and a concomitant wave of assimilationist programs designed to incorporate the colony as
a component of the fabric of the French interior.

One of the first critics to raise his voice against French Algerian practices
was the psychiatrist Auguste Voisin. In 1873 he wrote of the lunatic ward at the
Hôpital Civil d'Alger that "one imagines this ward is the most insufficient, the
most defective, and the most elementary in the world." The facility "recalled
lunatic establishments . . . in France before the charitable reforms of Pinel."
Agitated patients here were "fixed to their beds day and night," and because
the facility was insufficiently equipped for them, they were transported to
metropolitan asylums as soon as possible.[70]

The transportation of patients to metropolitan facilities constituted the
official response to insanity in Algeria for decades. Military men who came
unhinged in the course of duty were treated at Val-de-Grâce in Paris, but colonial authorities shipped civilians and even indigenous Algerians who posed
a significant danger to public safety to asylums in Marseille, Montpellier, and
Aix-en-Provence. Most critics agreed this was only a makeshift solution, pointing in particular to the 49 percent annual mortality rate suffered by Muslim
patients in the asylums (mostly due to tuberculosis and exposure).[71] Yet the
phenomenon of transportation rendered the Algerian situation somewhat

unique, even inspiring potential solutions to the problem of caring for the insane. A French Algerian physician named Barbier proposed a particularly fantastic idea. Barbier had learned from a colleague who had escorted Algerian mental patients to Aix that the insane never suffered from seasickness. Even in "atrocious weather, when everyone was sick . . . and when all one heard was retching, my madmen were calm, relaxed, eating well, and not saying a word." It was only upon landing at Marseille that the patients "renewed their most beautiful screams and frolics." Reflecting on this information, Barbier asked "if a passage of 30 hours is a means of calming lunatics, what might a journey of 30 days or more do for them?" Barbier proposed the establishment of floating colonies for the mad in the Mediterranean, where patients would remain for weeks or months to test the soothing influence of the sea's motion: "before being thrown in the wastebasket, this deserves to be taken into serious consideration."[72]

Stultifera navis: alongside the Pinel legend, another myth in the history of insanity reemerges in the colonial context—the Ship of Fools that Foucault employs as a rhetorical foil for the modern management of unreason in his *Histoire de la folie.*[73] Barbier's outlandish solution never drew serious attention. Yet the proposal itself suggests that all manner of hypotheses were considered for a very real problem. Most critics of the regime lobbied to revise the 1838 law in order to ensure its promulgation throughout the colonial domain. Paul Gérente, a psychiatrist and Algerian senator, brought this inconsistency to public attention in Paris, proposing the law's complete revision.[74] Acknowledging that "Pinel elevated the lunatic to the dignity of the patient," he regretfully noted that "we are far from the day when this concept will be universally admitted." The new law proposed to reduce bureaucracy and to protect patients' rights, in part by incorporating Algeria in its purview, as the colony "should possess on its territory the necessary establishments for the treatment of patients suffering from mental disorders."[75]

The law never passed the conservative Senate. Meanwhile, criticism of transportation reached a fever pitch. A former director of the Aix asylum published an extensive article in the *Annales médico-psychologiques* in 1896 titled "Mental Illness in Arabs," in which he argued that continued transportation greatly hindered the treatment of Algerian Muslim patients. Economically "onerous," the treatment of patients in Aix also constituted a veritable pathogen: the patient spent several days in the "awful cells at the Mustapha hospital" and then crossed the Mediterranean packed in steerage. Once in Aix several days later, the patient was forced to change from a loose-fitting *burnous* into the asylum uniform, which "would quickly be reduced to tatters," and had to adapt immediately to a diet that included pork and wine. There were no Muslim religious facilities in the asylum, and there was no Arabic interpreter.

The complete absence of family and a new climate compounded linguistic and cultural differences to render a cure practically impossible.[76]

Other critics indicated that the procedural abuses inherent in the transportation system were just as brutal as the chains of the *maristans*. In an imaginative critique published in the *Annales* in 1909, another psychiatrist from Aix followed a hypothetical patient from capture in Algeria to his invariable death from tuberculosis in a French asylum. The problems began with a misdiagnosis by poorly trained physicians in Algiers: "Let us not forget that in France it is the most scientifically qualified among us who are charged with this delicate service." Patients were then "confined in narrow cages" in a "hold near the engines" and usually straitjacketed. Guards often abandoned their charges while they drank and socialized, recklessly endangering them. Corrupt guards also frequently smuggled contraband under patients' straitjackets as a means of passing through customs unquestioned. Once in France conditions were not much better than in North African *maristans*, especially in Aix's "Arab ward," which was populated with "violent, vicious, noisy" patients. In addition to the culture shock of the French asylum, physical illness was rampant, and inmates tended to die quickly. Miserable deaths were only the penultimate insult: in violation of Qur'anic principles, asylums sold the patients' bodies to the Montpellier Medical Faculty for anatomical study, a "macabre profit" that the author criticized as "cynical and amoral."[77]

Louis Livet, a French Algerian medical student, built on this attack, calling the transportation system "expensive, inhumane, and antiscientific." Livet accused authorities of ill-will toward the insane: where modern psychiatry considered the mentally ill "patients," the colonial administration considered them "beings who deserved confinement when they became dangerous for the public well-being." Patients paid the price for this bureaucratic callousness. Livet described the arrival of three Algerian patients in Marseille to demonstrate this point:

> Three lunatics, a man, a woman, and a ten-year-old boy, arrived last night from Algiers. . . . The woman was in a state of undress which was painful to see, without stockings or shoes, covered only with some formless rags, without resemblance to any piece of clothing whatsoever. Every one of this unfortunate woman's limbs was shivering, and she was crying, even sobbing from the cold. There is an absolute absence of humanity in making a human being travel in these conditions.[78]

Livet and other reformist psychiatrists also played to public fears by noting what they considered to be a disproportionate propensity for violence in these patients.[79] Some found it a racial issue, arguing that Arabs were predisposed to violent crime, while others argued that psychiatrists only came into contact with dangerous patients—the ones most likely to draw police attention.[80] They cited the cases of a number of Algerian patients given to sexual violence, including one "whose hashish-inspired delirium developed his considerable unnatural instincts," leading him to assault European patients on the wards. Another example was an "indigenous sodomite"—a commonplace accusation of French settlers toward Arabs—who "constituted a great danger for people and children he met."[81] Another still was a paranoid "lunatic of many years" who had murdered, assaulted, and defamed a number of Arabs, Europeans, and even family members for stealing his imaginary goats. Yet these patients went free, relieved of responsibility because of their mental state.[82]

The threat to public safety posed by unhospitalized patients resonated powerfully in Algeria's vast settler community. All of these cases pointed to a need for confinement facilities in Algeria as a matter of preserving public safety.[83] Yet proposal after proposal to rectify the situation foundered. From the 1870s, institutions had been proposed virtually every three to five years, only to meet rejection on budgetary grounds. It was only after the Tunis Congress in 1912 shed a powerful light on France's failures to provide for either the needs of colonial patients or the safety of its colonial settlers that administrators engaged in a sustained campaign to build a local institution in Algeria.

The most significant proponent of the Hôpital Psychiatrique de Blida-Joinville was Antoine Porot, the psychiatric professor from Lyon who had opened a small neuropsychiatric clinic for European patients in Tunis in 1911 and who emerged in the interwar period as Algerian psychiatry's leading advocate. Infamous from Frantz Fanon's excoriation of his racist pronouncements about Algerian mental inferiority, Porot is less well known as the principal architect of French Algeria's network for psychiatric care.[84] In 1925, Porot received a chair in psychiatry at the Algiers medical faculty, and from this point he lobbied tirelessly for the construction of a state-of-the-art psychiatric hospital near Algiers, engaging his students in the struggle as well. Paul Sauzay, for example, one of Porot's first students, used his medical thesis to attack opponents who blocked the financing of the Blida hospital, accusing the Algerian Fiscal Assemblies of "ignorance" and "seeking to protect personal interest to the detriment of the general interest."[85] In 1926, Don Côme Arrii, another Porot student, published a thesis about the "criminal impulsiveness of the indigenous Algerian" that lent empirical weight to assertions about roving madmen and the danger they posed to Algerian public safety. Extensive documentation of twenty case studies showed that "too many lunatics still wander freely in the Algerian interior, free to indulge in all the murderous consequences of their impulsiveness. [Their] families . . . fetter them with leg-irons, which does not always suffice for warding off the danger of murder." Arrii proposed a ready solution in his conclusion: "Let this new cry of alarm accelerate the assistance movement that finally seems to be taking shape!"[86]

The political infighting that surrounded the Blida project from the mid-1920s to its 1938 inauguration is a study in itself, as the next chapter details. The crucial matter here is that even when the major obstacle to psychiatric reform was government inefficiency rather than indigenous traditions, salvos attacking the status quo appeared virtually identical. Critics of French Algerian policy found the chains of Bicêtre transformed into bureaucratic chains of command that inhibited the proper care of the insane. Both the colonial and metropolitan psychiatric communities argued that transportation and the concomitant "deculturation" of the Algerian amounted to a life sentence of insanity or a death sentence of tuberculosis, and they called for the termination of the process on humanitarian grounds. At the same time, they employed the powerful rhetoric of public endangerment as a means of facilitating the establishment of local facilities in Algeria and expanding psychiatric power into the colonies. Unlike the case in Morocco, where the doctrine of "indirect rule" tolerated some degree of indigenous autonomy in culturally bound approaches to healing, critics in Algeria insisted that the medical infrastructure—like the colony itself—required complete assimilation to a French model.

...

A constant retreat to the Pinel myth's dual emphasis on humanitarian reform and protective confinement framed the debate over colonial psychiatry in the terms of the French clinical tradition. And the Pinel myth continued to inform the ways French psychiatrists reflected on their efforts, even after colonial psychiatric hospitals began operation. In a 1935 thesis titled "Medical Welfare for Psychopaths in Tunisia," a French medical student wrote of conditions in *maristans* that "one thinks of Pinel and of the state in which he found the lunatics of Bicêtre. . . . Certainly, the Tékia's patients were not treated better than Bicêtre's lunatics of that era."[87] For the Blida hospital's official inauguration in 1938, two psychiatrists prepared a study of the history of Arab medicine and the psychiatric reform movement in Algeria since French conquest that addressed the heroic efforts of French psychiatrists in their struggles against barbaric practices in North Africa.[88] As late as the 1950s colonial psychiatrists still illustrated their history through the myth: the psychiatrist Pierre Maréschal, director of the Manouba hospital, described the Tékia's conditions as "exactly those of Bicêtre before Pinel."[89]

Critics' emphasis on the poor conditions in the *maristans* and the abysmal treatment of the insane shows a consensus that is too strong to be purely coincidental. Observations unanimously detail wretched conditions that must have shocked the sensibilities of a professionalized psychiatric discipline that founded itself on the elimination of precisely these abuses. Yet the political motives of this rhetoric are unmistakable. The overwhelming consensus on the need for psychiatric reform in the European model tells us as much about the French psychiatric profession as it does about actual conditions for the insane in the Maghreb: the observations indicate above all that the persistence of chains in the *maristans* astonished figures who upheld their profession's legitimacy by constantly emphasizing psychiatry's "elevation of the madman to the dignity of the patient." This concern with psychiatric reform in France's North African colonies reflects the emphasis many French psychiatrists placed on the professionalization of their often maligned yet still influential discipline. Certainly, the Moroccan, Tunisian, and Algerian cases presented important contextual differences. But the similarity of psychiatrists' responses outweighed these differences, reflecting the nature of the discipline more than any shared geographic, cultural, or administrative traits of the North African colonies.

Like any origin myth, the Pinel legend derived its power from its constant invocation as a near-magical incantation. It is interesting to note that the myth became more insistent in its North African application at precisely the moment when an entrenched French psychiatric profession found itself under siege. With the turn of the twentieth century, the influence of French alienism was under attack on all fronts: German psychiatrists made considerable advances on French technological innovations, Freudian psychoanalysis threatened the power dynamics of the asylum structure, and an increasingly powerful psychological science in France questioned the "sterile nosology" that characterized the French psychiatric tradition.[90]

Since Frantz Fanon's powerful critique of colonial psychiatry, historians have emphasized the uses of mental medicine in the service of colonial racism. The abuse of medical authority was clearly an established tradition in much of colonial medicine, where practitioners frequently defended settlers' interests above those of their patients. Yet historians have largely ignored the professional impetus behind the movement for colonial psychiatric reform. In the case of French North Africa, psychiatrists recalled their discipline's foundational legend as a call for professional renewal in colonial territory. The temptation to bring the Pinel myth to bear on North Africa was too great to resist: both the *maristans* and callous colonial administrators in Tunisia, Morocco, and Algeria proved to be excellent foils for renewing French claims to progressive clinical science in the face of superstitious ignorance by rebuilding the psychiatric profession on foreign soil.

2 The Shaping of Colonial Psychiatry
Geographies of Innovation and Economies of Care

Some fifty kilometers southwest of Algiers, Blida, known as the "city of roses," sits against the majestic backdrop of the Atlas Mountains in the fertile Mitidja plain. Although the Ottomans had settled the region as early as the seventeenth century, French Algerians considered Blida to be a project of their own making. With its street markets and festivals, its mild winters and hot summers, the city inspired easy comparisons to Provençal villages.[1] Blida was also unmistakably a colonial city. For Jeanne Cheula, a settler from Algiers who lived there in the 1920s, several characteristics indelibly marked Blida. Blida was the "pride" of French Algeria, an "orchard without limits": the "exquisite taste" of its fresh water and the "unforgettable scent" of its orange trees, jasmine flowers, and roses made of Blida an "enchanted garden"—a testament to "the tireless labor and the endless sacrifices" of the region's first French settlers in the mid-nineteenth century.[2] Yet Blida was a city divided by culture, religion, and politics. Settlers in the European quarter were farmers and citizens, but they were also soldiers in a colonial outpost that abutted an Arab city. The existence of the dusty Arab medina, with its poverty and its decaying buildings, side-by-side with the wide avenues, fountains, and regular military processions of a garrison town with some eighty thousand Europeans, exemplified for many settlers the contrast between what they considered to be French dynamism and Algerian torpor. Here a flourishing settlement, forged out of a fetid swamp, sat next to a decadent remnant of the era before French conquest.

That Blida was also the subject of contentious debates over the nature and extent of French medicine's civilizing mission is fitting. The city was the site of North Africa's largest psychiatric hospital. First proposed in 1912, the hospital broke ground in the late 1920s and became a vast campus whose dozens of pavilions housed over two thousand patients by the 1950s; as with Bedlam, the name Blida became synonymous with insanity in settler circles.[3] The Hôpital Psychiatrique de Blida-Joinville, like the settlement of Blida itself, represented an enormous and tangible achievement for colonial development. Yet the institution faced intransigent opposition from the moment its designers proposed its construction. Despite recognition that Algeria faced a crisis of madness, plans to ameliorate that crisis engendered fierce arguments over what constituted an appropriate response to mental illness in colonial settings. The Blida hospital served as a vessel for impassioned discussions over the relationship between colonialism and medicine, and over the nature of the French colonial project in Algeria itself.

At the heart of political debates over funding for psychiatric facilities in Algeria were questions pertinent not only to psychiatry in the colonies, but also to the future of the psychiatric profession in France. Most administrators and psychiatrists recognized the plight of the colonial insane and the failures of transporting patients to French asylums. Yet debates over what colonial institutions should look like and how they should function were fractious precisely because psychiatry itself was such a contentious field in the interwar period. For many, the proper solution lay in constructing a custodial asylum in Algeria for the confinement of the dangerous insane: what worked in France could work for the colonies. Yet for others, this proposition threatened to perpetuate a malfunctioning system. For those who had employed the language of the Pinel legend as a means of mobilizing sympathy for the colonial insane, the construction of psychiatric institutions in the Maghreb presented an opportunity as well as a challenge. Indeed, in many ways the legacy of Pinel resonated more strongly among colonial psychiatrists than with their colleagues in France, where complacency dogged reform efforts. The rhetoric of reform in the colonial sphere implied a desperate need for professional renewal by highlighting the ossification of asylum psychiatry in France as well as the suffering of the colonial insane and demanded an innovative response.

Institutions for the insane represented a smaller fraction of the colonial budget than other projects deemed to further the civilizing mission, such as railroads and schools. Yet discussions about them in administrative and medical circles reveal similar concerns. Questions about what shape colonial development should take—and what role science should play in colonial investment—were central to the debate. At stake were not only the fates of thousands of colonial patients, but also the future of French Algeria. For those who measured colonial progress solely in terms of financial gain, colonial development implied a transfer of proven technology to new terrains. For those who saw in imperialism an obligation to renew colonial space, *mise en valeur*, or the improvement of a decadent terrain, necessitated geographically and culturally specific innovation. Similar contests played out in the struggles to build psychiatric institutions in Tunisia and Morocco, yet it was in Algeria, the keystone of the French empire and the principal showcase of French colonial development, that the debate over colonial psychiatry had the greatest resonance. Although the provision of psychiatric care provided the central language of the debate in Algeria, its implications concerned an elaborate calculus at the core of interwar French colonialism, one in which material economies of development figured in tandem with moral economies of care.

Hygienic Technologies and the Geographies of Innovation: Reimagining the Asylum

Algeria's contest over mental assistance in the 1920s was nearly precluded in the prewar era. French colonial governments established several mental health programs with little or no controversy in the aftermath of the Congress of French and Francophone Alienists and Neurologists at Tunis in 1912. The meeting drew political attention to the crises posed by insanity in the colonies and prompted a wave of proposals for managing the problem. Most of these projects involved the construction of custodial asylums for the confinement of dangerous patients. Several such programs unfolded with little debate because the vast distances between these locales and metropolitan France rendered the transportation of patients to Europe largely impracticable.[4] In 1912 in Madagascar, for example, administrators opened an asylum that held roughly 180 patients at Anjanamasina.[5] The government-general in Indochina approved construction of an asylum at Bien-Hoa, near Saigon, in the same year; the asylum opened to some 140 patients in 1919.[6]

Algeria nearly followed a similar path. Théodore Steeg, the interior director of the Algerian government-general, became an enthusiastic partisan of the psychiatric reform movement in the aftermath of the Tunis congress. Steeg found the transportation system "contrary to principles of humanity and also to public order" and insisted that it was "unacceptable that Algeria, with its hospitals and its prisons, [had] no asylum, or even asylums."[7] With the Algerian governor-general, Charles Lutaud, he formed a planning committee headed by Joseph Saliège, a French physi-

cian from Algiers, and Henri Mabille, a psychiatrist and director of the
La Rochelle asylum who had directed several administrative inquiries of
psychiatric institutions in metropolitan France, to design a psychiatric
system for the colony.[8] Mabille and Saliège proposed the construction of
a facility at Blida that would be based on the model of the Sainte-Anne
asylum in Paris. The institution's twenty pavilions were designed to cor-
respond to patients' and administrators' needs, and included wards for
triage, for violent patients, and for the senile and bedridden, as well as an
"agricultural colony that would allow calm patients" to work and "to live in
relative freedom."[9] The model resembled many French institutions, with
one exception. Mabille acknowledged that designing a colonial asylum
was "more complex than in France," because such a facility had to care
for "not only European and [European-] Algerian lunatics, but also native
lunatics." Providing few specifics, Mabille noted that these patients would
most likely require "special infirmaries and sleeping quarters" that would
"respond in a quite particular way to their general behaviors, their mores,
and to their civilization."[10]

Because Blida lay a considerable distance from Algiers, some committee members objected that the site was less than ideal. Yet Blida made up
for its compromising location in other ways. Municipal authorities offered
the government-general a tract of eighty-seven hectares of arable land in
the Joinville subdivision on Blida's outskirts for the construction of the
asylum, including water and electrical service, shade trees for the facility,
and a tramway between the institution and the city. The gift promised to
keep projected costs for the asylum within reasonable limits, allowing the
committee to propose at the same time a training clinic at the Mustapha
hospital in Algiers.[11] But soon after the committee filed its report in 1914
the outbreak of war forced governments to redirect their resources, and
plans for colonial assistance programs fell by the wayside.

Algeria again took up the question of the insane in the war's aftermath. The project was particularly attractive to Steeg, who was appointed
governor-general in 1921. A member of France's Radical party, Steeg was
committed to advancing colonial goals through civilian instruments and to
furthering the benevolent image of French rule.[12] In 1923 Steeg submitted
an updated version of the Blida plan to Algeria's fiscal assemblies. Unlike
the rest of the French empire, whose budgets and taxation were determined by the ministry of colonies, control over Algeria's budget was held
by the assemblies. Governors-general were appointed by French presi-
dents and had authority over legislative policy, yet their hands were often
tied by the powerful settlers who populated the assemblies and generally
represented the interests of wealthy landholders.[13] Although the delegates

were not overtly hostile to funding medical assistance projects—indeed, many were physicians as well as landholders—they tended to privilege the colony's economic infrastructure "while according social problems low priority" in calculating Algeria's budget.[14] The assemblies were therefore somewhat cool to the administration's requests for funding for the Blida asylum. Although the delegates approved of this project in principle, they also requested more detailed plans before committing to funding the project so as to avoid "putting the cart before the horse." In one delegate's words, "I see the usefulness of the asylum in question, but I would like to know where we are headed."[15]

This request unleashed a series of unanticipated and contentious debates. Under the direction of Jean Lépine, a psychiatry professor at the Lyon medical faculty, a new advisory committee broke with its predecessor's recommendation and outlined an entirely new framework for psychiatric assistance in Algeria. Whereas Mabille and Saliège's report conformed to a prewar paradigm that privileged the asylum as the cornerstone of a mental health care system, the recommendations of Lépine's committee emerged from a psychiatric mindset that was new to France in the interwar period. Moreover, the Lépine report, in its reflection of new attitudes toward the place of science in France's colonial mission, contributed to an enduring dispute over the nature of France's colonial obligations.

...

At the turn of the twentieth century, a number of reform-minded French psychiatrists began to call some of their discipline's foundational principles into question. Since its inception, the French psychiatric profession had based its practices in the asylum. Pinel, of course, had contributed significantly to this tradition by implementing a series of reforms in asylum design in the early nineteenth century. The French law of 30 June 1838 codified many of these concepts. By mandating the construction of France's departmental asylum system and placing oversight for these institutions and the nascent psychiatric profession in the hands of the interior ministry, the law linked the profession inextricably both to the state and to the asylum as psychiatry's principal therapeutic instrument.[16]

By the end of the century an increasing number of reform-minded psychiatrists had begun to express grave doubts about both the asylum's efficacy and the state of psychiatric practice in France. Cure rates for asylum patients were extremely low. For Edouard Toulouse, a psychiatrist at the Villejuif asylum on the outskirts of Paris, French psychiatry's rigid commitment to the 1838 law and the asylum, an institution that itself unduly stigmatized patients with the badge of incurable madness, was to blame. In

1899 Toulouse questioned the inevitability of the "incessantly increasing number of lunatics held at public expense" in France.[17] Early observation and treatment of acutely afflicted patients outside of the asylum could prevent the onset of longer-lasting afflictions. Toulouse therefore advocated a compartmentalization of psychiatric treatment that would distinguish curable from incurable patients—a distinction that would serve both economic and therapeutic interests by saving acute patients from long-term confinement in the asylum, where their afflictions often became chronic.

Experiences during the First World War greatly reinforced Toulouse's convictions. During the war, the French army directed over twenty thousand shell-shocked soldiers to the Val-de-Grâce military hospital in Paris, where they overwhelmed the unit's psychiatric ward. Yet this adverse experience proved a crucible for innovation, showing the potential of new methods for processing insanity according to principles of scientific rationalization. Faced with such vast numbers, military psychiatrists borrowed from American and British experiments in mental hygiene and made careful distinctions between chronic and acute cases, interning only a quarter of their patients for long-term care in asylums. These figures suggested that internment was contraindicated for many cases and prompted deep reflection on the problems of the 1838 law in certain psychiatric circles. Although the law had been novel for its era and protected patients' rights, confinement tarnished even the mildly ill with the stigma of lunacy and therefore represented an obsolete code for patient care. In contrast with asylums, Toulouse declared, "open services would allow us to avoid the social taint of confinement for acute psychopaths for whom mixing with chronic patients actually hinders treatment."[18]

Citing this experience, Toulouse and his colleagues Georges Génil-Perrin and Roger Dupouy founded the Mental Hygiene and Prophylaxis League in 1920 with the goal of reforming the 1838 law. Like reformers in the colonies, mental hygienists such as Toulouse and Dupouy represented themselves as the true heirs of psychiatric enlightenment, arguing in one article that "Pinel's work has remained incomplete." The French asylum functioned more as a prison than as a hospital, meeting the needs of social protection more than those of the majority of miserable patients. "This is not what Pinel would have wanted," they insisted: as a "liberator of madmen, he wanted to deliver them not only from their chains, but also from their isolation and their confinement."[19]

The League proposed a technological rather than a theoretical solution to this problem, yet one that brought with it significant epistemological implications. The asylums at the core of the 1838 law drew clear lines between madness and reason, confining the former to protect the latter from insanity's physical, moral, and spiritual threats. What the League advocated was the development of a means of managing insanity that reflected a more flexible conception of the boundaries between normality and pathology. Based on the notion that "madness, in a great number of cases, was an avoidable and curable disease" and that decisive action could "prevent acute afflictions from becoming chronic," Toulouse and his colleagues embraced a philosophy of comprehensive prevention and rapid treatment.[20] The crucial response to the increasing prevalence of madness was therefore a reorganization of the nation's mental assistance network that placed the emphasis on prophylaxis and hygiene rather than the internment of chronic patients.

The League self-consciously modeled itself on groups dedicated to the struggles against cancer and tuberculosis. Yet the group also presented itself as a patently modern and scientific organization by borrowing heavily from the language of industrial rationalization. The League's ideals were steeped in the values of technological utopianism, which were spreading rapidly through interwar Europe.[21] The resemblance of the League's ideal hospital to the rationalized workplace was therefore no coincidence. The Hôpital Henri-Rousselle, opened in Paris in 1922, was a model for the modern health care facility based on the well-organized factory. An asylum without walls, Henri-Rousselle consisted of a series of tightly linked services and laboratories for the promotion of mental health and the quick repair of mental illness. A dispensary performed triage and outpatient treatment, sending some patients to the psychiatric hospital for more sustained observation. Social services extended the dispensary's reach into the public through surveillance of patients' homes, schools, workplaces, and homeless shelters. Finally, laboratories and research centers provided scientific backing for clinical diagnoses.[22] Toulouse proudly claimed that he had "borrowed this new hospital doctrine from industry, notably the rule of the division of labor and the discipline of collective work under a single scientific, medical, and administrative direction, as all converge toward the same end."[23] In Toulouse's opinion, the industrial organization of the Hôpital adapted it most effectively to contemporary psychopathological conditions. Whereas the asylum was still appropriate for "incurable or dangerous psychopaths," the open service provided more comprehensive care by allowing for careful distinctions between these and more minor afflictions and enhancing the possibility of rapid intervention.[24]

The experience at Henri-Rousselle reflected the League's efforts to bring psychiatry into parity with other medical specializations. Both the language of industrial rationalization and an emphasis on prophylaxis rather than rehabilitative treatment betray this intention. The transition

from a "lunatic asylum" to a "psychiatric hospital" entailed the implementation of a new therapeutic technology, one imagined as a set of interac-
tive components that comprised what François Béguin has called a "healing machine," and it offered a model that could be applied on a national
scale.[25] As much a spatial reorganization as a refinement of technical skill,
the renovation of psychiatry through the principles of mental hygiene involved a reconfiguration of mental health facilities with a new emphasis on
prevention. The new psychiatry sought to transform its institutions from
spaces of disease and suffering—warehouses of sickness—into units that
ameliorated madness through rapid therapeutic intervention.

Hygienists such as Toulouse and Dupouy also suggested the novelty
of their approach by adopting the language of microbiology. In addition
to modeling their work on (and coordinating with) leagues against tuberculosis and other scourges of urban modernity, Toulouse argued that
mental hygienists were effectively Pasteurians without microbes. His writings drew strong parallels between the risk of madness and that of infectious diseases such as tuberculosis, encephalitis, and syphilis in modern
industrial society, and he insisted that prophylactic living offered the most
effective means of ensuring mental and physical health.[26] Toulouse and his
colleagues went so far as to suggest that the new psychiatry was a *laboratory*
discipline. Although scholars in science studies have engaged in protracted
debates about the laboratory as a sign of scientific modernity, it is clear that
Toulouse and other mental hygienists perceived it as such.[27] Indeed, the
new field of "psychotechnics" boasted that the psychological laboratory
offered clear evidence of the efficacy of mental hygienic practices.[28] Just as
the Pasteur Institutes isolated the sources of disease and developed strategies to ward off sickness, the psychotechnical laboratory was, for Toulouse
and his collaborators, an obligatory point of passage for mental healing,
a space that rendered mental illness observable, mutable, and ultimately
preventable.

The League therefore attempted to recast psychiatry as an efficacious
profession operating explicitly in what Michel Foucault has called the field
of biopolitics. In his 1976 lectures at the Collège de France and later in the
first volume of his *History of Sexuality,* Foucault introduced the concept of
biopower as a complement to the disciplinary regimes he had outlined in
his earlier works. Whereas disciplinary institutions—the asylum, the hospital, the school, the factory, the prison—operate at the level of the body,
shaping behavior and molding individualized citizens into a coherent
whole, biopolitics, as a "new technology of power" more closely linked to
the state, operates at the level of populations. Biopolitics aims at sickness,
economics, and madness themselves in their aggregate forms, targeting

not the individual sick person, the vagrant, the madman, but endemicity, disability, and environment; its goals are the improvement of the population's collective life, the management of risk, and the preservation of health. Biopolitics thus acts at the level of statistics: rates of mortality and morbidity, yields of internment and rehabilitation, a taming of risk, and a maximization of reward are its principal registers.[29]

Merging techniques of individual discipline and the governance of populations, Toulouse's vision represents an instantiation of this politics in action. He dreamed of remaking France into what he called a "biocracy," or a "state in which the rules of social evolution would be directed by the life sciences."[30] As early as 1921, the Mental Hygiene League's organizational literature suggested that "the psychical life of individuals forms the essential condition for all social activity." Therefore, although physiological disabilities could often coexist with a "nearly normal professional life," any "defective mental state, even a slight one, entails the diminution or the stopping of productive activity." Signaling a clear link between "individual performance" and "national prosperity," Toulouse insisted that France, "impoverished and exhausted by the war, should, more than any other country, concentrate all its efforts on the reconstitution of its capital of psychical energy."[31]

In contrast to the asylum's power merely to confine, his reimagination of the psychiatric unit as an open service could organize life itself—of the healthy as well as the sick—according to the principles of sound mental hygiene. Such a program promised to raise the psychiatric profession's status by marking its commitment to progress and by improving the performance of mental medicine. As with the health of the population, the efficacy of the program could best be measured in its aggregate form: the dispensary accomplished its goals by increasing its production dramatically in its early years of operation, providing fourteen thousand consultations by 1928 and achieving an "amelioration" rate of 50 percent in the same period—a figure far superior to the 20 percent average for other institutions in the department.[32]

Despite such persuasive figures, the conservative French senate rejected a reform proposal that included these revisions.[33] Even the French psychiatric community as a whole found the reforms too threatening to the traditions of institutional power in the asylum; by the 1930s, some went so far as to propose Toulouse's expulsion from the Société Médico-Psychologique.[34] A number of reform-minded psychiatrists continued to mobilize for the rejuvenation of the field throughout the interwar period, yet the hygienists' program remained limited to a few clinics in France until well after the Second World War.

As Bruno Latour has argued, Pasteurian microbiology received a similarly cool reception among mainstream physicians in metropolitan France in the late nineteenth century. It was instead in the colonies that an international network of Pasteur Institutes took root and that the new discipline initially flourished. Close coordination between administrators who saw the utility of microbiological research for colonial public health and scientists who sought a free field for experimentation away from the scrutiny of an established medical profession allowed for the development of a symbiotic relationship between the Pasteurians and the stewards of empire.[35] A parallel situation marked the development of psychiatry in the interwar period. Debates about the establishment of mental health programs in the colonies suggested that North Africa might prove to be fertile ground for the implementation of an experimental psychiatric agenda. The colonies emerged as a key venue for staging a new biocracy, where the sciences of the mind could join forces with the civilizing mission in the interest of ensuring public safety by improving the public's mental health.

...

The deployment of psychiatry in Algeria reflected the biopolitical sensibilities of metropolitan reformers and adapted them to the colonial setting. The Lépine committee, which included Joseph Saliège, Algerian public health inspector-general Lucien Raynaud, and Lépine's former intern Antoine Porot, embraced the basic principles of modern mental hygiene. Yet the architects of Algerian psychiatry committed themselves to the notion that progressive scientific intervention held the key to not only a harmonious society, but also to effective colonial governance.

The Lépine committee's self-described charge was to "enlighten the Administration on the evolution of new ideas and notions of assistance to psychopaths."[36] It emphasized in its report that "internment in the asylum" was a "last resort," rather than the sole possibility for managing mental illness. Instead, the "crucial element" in mental health care was an open ward in a general hospital for the "early and opportunistic treatment" of acutely stricken patients, over 50 percent of whom the committee insisted were curable.[37] The new committee argued that Algeria's mental health needs could be best met with a two-line system for the care of the mentally ill: a smaller, seven-hundred-bed unit at Blida for chronic cases, combined with primary care wards in its major cities. Operating outside the purview of the 1838 law, the facilities would welcome patients for free consultations. Their location in general hospitals, rather than within or adjacent to a lunatic asylum, would help to avoid the stigma associated with madness in the general population, and would therefore facilitate cures by removing

the disincentives for voluntary early treatment of psychological disturbances. This reconfiguration of psychiatric infrastructure was "the absolute and essential condition" for "effective reform" of care for the mentally
ill in Algeria. Finally, the committee advocated the use of the departmental
open services as teaching centers. Psychiatry, the authors insisted, was an
essential part of modern medicine, and instead of producing just "a small
number of specialists," medical training should encourage all students to
develop a basic understanding of psychiatric principles: "like every human
endeavor, this reform will only reach its full potential through the continuous and enlightened effort of the men destined to apply themselves to
it."[38]

Although this program appeared to be a radical departure from established treatment patterns both to the fiscal assemblies in Algeria and to
many psychiatrists in France, its most novel element had been in use in
North Africa for over a decade. The committee's advocacy of an "open
service" as the foundation of Algeria's mental assistance network drew on
the experience of Antoine Porot's neuropsychiatric clinic in Tunis. Despite
its mere twenty-four beds, this clinic—and the career of its founder—remain touchstones for the history of French colonial psychiatry. Porot (figure 4) is best known as the founder of the Algiers School of French psychiatry and the target of Frantz Fanon's excoriation in *The Wretched of the
Earth*.[39] Fanon indicted Porot as the father of psychiatric racism in Algeria,
citing studies in which Porot and his students elaborated a collective diagnosis of the North African mind as primitive, criminally impulsive, and
feebleminded. Historians have since considered the works of Porot and the
Algiers School as little more than a pseudo-scientific support system for
colonial racism.[40]

Yet many of his contemporaries saw him as a progressive innovator.
Born in Chalons-sur-Saône in 1876, Porot studied under the psychiatrist
Jean Lépine at the Lyon medical faculty, where he completed his thesis on
mercury treatments for neurosyphilis.[41] In 1907, Porot moved to Tunisia,
where he soon began to lobby tirelessly for the construction of psychiatric institutions—work he developed prodigiously upon his enlistment as a
military psychiatrist during the First World War and his eventual posting
to Algiers's Maillot military hospital in 1916. Speaking of the Tunis clinic,
one of Porot's successors reminisced, "It was there that medical care was
given to lunatics and that we really performed psychiatry for the first time
in Tunisia."[42] Upon Porot's death in 1965, Léon Michaux, president of the
French Medico-Psychological Society, described him as "one of the great
modern French psychiatrists": in addition crediting him with the "revolutionary innovation" of establishing "psychiatry's first open service" at

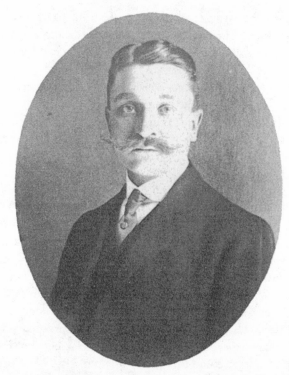

Figure 4.   Antoine Porot in 1912. From *L'informateur des aliénistes et neurologistes* 7 (1912). Reproduction courtesy of the Ebling Health Sciences Library, University of Wisconsin–Madison. Reprinted by permission of Bibliothèque nationale de France.

the ward in Tunis, he was also the director of a "brilliant school" and the "creator of psychiatric care in Algeria."[43] Even the current edition of the *Manuel alphabétique de psychiatrie*—a sort of *Diagnostic and Statistical Manual* for French medical students—describes Porot's clinic in Tunis as indeed the first truly open service in the French dominion, followed much later by similar endeavors in France.[44]

The ward was certainly the first of its kind in North Africa (see figure 5) and was among the first in any French-speaking terrain. Although it had only twenty-four beds and served only the city's European population, Porot rated the ward an unqualified success in treating "the entire gamut of patients, from the calmest to the most violent." Taking the hospital rather than the asylum as its model, Porot's facility provided "simple, necessary, and sufficient" care for the mentally ill in the absence of an asylum. Unlike most French psychiatric institutions, which were supervised by departmental prefectures, Porot's ward invested the physician with complete autonomy. By paring bureaucracy to a minimum, Porot created an open

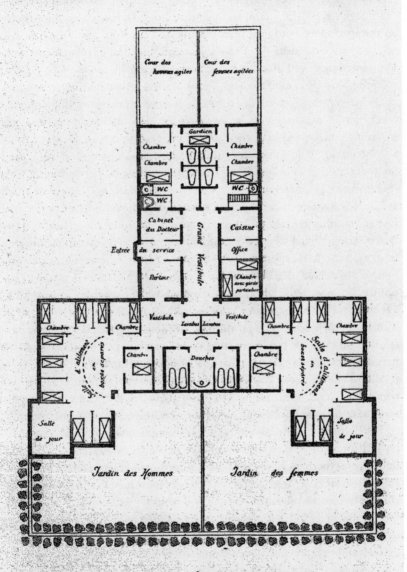

Ville de Tunis.   Hôpital civil français.

PLAN DU NOUVEAU PAVILLON D'OBSERVATION ET DE TRAITEMENT
PSYCHIATRIQUE
(Service du docteur Porot)

Figure 5.   Floor plan of Porot's Neuro-Psychiatric Ward at the Hôpital Civil de Tunis, 1912. From *L'informateur des aliénistes et neurologistes* 7 (1912). Reproduction courtesy of the Ebling Health Sciences Library, University of Wisconsin–Madison. Reprint by permission of Bibliothèque nationale de France.

facility that departed from the asylum's traditions of concealment and confinement. The service enjoyed a good reputation in public opinion because
of this openness—for example, in contrast to most French asylums, Porot
encouraged families to visit their hospitalized relatives—and the unit also
achieved strong results. By Porot's account, over half of his patients were
discharged as cured after less than a month, and fewer than 10 percent
required long-term confinement. Porot offered little detail regarding precisely how a "cure" was defined; yet his accomplishments stood in marked
contrast with most asylums, whose own statistics attributed lasting cures
to fewer than 10 percent of their patients.[45]

The clinic, which Porot administered from its opening in 1911 until
his move to the Maillot military hospital during the First World War,
shared many characteristics with open services such as Toulouse's clinic
at Henri-Rousselle: indeed, André Antheaume, the founder of the journal
Hygiène mentale, cited Porot's ward, among a few others, as a pathbreaking
facility and a model for metropolitan reform.[46] Yet Porot's efforts differed
from metropolitan experiments with open services in several crucial ways.
French physicians such as Toulouse who tinkered with administrative procedure did so with the safety net of an established psychiatric network below them. By contrast, Porot built his service to fill a psychiatric void in
Tunisia. French doctors had the luxury of choosing patients who were particularly suitable for treatment in open services. Porot's ward accepted all
patients, serving the colony in isolation. But on one important level, the metropolitan experiments and the Tunis ward shared a similarity: their patients were all Europeans. From 1911 to 1915, when Porot administered his
service, indigenous Tunisians still relied on family care or the *maristans*.[47]

For Porot and many contemporaries, the clinic pointed toward psychiatry's future in the metropole as well as in the colonies. Even as the unit was
under construction, Henry Bouquet, a medical student from Lyon, her-
alded the facility as "inspired" by "the most recent medical principles." The
clinic offered both physical and symbolic signs of medical progressivism. In
the naming of its wards, it substituted terms such as "nervous illnesses" for
more archaic ones such as "lunacy"; in its practices, it abandoned mechanical restraint in favor of close observation of patients.[48] Visiting psychiatrists
who celebrated the inauguration of Porot's "beautiful pavilion" during the
Tunis meeting of the Congress of French Alienists lauded his accomplishments more fully.[49] Coverage of the inauguration in the medical press emphasized how the clinic demonstrated the possibilities for "economically
solving the problem of assistance for lunatics" in the colonies by employing
a general hospital setting for the prompt treatment of acute cases, avoiding
the need to intern such patients in asylums, at great cost.[50]

Porot saw his clinic as an initial step toward the development of a comprehensive psychiatric network in the Maghreb and implored authorities to offer such services to Tunisia's native population, "whom France has the duty to protect."[51] In his report titled "Assistance to Lunatics in the Colonies," the Bordeaux professor Emmanuel Régis agreed, describing the ward as a prototype to be replicated throughout the French empire. Following the initial successes of Porot's regime, Régis proposed the implementation of a two-line system of defense against mental illness in the colonies, similar to the program outlined by the Lépine commission. A "first line of assistance," modeled on the Tunis clinic, would serve acutely ill patients. Those who suffered from incidental crises such as alcohol- or fever-induced deliria—not uncommon in colonial settings—could be easily distinguished from those afflicted with chronic mental illnesses such as dementia praecox or manic-depressive psychosis. The latter might be treated in the clinic as well but would likely require long-term hospitalization in an asylum, the second line of assistance. By operating outside the purview of the 1838 law, this new system would avoid the slow-moving machinery of institutional bureaucracy by placing the hospital, rather than the asylum, at the center of mental health management. "This," Régis argued, "is just what Doctor Porot understood and accomplished in his pavilion at the French hospital in Tunis."[52]

Such sentiments hint at the ways in which the Tunis clinic and the designing of a new Algerian psychiatry were microcosms of the colonial project as imagined by an emerging cohort of progressivist settlers. They represented the possibility for remaking, renewing, and regenerating French ideas in what many colonists imagined were scientifically devoid settings. As Porot saw it, North Africa represented a psychiatric "blank slate." The decaying vestiges of Islam's illustrious medical past—the overcrowded and brutal *maristans,* pilgrimage sites, healing rites performed by wandering *marabouts*—only highlighted the absence of medical modernity in the region. Speaking of his work at the Tunis clinic, Porot argued that such conditions made it "easy, as well as necessary, to innovate."[53] If psychiatry was to be remade as a technology of public health, the colonies, unencumbered by a commitment to the asylum and yet saddled with a population that demanded regulation and organization, offered a critical site for its redevelopment.

As progressive as these services appeared to their advocates, they also generated enormous controversy among psychiatrists and colonial authorities. The appropriate format for psychiatric renewal rapidly became a venue for a much larger debate over France's obligations to its colonies. Mental health reform in interwar North Africa was a central theme in an escalating argument about the roles of science and medicine in colonial administration. For those who saw French colonialism as a civilizing force for progressive good, the successes of Porot's clinic in Tunis demonstrated how the colonies could be a crucible for innovation, ameliorating a crisis in colonial rule and simultaneously modeling a new future for a profession in the metropole. Yet others, who saw colonialism as a source of wealth rather than a space of investment, found this emphasis on innovation too experimental to justify its expense. The debate over psychiatric reform in Algeria effectively polarized colonial administrators into two camps: those who saw in colonial obligations a moral economy of care versus those who plotted colonial administration according to material economies of production.

Colonial Biopolitics and Economies of Care: Financing Reform in Algeria

Debates over the management of mental illness in the Algerian Fiscal Assemblies revealed this polarization clearly. Many in the Algerian administration and in the assemblies themselves were persuaded by the resuscitation of the "Pinel myth," which characterized the rhetoric of colonial psychiatric reform in the early twentieth century. As he presented the government-general's funding request to the assemblies in 1923, the Algerian interior director spoke of the "unfortunate conditions" in which Algeria's patients languished in French asylums, describing them as "contrary to humanitarian principles."[54] Some Muslim delegates—in addition to the forty-eight French delegates who represented Algeria's roughly 700,000 settlers in the interwar period, Algeria's 5 million Muslims indirectly elected twenty-one representatives—agreed with this view, calling attention to the "suffering and isolation" of the insane in the absence of local care.[55] Boldly speaking for all his colleagues, one European delegate from Oran argued that "we only want one thing: to accomplish a humanitarian project."[56]

Others, however, placed immediate economic concerns in the foreground. Whereas mental hygienists in France saw such spending as an investment in the nation's workforce, and therefore its productive industrial yield, many settler delegates found spending dedicated to the mentally ill a tragic waste of funds in an era of postwar recovery. Insisting that any Algerian facility must necessarily draw fewer resources than transporting patients to French asylums, several delegates noted that any alternative made poor economic sense. Fees for maintaining patients in France totaled roughly 50,000 francs per year; even after spending twelve million francs to build an asylum in Algeria, the colony would incur the same costs for care per patient, while also paying nearly a million francs in annual interest on the construction costs.[57] The following year, when the Lépine committee's report outlined not an asylum but a network of institutions for psychiatric care at unknown—yet certainly higher—operating and construction costs, a growing roster of fiscal conservatives sought to quash the proposal definitively in order to reserve these funds for more "practical" uses, such as the treatment of tubercular patients.

The debate highlighted a clear rift in styles of colonial administration by revealing the two fundamental aspects of mental assistance in Algeria. To cite one official, "two questions" were at stake, "one of a moral order and one of a material order."[58] Proponents of reform responded by appropriating the economic rhetoric of their colleagues. Some argued that implementing a novel psychiatric program with a more effective cure rate would result in "a real savings." If open services could achieve a 50 to 60 percent cure rate, as estimated by Lépine, costs would ultimately amount to far less than the current rates of 10 percent achieved by French asylums "where the unfortunate patients remain indefinitely." These asylums merited the condemnation that "Dante wrote on the gates of Hell: 'Abandon all hope here.'"[59] Others inverted economic logic by arguing that a moral calculus of obligation to France's *protégés* in the colonies superseded fiscal concerns. According to one delegate in 1925, the honor of the colony was at stake: "a country's prosperity loses the greatest part of its significance if it does not have the capacity to satisfy social needs of this magnitude." It was "not only a matter of morality, but of honor" that Algeria establish modern mental institutions worthy of the name. Insisting that his colleagues were "ignoring their moral obligations," the delegate rhetorically asked them to predict at what point "Algeria's fortune will be sufficient to free yourselves from the sole care of seeking prosperity."[60] Many colleagues agreed that amassing moral capital was as central to national prosperity as the securing of wealth. One of Porot's closest allies in the assemblies invoked common themes of honor and independence from France, arguing that "a country . . . is not only great when its material riches are great; it is all the greater, it is all the more honorable, when it adds to its intellectual and moral worth institutions whose entirely humanitarian function comprises at once its independence and its beauty."[61] Implementing a comprehensive mental health system held the possibility of putting Algeria on the leading edge of medical reform, rather than keeping it merely a "tributary of France."

By 1925 those who argued that "the moral point of view trumped everything" had gained an important ally in the Socialist governor-general Maurice Viollette.[62] Best known for his failed efforts to expand freedoms for Muslim Algerians during his subsequent tenure in Léon Blum's Popular Front government, Viollette had attempted to liberalize the Algerian regime since his days as a senator and as governor-general. As Benjamin Stora and other historians have pointed out, Socialists in the interwar era adopted a genuinely assimilationist position by seeking to implement colonial reforms through the extension of French civilization's benefits to the colonized. Significant investment in colonial infrastructure was central to the plan: schools, clinics, and model villages were among the massive public works projects touted by SFIO stalwarts such as Jean Jaurès and Guy Moutet.[63] For Viollette, cold demographic logic as well as ideology necessitated such programs: seeing the prospect of "ten million Algerians" in the near future, he asserted that reforms could make them "Frenchmen" rather than "revolutionaries."[64]

Such perspectives contributed to a growing rift in styles of colonial administration between metropolitan and settler authorities. Although Algeria was an assimilationist regime in theory—with the expectation that male Algerians would eventually attain French citizenship—this notion was widely rejected by settlers, who sought to maintain insurmountable barriers between colonizing and colonized populations.[65] By the turn of the twentieth century, settlement had increased dramatically in port cities such as Oran, Algiers, and Bône, while, at the same time, appropriation of arable land forced many Algerian peasants into the same urban settings.[66] Historians have documented a strong connection between this phenomenon and a move away from the assimilationist policies of the early administration of Algeria.[67] Although assimilation remained official policy through the end of French rule, increasing tension between Europeans and Algerians as well as the entrenchment of a new settler identity encouraged policies that emphasized difference. Although the French never ruled in Algeria according to an "associationist" policy, these notions of difference fostered the divergent governance of native and settler populations.[68] In addition to dramatic disparities in political representation for settlers and Algerian Muslims in institutions such as the fiscal assemblies, the Code de l'Indigénat, a legal system that officially established divergent penalties for criminal offenses committed by Europeans and Muslim Algerians respectively, offers a chief example of these policies of difference.

By contrast, many administrators from metropolitan France—including Viollette and his successor Jules Carde—subscribed to an explicitly assimilationist view. Adopting the emerging technocratic spirit of the interwar era, these figures seized on scientific and medical achievements as key symbols of French civilization's greatness and as powerful ideological instruments for the remaking of the colonies, and indeed France itself. The elaborate conjunction of a new appreciation for the uses of science for the state, an awareness of the continued importance of maintaining imperial hegemony, and a pervasive sense of economic and social crisis in interwar France set the stage for a new consideration of colonial development, or *mise en valeur*. In the wake of the First World War's economic and demographic devastation of France, the empire took on a renewed importance. Colonial manpower and matériel had been decisive factors in securing France's slim margin of victory; many centrist and left-leaning thinkers imagined the colonies to hold solutions to the crises that the nation faced in the aftermath of war as well. A reconfiguration of the "civilizing" programs of the early Third Republic—one relying on intense application of the social and exact sciences to develop the "rational exploitation" of colonial production at all levels—held the potential of what the historian Christophe Bonneuil has called a "miracle cure" for France's interwar woes.[69]

These convictions formed the ideological backbone of a program that aimed at the biopolitical remaking of the French empire. Just as Toulouse emphasized the limitless social possibilities of a biocratic state, colonial administrators sought to direct life toward productivity. Emerging nationalisms among disaffected colonial intellectual groups only encouraged this development. As Alice Conklin has argued, fields such as eugenics and social hygiene took on increasing importance for the "biological regeneration" of France and its colonies in a period of perceived degeneration and decline.[70] The growing importance of these forms of social scientific expertise often had the psychological effect of hardening racial boundaries by exposing the biological instability of whiteness and thereby threatening the racial security. Yet such ideas could equally reinforce assimilationist programs that sought to preserve (or develop) colonial hegemony through practices of investment and discourses of inclusion, or what David Scott has termed the "political rationalities" of colonial rule. According to this logic, the deployment of social and behavioral scientific knowledge as a means of reorganizing colonial life pointed to the promise of the nation's future.[71]

Algeria, as the cornerstone of the empire and home to France's largest overseas population, was a crucial space for the elaboration of these political rationalities, especially in the domains of public health and medicine. For those such as Viollette who saw the colonies as an experimental laboratory for the modernization of France, medical infrastructure provided an institutional mechanism for the redirection of Algerian life. In addition to its uses for preserving the health security of the empire, sanitary policing served a project of colonial governmentality by rendering populations visible and knowable in their aggregate forms. A massive upsurge of medical activity in Algeria in the 1920s and early 1930s, manifested in

concrete structures and programs that aimed at the "knowledge and regulation of the other" through its inclusion in the medical state, facilitated
this end.[72] In 1923, for example, the Algiers medical faculty established an
Institute for Colonial Medicine and Hygiene that served as a foundation
for Viollette's creation of a central medical and public health office in 1927.
Under Viollette's direction, the government-general also implemented a
welfare program for the assistance of new mothers and nursing infants. By
1932 the successes and promise of such programs influenced a complete
reorganisation sanitaire in the colony, undertaken as part of the centenary
celebration of French Algeria.[73]

This setting provided a fertile environment for development of a reciprocal relationship between mental hygiene initiatives and the biological
rationalities of colonial rule. Because of its explicit connections to eugenics and its apparently predictive capacity to analyze human behavior and
sociability, psychiatry was central to concerns about population health and
the preservation of social order in Algeria. The Commission Coloniale
d'Hygiène Mentale, created in 1924, points to this intersection. As the
French Mental Hygiene League's efforts hit impasses in the senate, this
committee sought applications for new forms of psychiatric organization
in the service of colonial expansion. The committee's charter indicated its
concern with bringing expertise to the "organization of psychiatric services
deserving of the name in the French colonies" as well as the development
of mental hygiene programs and the recruitment of psychiatric personnel
for colonial service.[74] The program aimed at far more than the extension
of a European model into colonial space. Critical among the charges of
meaningful mental hygiene was outreach into colonial society. In addition
to strengthening the "struggle against alcoholism and diverse addictions,"
the group promised to "struggle against local superstitions" in the promotion of sound mental health in colonial settings. Finally, the committee
pledged to analyze the "normal and pathological psychology of indigenous
populations," promising to amass this information with the goal of shaping
"methods of colonization as well as individual and collective professional
orientation" of native societies.

Yet far from a clear imposition of a metropolitan agenda on colonial
health services, the committee's program derived heavily from antecedents and contemporary initiatives in North Africa. At the time of the
committee's creation in 1924, Porot's work in Tunis represented the only
existing model for an effective colonial psychiatric service, and the Lépine
commission had already proposed a similar program in Algeria. Indeed,
Porot's and Lépine's advocacy for a complete network of psychiatric assistance in North Africa provided an essential catalyst for building such

a program. Despite the opening of colonial psychiatric facilities in Indochina, Madagascar, and West Africa, the Maghreb was the only site where programs such as those the committee envisioned were ever implemented, demonstrating the importance of Porot's energetic lobbying and interest in the project among influential settlers over the imposition of metropolitan authority. Porot's efforts in particular exemplified the concern with designing a new form of colonial mental expertise, one that tailored modern mental health systems to suit the needs of colonial settings. With its appreciation for practical matters such as appropriate architectural design for the Algerian climate and the capacity to situate local pathologies in an existing nosological order, Porot's model for colonial psychiatry thus emerged alongside the subtle new imaginings of colonial governance that characterized the interwar period.

Social engineering through psychiatry came at a high cost, however, which proved the source of volatile debates in Algeria's fiscal assemblies. Although Porot and Lépine's progressivist plan held significant promise for remaking Algeria, colonial psychiatry itself was an untested system. As one delegate exclaimed in 1923, the government-general was "launching into the unknown!"[75] Even those who agreed in principle that medicine was of critical importance to the political economy of colonial rule found the hygienists' claims far-fetched. A doctor named Bordères, a member of the delegation of Colons from Oran, argued repeatedly that precious hospital funds should be used for tubercular patients rather than the mentally ill. "In the current state of medical science," he noted, "madness is not always something curable."[76] If the government-general really cared about "social yield," it should "concern itself first with patients who can be brought back as quickly as possible to life and to work"—those who suffered from "much more serious and much more curable sicknesses" than madness, including malaria, syphilis, and tuberculosis.[77]

As the fiscal assemblies ran into repeated impasses over the role of government in provision for the insane, Viollette initiated construction on the Blida project. Viollette and his cabinet subsequently portrayed this move as one of decisive action in the face of the assemblies' dithering.[78] Others considered the action a classic example of Viollette's quixotic manner. Armand Maurin, a doctor who was a child in Algeria during Viollette's tenure, saw Viollette's ideas as "generous" in spirit and noted that his style "fortunately departed from the racist egotism that dominated Algerian politics." Yet this "new Governor was unfamiliar with the country": he "lacked experience," and his "humanitarian initiatives" became "absurd realizations in their application."[79] The Blida constructions undertaken in 1926 and 1927 represent classic examples. Construction costs quickly surpassed their budget, and faulty building and site mismanagement introduced new problems. Suffering from financial difficulties, the city of Blida found itself unable to supply the water and power lines and shade trees it had promised in 1912. According to two consultants called in to view the work in 1927—Porot and Raphaël Lalanne, director of an asylum at Maréville—the design of the buildings itself presented significant problems: "Everything has been reduced to vast, very bright dormitories (too bright, perhaps, and without shelter from the sunlight, particularly troublesome in this bare plain with no trees)." Such a facility suited only "absolutely tranquil subjects, capable of living in common, which is a minimal portion of the lunatic population." The severe sunlight of the Algerian climate could easily aggravate violent patients' conditions; installing curtains posed a suicide risk.[80] Opponents of the hospital in the assemblies pounced on these gaffes. One delegate described the hospital as covered by a "shadow": "not that of the trees, but of ill will and poor direction. Perhaps this would be sufficient to protect everyone from the heat of the sun!"[81] Another argued that even "if there are no madmen at Blida, we should recognize that an act of insanity has certainly been committed: that of the constructions."[82]

These blunders called attention to the need for new forms of expertise in the management of insanity. Testifying before the assemblies, Porot asserted that the "constant collaboration of a specialist physician and the architect" represented the only solution to Algeria's problems. Between 1927 and 1929, Porot worked closely with the government-general's official architect, M. Garnier, to build a feasible psychiatric system for Algeria. From the outset Porot and Garnier announced that creating an assistance program "ex nihilo" presented "a horde of problems"; at the same time, it is clear Porot seized this opportunity to implement radical reforms in the technology of mental health management alongside an adaptation of modern forms to suit colonial needs.

The issue of adaptation deeply informed debates surrounding colonial planning in a range of contexts, raising questions about the colonized environment as well as the assimilation of space and population into the colonizing culture. A growing literature has begun exploring the inherent tensions of colonial architecture and urbanism, for example, focusing on the problematic intersections of the organization of space, governmentality, and the dilemmas of colonial modernization. The interwar period in particular was marked by profound consternation over the apparent paradoxes of assimilation and domination through architectural and urban forms. As Patricia Morton has argued, colonial architecture was commanded to enact two opposing "scopic principles" that mirrored the contradictory goals of the interwar civilizing mission. On the one hand, commercial and residential architecture sought to reinforce the social hierarchies of colonialism through a segregation of urban space; on the other, the same forms were required to reflect a seamless integration of colonial and metropolitan worlds.[83] A Europeanization of space thus also demanded a rigid distinction between the European and the local in an ideologically fractured environment, a new manifestation of the disciplinary geography that characterized the nineteenth-century colonial city.[84] Chief examples of the resultant tensions in these hybrid forms are found both in the layout of the Paris Colonial Exposition of 1931 and in Lyautey's Morocco.[85]

Interwar Algeria offered a theater for a parallel performance, characterized by an effort to undo the errors of the past through effective programs to reconfigure urban environments. Regret over the bludgeoning of the city of Algiers through the nineteenth century—characterized by a ham-fisted bulldozing of Arab quarters and the erection of aesthetically thoughtless and substandard European neighborhoods—informed programs of urban renewal that aimed simultaneously at restoration and modernization. Architects and planners in the 1930s produced a hybridized schema for indigenous housing in Algiers, for example, that experimented with both stylized Islamic forms and modernist-rationalist structures, toward the end of portraying the incompatible traits of sensitivity toward local culture and colonial grandeur. By offering "hygiene, well-being, and aesthetics" to the colonized, they promised effective management of urban populations and problems while introducing "a higher degree of civilization" through external forms, in the words of the president of Algiers's Chamber of Commerce in 1930.[86]

On a smaller scale, individual buildings and institutions performed a similar role as repositories of these tensions of hybridity. Hospitals were no exception. Their construction demonstrated the colonial administration's commitment to its indigenous *protégés*, yet also literally concretized the tensions of the civilizing mission. Like the colonial city, with its endemic typhus, plague, and cholera, the hospital had specific hygienic requirements that demanded the implementation of modern sanitation. Yet the provision of care mandated a sort of fragmentation in this design through its need for a segregated environment, one effectively suited to the housing and maintenance of settler and indigenous populations. An Algerian public health official pointed to these tensions in 1940, noting that "the development of hospital welfare [in Algeria] has had to account for two clearly established principles." First, giving Algeria its rightful "European character"—assimilating space and modernizing care—required that hospital structures be "analogous to those existing in the Metropole." Yet at

the same time, Algeria's "colonial character" required "a special hospital and medical organization"—the compartmentalization of hospitalized
populations by ethnicity and adaptation to local circumstances.[87]

These ambivalent ideals—a simultaneous civilization of space and differentiation of populations—informed attempts to develop a modern colonial psychiatry in Algeria. As early as 1923, officials in the government-
general made clear that "servile" replications of European asylums would
not be acceptable for Algeria's circumstances.[88] This concern is paramount
in Porot's accounts of how to design a colonial psychiatric framework in
the late 1920s and early 1930s (figure 6). It was clear to Porot that even
outside the colonial context, psychiatric hospital design presented important complications absent from other health care formats. Speaking of the
development of a first-line ward at the Mustapha hospital in Algiers, Porot
argued that an effective service necessitated "a specialized hospital organization" and a "general economy" that was carefully planned "from the
outset." Above all, attention had to be focused on the classification of patients. "The ward must be compartmentalized according to several coef-
ficients at play simultaneously: separation by sex, race, and the reactions of
patients (calm, semi-calm, and violent)." These concerns necessitated not
a modification, but a "complete remodeling" of a standard ward. Attempting to do so on the cheap constituted "a danger that cannot be protested
too much": it threatened to "reduce [the ward] to impotence." The colonial context for such a ward compounded these requirements. In addition
to mandating a further degree of separation by ethnicity, the absence of
sufficient psychiatric services in Algeria meant that each existing ward
had to perform additional duties that were unnecessary in many metropolitan wards. Each colonial service had to be both large and flexible at
the outset, allowing for future expansion, because of the need "to account
for the rapid development of Algiers" and other colonial cities. Moreover,
such wards also had to incorporate a teaching service to train physicians
to recognize and treat mental disorders in small hospital units distributed
throughout the colony, at least at the level of triage.[89]

The construction of a large new hospital to serve "second-line" functions in Algeria added further complications and demanded clear attention to colonial needs in its earliest stages of design. As the failed early
construction work at Blida made clear, such apparently mundane concerns
as climate were critical to effective hospital design. Even in metropolitan hospitals, attention to climate had been paramount since the hospital
reached its earliest recognizably modern incarnation in the late eighteenth
century; in the colonial setting, ethnic divisions, the conditions of colonial labor, and cultural differences compounded factors such as the

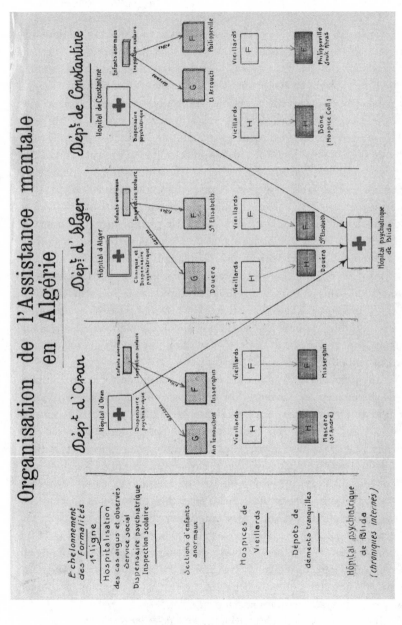

Figure 6. Organization of Mental Assistance in Algeria. From "Organisation de l'Assistance Mentale," Algérie, GGA 9 X 184, Centre des Archives d'Outre-Mer, Aix-en-Provence.

unforgiving North African sun to elevate the specifics of place to primary importance.[90]

The ideal of sensitively adapting a model hospital to the Algerian social, economic, and geographic environment saturates Porot and Garnier's plans for the Blida project, as presented both to the Algerian administration and to medical audiences. Yet they went far beyond merely adapting a metropolitan model to the colonial context. Instead, the psychiatrist and the architect sought to avoid what they considered the grievous errors of the typical nineteenth-century asylum in producing a facility that would raise the accepted standard for mental institutions in Europe as well as in the colonies. As a means of "sparing" patients and families from the "false and outdated conception" of and "popular prejudices toward madness" that were inextricable from "the old term 'Lunatic Asylum,'" with its evocations of "social protection from deranged and dangerous individuals," the facility was a "Psychiatric Hospital," which signaled instead the idea of patients "deserving of medical care and active therapeutics, but in a specially designed setting." The typical asylum's "symmetry" and "rigidity" had a "monotonous and depressing effect on patients in barracks houses." In contrast, Porot and Garnier strived to provide "extended views" over the hospital campus and its gardens through east-facing windows as a means of providing a calming setting while avoiding the most brutal effects of the sun.[91] As with any modern hospital, the plan included a range of psychiatric and medical services in addition to places of recreation and worship for both Catholics and Muslims.

Yet the psychiatric hospital did need to serve the protective role inherent to the concept of "asylum" for both patients and society even as it attempted to jettison the term's stigma. The general plan of the campus (figure 7) and the design of individual buildings (figure 8) reflected this tension. The adaptation of each building to the protection of its patient population was essential; thus, "no multi-storied buildings for those obsessed with suicide, for whom the window or the stairwell would be an easy temptation." In the case of those "who need close attention at all times," a design with limited exits and "panoramic surveillance" was essential. Yet the preservation of public safety, also among the hospital's most important missions, required a lockdown facility, the *quartier pénétentiaire* in addition to other units, especially given Blida's role as the colony's only comprehensive mental hospital: "Algeria, departing from a *table rase*, must not forget this special unit, so useful for social protection."[92]

This was especially the case given the violence that psychiatrists such as Porot deemed specific to the Algerian Muslim patient, attention to which marked every aspect of Blida's design.[93] Whereas European hospitals, for

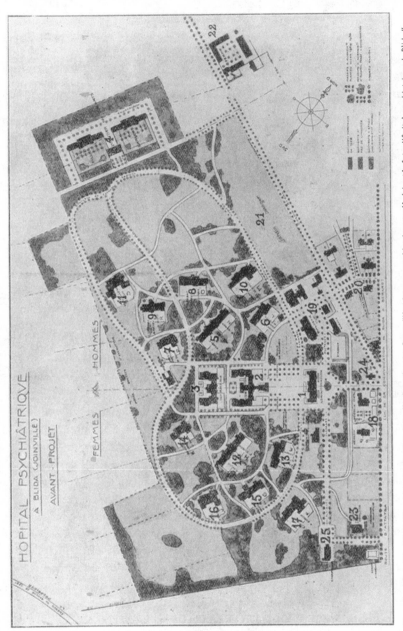

Figure 7. Plan of the Hôpital Psychiatrique de Blida-Joinville. From Antoine Porot, "L'assistance psychiatrique en Algérie et le futur Hôpital psychiatrique de Blida," *Algérie médicale* 65 (1933). Reprinted by permission of Bibliothèque nationale de France.

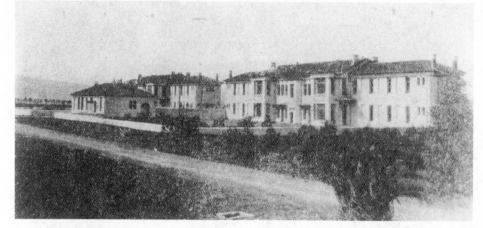

Figure 8.   Pavilions at Blida, 1933. From Antoine Porot, "L'assistance psychiatrique en Algérie et le futur Hôpital psychiatrique de Blida," *Algérie médicale* 65 (1933). Reprinted by permission of Bibliothèque nationale de France.

example, required only two principal sections for patients—to separate men and women—the colonial hospital required four to allow segregation by ethnicity as well. Most general hospitals in Algeria housed patients in an ethnically mixed environment. But the volatile conditions in a mental facility did not allow for a similar sense of "hospital community." Racial tensions in Algeria that simmered below the surface could easily rise in the heated atmosphere of the mental ward. Drawing on a growing body of knowledge about the spontaneous violence of the North African madman, Porot warned of potential situations in which "disordered minds, divergences in moral conceptions and social conceptions, and latent impulsivity could at any instant rupture the essential calm, stoke deliriums, and give rise to or create dangerous reactions in such an eminently inflammable milieu."[94] The "complete separation (with few exceptions) of Europeans from natives" was thus "indispensable" at Blida, where "the patients' morbid mentality could give rise to situations that we must avoid at all cost."[95] Concern about the potential disruption caused by Muslim patients was also reflected in the relative sizes of wards designed for violent and calm patients. Despite lower anticipated numbers of Muslim patients in the initial population—Porot planned for 135 Muslim men and 70 Muslim women versus 195 European men and 200 European women—the same number of beds was dedicated to violent patients in each pool.[96]

Above all, the novelty of a modern psychiatry in Algeria and its effects on labor and culture raised important questions and dictated important elements of the hospital's design. The absence of a psychiatric tradition in North Africa meant that the "recruitment and training of the nursing staff [would] be particularly difficult in this country." Architectural finesse posed solutions to both problems: it was possible to "make up for the relative deficiency" of the staff "through a carefully studied arrangement" of the wards.[97] Most important, the experimental nature of the facility demanded flexibility. Even with the most careful planning, it was unclear what proportions of men, women, Europeans, Muslims, voluntary admissions, administrative confinements, calm patients, and violent cases the hospital would actually serve in practice. Algeria's Muslims presented the most variables: Porot argued that there was no way to tell how they would react to a hospital that respected Muslim customs. Blida might thus receive such patients only by administrative orders, but he felt confident that "little by little," it would welcome Muslims, "even women, in rather high numbers, sent by their families."[98]

The project was utopian in its conception. It would solve the problem of madness in Algeria through the provision of first-rate care in situ. The plan also opened the possibility of placing the colony at the forefront of mental science by creating a new center for the study of psychology and ethnicity in Algeria. Finally, through the sensitivity of its design, the hospital promised to open a new avenue of communication between Algeria's Muslim and European communities through the apparently universal applicability of scientific medicine. Yet two major obstacles stood between Porot and Garnier's design and the project's implementation: Algerian law and Algerian finances. The legal problem proved the less daunting of the two. The law of 1838 had been promulgated in Algeria in the late nineteenth century; therefore, the two-line system that Porot had proposed was technically illegal. With his history of supporting public hygiene measures during his tenure as governor-general in French West Africa from 1923 to 1930, Jules Carde, Viollette's successor, proved a strong ally to Porot. In Algeria he oversaw a complete reorganization of the public health system that unfolded in the early 1930s, involving the creation of a public health ministry, the opening of two dozen new hospitals and clinics, and the implementation of a massive social medicine program for outreach into Algeria's Muslim population.[99] In the words of the physician and public health director Alexandre Lasnet, the program could ideally force Muslim society to "cast off its atavistic prejudices and to habituate it little by little to essential notions for preserving itself from preventable disease and in particular from those that weigh heavily on newborns."[100] The reorganization held important implications for psychiatry. For Carde, the two-line system of defense against mental illness represented "an extensive application of scientific and therapeutic progress from which mental medicine has so strongly benefited in recent years." In 1934 he issued a general instruction that organized the operation of the first-line services. This document legally assured the operation of these centers outside the rubric of the 1838 law and served as a model for the French memorandum of 13 August 1937 that proposed similar regulations.[101]

The instruction, which had the force of law, pointed to the opportunities for innovation that were inherent to the colonial scientific environment. Whereas psychiatrists in France had rejected similar reforms through the 1920s, in Algeria the close cooperation of a small cluster of psychiatrists working with Porot and the government-general allowed for pathbreaking legislation. The document streamlined the legal requirements for psychiatric hospitalization by stipulating that services could receive "any and all patients afflicted with psychic or psychoneurological disorders . . . under the same conditions as other wards, at the patient's or his family's request." Other hospital services could also transfer patients showing psychological manifestations into psychiatric wards with the psychiatrist's approval. Patient releases became as unrestricted as admissions. Given the physician's prior approval, and provided they posed no danger to themselves or others, families could claim voluntarily placed patients at any time; the 1838 law pertained only in cases involving patently dangerous patients.[102] Virtually all control over patient admissions, releases, and treatment regulations (including diet, recreation, visitation, and religious observance) remained in the physician's hands, granting Porot "permanent technical control over psychiatric wards established by the Direction of Public Health of the General Government of Algeria," a power that "extended to all existing psychiatric services in the hospitals of the Colony."[103]

Debates over the financing of the new system proved more contentious. The "progressive" design of the Blida Psychiatric Hospital also entailed a high price tag: Porot estimated total costs to run to three times the amount envisioned by the fiscal assemblies. The proposed plans provoked a new outburst of heated discussions in the fiscal assemblies about the role of medicine in the colonial state and vice versa. The more fiscally conservative delegation of Colons sought to bury the project without further "tiresome" debate, because "this comedy should come to an end."[104] Declaring his "firm intention to lay this issue to rest definitively," one delegate declared that Algeria's "lunatics" were "already cared for as they should be."[105] The same delegate had rejected the idea of the Blida hospital outright a year earlier as well on humanitarian grounds, asking his colleagues if "it is really truly humane for a family to go see one of its members completely deprived of reason, who doesn't even recognize them? Quite the contrary, I think it's heartbreaking for the family, and that it is even more painful at times to go see one of one's own in this state than to cry over a tomb."[106] The more "humane" solution of transportation to metropolitan asylums both mercifully removed the patient from the family's view and met the colony's needs at a fair price.

Yet the notion of a moral economy of care proved more persuasive to the assemblies as a whole. In 1929 one of Blida's representatives in the delegation of Non Colons, the newly elected Marcel Duclos, launched into an impassioned discussion about Algeria's obligations to its subjects. "Algeria is a new country, a young country, an eager and rich country; the generous ideas of social assistance and welfare that nourish the Metropole and that are in full bloom through admirable projects, should they be lacking in its most beautiful colony? This cannot be." Reminding his fellow settlers about the scrutiny to which Algeria would soon be subjected, Duclos argued that "this cannot be even more so, gentlemen, on the eve of this grandiose spectacle that will constitute the Centenary," the coming celebration of the hundredth anniversary of the conquest of Algiers. Without investing in such assistance projects as the Blida hospital, Duclos insisted, "*we* will be impoverished by not enriching the means that are at our disposal and to which our hearts should devote themselves." It was "toward this goal, so close to us, refined and altruistic, that we should reach," and not to the easy and cruel solution of continued transportation to metropolitan asylums.[107]

By raising the specter of the looming centenary celebration, Duclos forced a reconsideration of the project. More than a solution to Algeria's madness problem, a first-rate psychiatric system was a testament to the "generous and humane spirit of Algeria." The centenary—coinciding closely with the 1931 Colonial Exposition in Paris—prompted French Algerians to reconsider their role in "civilizing" the colony. Historians such as David Prochaska have argued that it was the presence of European settlers and their political and economic agendas that "made Algeria French." But major "civilizing" endeavors that emphasized scientific and technological innovation provided opportunities not only to demonstrate a commitment to colonization as a project, but also to outshine metropolitan programs and demonstrate the capacity of colonialism to rejuvenate a society. As Waltraud Ernst has suggested for the context of British India, massive public institutions served an important colonial role, not so much in their actual operation as in their symbolic function. Institutions such as hospitals, prisons, highways, railways, schools, universities, museums, and of course asylums were expensive projects—usually far more costly in colonies than at home—that paid off by making the colonizer's benevolence visible, even prominent. Whether they facilitated social control or not, whether they promoted indigenous advancement or not, public institutions left indelible marks of colonial governance, symbols of national prestige and power that garnered public attention and occupied prominent places both visually and in public opinion.[108] An institution such as Blida could add to the prestige of French Algeria in its hundredth year, demonstrating for the French and indigenous public the government's commitment to its people and the positive impact French civilization could make. Responding to Duclos's rhetoric, the fiscal assemblies adopted the project in principle, but demanded that it be restrained to twenty-five million francs.

Healthy Babies and Monkey's Lanterns

Presenting the newly opened Hôpital Psychiatrique de Blida to the readers of *Algérie médicale* in 1933, Antoine Porot acknowledged that "there is always some satisfaction, for a doctor, to bring a healthy newborn to term after a series of stillbirths and abortions."[109] His celebratory rhetoric acknowledged that the history of psychiatric planning in Algeria had been "anguishing," but emphasized that the achievement of such an innovative facility in a region with no existing public institutions for managing mental illness had rendered the political infighting and consequent delays that marked the budgetary struggle over Blida worthwhile. According to Porot and his colleagues, the very conception of the Blida hospital represented a significant step forward in the fight against mental illness not only in Algeria, but in metropolitan France as well. As Pinel had "elevated the madman to the dignity of the patient" in unchaining the inmates at Bicêtre, so Blida elevated the asylum to the dignity of the hospital.

A celebration of modernity accompanied the inauguration of psychiatric hospitals in French North Africa through the 1930s. Although the French had already opened custodial facilities in other overseas possessions, the advent of the North African institutions marked a turning point in colonial and metropolitan mental health care. Standard interpretations of colonial psychiatric institutions stem from Frantz Fanon's accounts of Blida's overwhelming patient loads and his indictment of French medical racism in *The Wretched of the Earth* and *A Dying Colonialism*. Although these assessments remain valid for the postwar era, it would be a mistake to assume from such accounts that French psychiatric hospitals in the Maghreb had always been decrepit, makeshift solutions for the confinement of social and political deviants. These institutions—not only the hospitals and clinics, but also the legal structures that regulated these networks of psychiatric assistance—brought important innovations to French psychiatry. Reformers' invocation of Pinel's legacy both prompted political action aimed at humanitarian reform and social control and also mandated that the resulting institutions employ progressivist technologies for managing mental illness. In contrast with the dismal institutions the British had built in their African colonies, the constructions in French North Africa were, in the eyes of their creators, modern facilities that applied the principles of mental hygiene and scientific rationalization to psychiatric care.

With its commitment to innovation, the Blida hospital, along with its satellite network for psychiatric care, contrasts markedly with the model of scientific diffusionism from a metropolitan core. It instead echoes the model that Bruno Latour outlined for the acceptance of the Pasteurian doctrine in the colonies rather than the hexagon, suggesting the possibilities for the implementation of a "progressivist" program in a colonial terrain, outside of the supervision and control of a professional metropolitan elite with a vested interest in the status quo.[110] Blida was also a useful symbol for those who sought to renew France's colonial mission through scientific investment and modernization. The acrimonious debates that surrounded funding allocations for Blida and other psychiatric units therefore orbited around the basic question of France's obligations to its colonies. By engaging the idea of moral versus material economies of colonial rule, officials used psychiatry as a tool for debating whether colonialism was a project or merely a system for exploitation. Such logic also often overlapped. Most agreed that care for the insane could be better in Algeria, and that in an ideal world the mentally ill deserved the best that France could provide: few saw investment in psychiatry as simply throwing good money after bad. Others saw psychiatry not only as a moral obligation, but also as a means of preserving public safety and Algeria's eugenic future: in Duclos's words, to abandon such patients to their own devices was to "prepare the army of crime."[111]

Innovative management of colonial madness thus constituted a critical venue for the deployment of a biopolitical agenda. Efforts to remake psychiatry as a form of population health and hygiene were not new in the late 1920s, as the efforts of France's Mental Hygiene League make clear. Yet these efforts found much greater success in North Africa than they did in France. Whereas Toulouse and his colleagues succeeded in opening a handful of clinics in metropolitan sites, Porot and the Algerian government-general founded an entire network of psychiatric care based on these principles. Part of the reason the colonies served as a crucible for psychiatric innovation was the absence of any recognizably modern psychiatric system in North Africa: the "blank slate" described by Porot and his colleagues. Yet more than the offspring of necessity, innovation merged with a new political imagination that linked colonial regeneration with medical investment.

In metropolitan France, mental hygiene was one of many discourses of recovery for a nation devastated by war. The "reconstitution of its capital of psychic energy" that Toulouse urged was a low priority for a nation engaged in the impossible project of attempting to return to the imaginary past of its mythical *belle époque*.[112] By contrast, in the colonies the new psychiatry was part of a coherent program of building and investing in the new, rather than recovering what had been lost. Psychiatry formed an essential component of a new order of colonial biopolitics, linked to optimism about medicine's capacity to shape a new and productive colonial future. As Algeria's director of public health testified before the fiscal assemblies, France's work in this domain "was considerable . . . and I am convinced that Algeria will be one of the first countries in the world endowed with a solid sanitary organization."[113]

The Pinel legend was in this way more suitable to efforts to develop a colonial psychiatry than it was to remaking the metropolitan asylum. The wretchedness of colonial *maristans* more closely fit its rhetoric and suggested the ways in which French medical science could develop a "barbaric" terrain. But it is also the optimism inherent in these colonial projects that informed their eventual warm reception. Colonial psychiatry promised both to regulate public order and to remake indigenous subjects through its "struggle against local superstitions."

As with other components of colonial *mise en valeur*, efforts to make a colonial psychiatry in interwar Algeria were more complicated than the Manichaean characterization that Fanon ascribed to the colonial project. With its emphasis on reform and professional reorganization, the progressivist rhetoric that surrounded colonial psychiatry testified to the ways in which colonialism was about science, modernization, development, and process as much as it was about exploitation: indeed, exploitation was inherent in the project of developing colonial space and managing colonial populations. Colonial psychiatry employed the redemptive language of biopolitics, which linked it closely to the visions of administrators such as Maurice Viollette, who saw Algeria as the site for the advancement of an assimilationist agenda. Yet as the following chapters show, such programs were based in a powerful epistemic violence, one that subsumed the subjectivity and the agency of the colonized in its effort to remake colonial space in a European mold.

The story of psychiatry's development in Algeria reveals clearly that "progressivism," of course, does not always mean "progress." Algeria's psychiatric units and others throughout the Maghreb were besieged with operational difficulties in their early years when the challenges of practice in a politically and culturally charged colonial environment became obvious. As Porot argued in 1933, a technologically sophisticated hospital environment constituted only one step toward the implementation of a successful mental assistance program; "qualified specialists and specialized personnel" were the essential core that could enable such technology to reach its full potential. Porot noted that all Algeria's exertion would amount to "a sterile effort and a waste of millions" if the colony did not complete the project by ensuring its smooth function and continuing support. Referring to the French children's story about how the promise of wonder leads to neglect of practical necessities, he argued that without this continued effort, "we would have only to reflect sadly on the timeless fable of the 'Monkey and the Magic Lantern'!"[114]

3

Spaces of Experimentation, Sites of Contestation
Doctors, Patients, and Treatments

As new hospitals across the Maghreb welcomed their charges, the French press sounded notes of both infectious pride and somber ambivalence. Journalists who gathered at psychiatric conferences and hospital inaugurations argued that the new institutions represented an important step forward for both patients and practitioners. The North African insane could now seek care "in the best conditions of hygiene, tranquility, and security" in these "model establishments for lunatics," while the new hospitals provided psychiatrists with a showcase for institutional reform in a colonial terrain.[1] Yet the mission of these hospitals also recalled the lowest depths of human misery, tingeing celebration with sadness.

The Blida hospital epitomized this paradox. For *La dépêche algérienne*'s reporter, who covered Blida's official opening in 1938, the hospital was more like a "pleasant estate" than a madhouse: its "charming pavilions, cheerful gardens, [and] wide pathways planted with young and beautiful trees" promised a "calm and joyful retreat." A decade later, *Alger républicain* described the hospital as a "veritable small city," its "delightful pavilions" and its "lawns and flowers" making up an "attractive community." Yet if it was a "paradise," it was one "stalked by wandering, soulless bodies."[2] The journalist from the *Dépêche* was struck by a profound sadness. The hospital's grounds were quite pleasant, but it was "cruel to speak of pleasure when one has just stood next to one of the most tragic aspects of human misery, seen a revolting face through the bars of a courtyard, heard a soulless scream mount toward the clear heavens on a beautiful morning, and remembered the poignant

Baudelairean prayer: 'Lord, have pity on the madmen and madwomen.'"[3] Regardless of the beauty of its setting and the efficiency of its operation, Blida's very existence recalled the depths of human unreason.

Reforming the Maghreb's institutions of madness represented a major accomplishment for the mission to "civilize" North Africa—"a great and beautiful French achievement," according to the press.[4] The hospitals encompassed the idealism that reformers brought to the colonial psychiatric project and represented the ways in which a psychiatry unencumbered by traditional institutions could revolutionize the discipline. A range of papers from the 1930s and 1940s emphasizes the accomplishments of colonial psychiatric pioneers, constantly underscoring the efficiency of the new institutions' operation as well as the capacity of colonial hospitals to place French psychiatry on the cutting edge of therapeutic practice. Yet this success was often illusory, and it entailed a high cost. The smooth, efficient operation psychiatrists celebrated was in many ways an artifact of confinement patterns rather than a measure of effective treatment. The increasing reach of networks for psychiatric internment also meant that exponentially higher numbers of patients entered the fold of state mental assistance in the Maghreb. As these waves of confinement filled their institutions to capacity, the hospitals designed to alleviate the burden of colonial madness themselves became overwhelmed, which provided the impetus for implementing innovative therapies. Such innovations bolstered the claim that the colonies constituted a new center for scientific development, yet they did so at the expense of alienating patients.

The stories of the hundreds of patients at Blida, Manouba, and Berrechid reflect the ambivalence that plagued psychiatric progressivism in the mid-twentieth century. At the same moment that new confinement mechanisms clogged hospitals, novel procedures offered a solution to the mounting crisis. Such therapies promised finally to bring psychiatry into parity with other medical specializations, but they did so at an often painful cost to the patient populations of the Maghreb. The "softer" treatments advocated by reformers in the 1920s—mental hygiene and social work programs—were implemented to great effect in Algeria's European enclaves. Yet psychiatrists also saw their North African Muslim patients as a data set for testing the efficacy and safety of increasingly invasive treatments in the hope of complementing institutional progressivism with new technologies for healing.

French psychiatrists understood the Maghreb and its subjects as a space of experimentation. A social history of institutionalization highlights the differences between local and European conceptions of mental illness and its treatment by detailing patients' reactions to confinement in a colonial regime. It also draws attention to the ways in which medicine constituted a site for negotiation between doctors and their patients and a location for contesting medical epistemologies. Rather than retrodiagnosing colonial patients through glimpses and gaps in their stories—was this one a paranoid schizophrenic? did that one suffer major depressive psychosis? was a third borderline?—examining the ways in which doctors delivered diagnoses and patients experienced them offers a methodological pathway into the powers and persuasions of colonial psychiatry. In French North Africa, patients clung to local beliefs in defiance of classification and treatment within European paradigms. But they did so neither as a form of reflexive resistance to colonial authority, nor because their illnesses were colonial fabrications. Instead, psychiatrists and patients engaged in a protracted argument about incompatible philosophies of sickness and healing. Exploring the different experiences of confinement, diagnosis, and treatment for European and Muslim patients exposes the ways in which the colonial situation complicated the already fraught relationship between psychiatrist and patient and points to the ways in which the clinical relationship often unfolded as a contest over hegemony.

Celebrating Modernity: Institutional Efficacy and Models of Confinement

Patients enter psychiatric confinement in many ways. Family or neighbors complain to authorities, whereupon an isolated disturbance becomes a judicial procedure. Criminals pass through psychiatric examinations when circumstances indicate their necessity. Police encounter individuals menacing public safety; a doctor's examination brings them into a medical, rather than a carceral fold. A homeless person fighting addiction becomes unruly and is brought into custody and goes from there into psychiatric confinement. Yet internment's inherent constraint of liberty and disparities of power—often tracking axes of race, gender, and social class—means that confinement is rarely a simple procedure. In the colonial setting, the politics of European rule further complicated psychiatric interventions. Despite great acclaim for the smooth operation of new psychiatric hospitals, the association of medical and state authority with European domination and conflicts between the persistence of local knowledge about mental illness and the imposition of biomedical models of treatment raised powerful tensions that exacerbated common strains between psychiatrist and patient.

Mechanisms of confinement in the Maghreb were shaped by the legal, geographical, and social context of French colonialism. Violent behavior, disciplinary infraction, addiction, physical illness, and cultural misunderstanding brought patients to the attention of colonial authorities, where the institutional apparatus of colonial psychiatry initiated a careful process of registration, tracking, internment, and treatment. Conforming to the model of industrial efficiency that mental hygienists and psychiatric reformers had adopted in advocating the new system, patients were managed and processed as much as they were healed. Conforming to colonial psychiatrists' efforts to promote North Africa as a center for scientific production, patients were exposed to a bewildering array of treatments geared at demonstrating the novelty and modernity of psychiatric medicine.

Before the advent of colonial psychiatric hospitals in the 1930s, internments were rare. The cost and logistics of transporting patients to French asylums meant that only patients who posed extreme social danger—often recidivists—entered official custody. The case of Mohamed ben Abed K., an Algerian who had spent time in two French asylums during the First World War, is representative.[5] Apparently cured of his dementia praecox and melancholic depression, he was released and returned to Algeria in 1925, where he inexplicably killed his wife. Victor Dechaux, a prison doctor who examined Mohamed, concluded that he suffered from a "hallucination of an impulsive character" that motivated his crime and ordered him back to the Aix asylum.[6]

At the end of 1933 French asylums contained over 1,300 North African inmates like Mohamed. Over half of the colonial patients in French asylums were of European rather than Muslim origin—an unsurprising demographic, given that families with roots in Europe were generally more likely to send relatives to French institutions and that colonial authorities were generally more willing to return all but the most dangerous Muslim patients to their families.[7] In theory, the establishment of local facilities would permit the internment, observation, and treatment of less serious cases, and more of them.

By the mid-1930s the Maghreb's new psychiatric networks appeared to have facilitated medical production and rationalized psychiatric care. Between 1933 and 1935, for example, the neuropsychiatric clinic at the Mustapha hospital in Algiers more than doubled its admissions, as did the clinic in Oran. More important, efficient early treatment alleviated the overcrowding that plagued so many other facilities and encouraged voluntary admissions: more than half of the patients at Algiers and Oran entered the state's care of their own volition. Plunging mortality rates, drastically reduced stays, and significant cure rates also characterized the new wards, with nearly half of their patients deemed sufficiently recuperated to return home within three months.

We must view these self-reported results with a skeptical eye: the elusive psychiatric "cure" operates on a sliding scale and is open to wide-ranging interpretation. But colonial practitioners used these figures to suggest that the technological modernization of madness through efficient management held the key to success. For Porot, colonial psychiatrists, unlike their metropolitan forebears, were not "handicapped by antiquated formulae and traditions" and had thus incorporated "modern conceptualizations of assistance and scientific data" in their program design. The early achievements of colonial programs such as Porot's own clinic in Tunis and Algeria's new network of care constituted strong evidence in favor of using these principles to modernize psychiatry globally. "Everywhere," Porot insisted, "where there is a large population and a large General Hospital, there should be a Psychiatric service, a *totalitarian* service, to use a fashionable expression, not only for temporary and intermittent afflictions that can arise in all services, but *for all currents of Psychiatry*." This "totalitarian" system mandated "an observation and treatment service" as well as a social work program and a teaching service, and, Porot argued, it "came naturally to mind and imposed itself where, departing from a *tabula rasa*, we had to create an entire psychiatric apparatus."[8]

Administrators, physicians, and urban planners saw colonial terrains as blank slates, experimental fields for creating and testing new scientific systems in a vacuum that could then be transported into the metropole. Scholars such as Paul Rabinow and Gwendolyn Wright have noted that colonial administrators saw overseas possessions as ideal testing grounds for "working out solutions to some of the political, social, and aesthetic problems which plagued France."[9] Yet the colonial Maghreb was surely anything but a blank slate. Local knowledge about suffering and healing proved resilient when faced with a modernizing psychiatry imposed from without. The resulting tension between a medicine that branded itself as a pathbreaking model for global psychiatric reform, on the one hand, and local ideas about mental sickness and health, on the other, made the clinic a critical site of contestation over the right to heal and in turn, over central aspects of the colonial project.

Visitors, administrators, and physicians consistently emphasized the luxurious aspects of the new installations. The travel writer Marise Périale signaled Berrechid in Morocco as a potential tourist destination that demonstrated France's commitment to the downtrodden, asserting that the hospital left "nothing to be desired and offer[ed] the maximum of well-being and comfort in an agreeable location for the patients."[10] A medical student echoed this sentiment in regard to Tunisia's new hospital at Manouba, arguing that "our protectorate can serve as a model for other colonies for the assistance of the psychopathological" because one could find "no better [example] in this domain," even in the metropole.[11] Ma-

nouba, with its "modern advances," was plush to a fault, according to critics: Muslim patients would be "transported from the slums . . . to a palace
from the *Thousand and One Nights*."[12] And Blida, as the keystone of colonial mental assistance, was for one journalist "a model of the genre in its
modern perfection."[13] Algerian fiscal delegates agreed that "the only thing
we can reproach the [Blida] hospital for is being very beautiful, very large,
and having cost the colony a great deal of money." The hospital was "from
the first glance" a "luxurious organization."[14]

Early reports celebrated not only the luxury, but also the efficacy of
these new models for care. After initial complaints of overcrowding, by
1936 Algeria was experiencing "the nearly normal and complete operation
of the different recently organized services on our two lines of assistance"
and was finally meeting "the real needs of mental welfare in this country."
Open wards in the cities allowed for the hospitalization of "an entirely new
category of patients"—acutely afflicted psychopaths—enabling them to
"benefit from a more liberal regime." This combination augured strong
economic benefits for the administration: of nearly a thousand new patients, only a third went on to long-term confinement at Blida, demonstrating that "early care and a better filtration after competent observation" left
"only the inevitable minimum of patients." Even Blida showed promising
results, releasing nearly 10 percent of its patients as cured in 1936, a high
proportion considering the "filtration" of most easily curable patients at
the departmental level.[15]

Smaller but similar programs also opened in the Moroccan and Tunisian protectorates in the same period, which experienced similar performance. In Tunisia, Manouba also had begun operation by the mid-1930s
in conjunction with the neuropsychiatric pavilion at Tunis's public hospital. In 1936 only 20 percent of the patients who passed through the pavilion were admitted to Manouba, while nearly 60 percent were released.[16]
Morocco's network of facilities handled similar numbers in the mid-1930s,
with some 350 patients (both European and Muslim) admitted to the Berrechid hospital in 1937 alone, along with several dozen Europeans passing
through an open ward at Casablanca's public hospital.[17]

Psychiatrists and public health officials consistently invoked the operation of the new hospitals "at full yield" and in equilibrium as a means of
demonstrating their effectiveness and justifying investments in colonial
mental health. Such figures, however, are illusory and incomplete. They
are more clearly an artifact of patient demographics and the chief pathways
to confinement than they are a measure of institutional efficacy. Patients'
ethnicities, as well as the afflictions from which they suffered and the treatments they received, correlated closely to the length of their confinements

and contributed to uneven patterns of movement, distribution, internment, and recuperation. These social and medical factors belied any notion of an "average" internment and point to the importance of contextualizing diagnoses and individual patients' experiences. Certain patients—indeed entire groups of patients—did far better than others in the new hospitals, and confinement for certain afflictions yielded far quicker releases, both of which shaped an artificial aggregate picture of institutional progress.

Although they rarely figured in psychiatrists' writings or in official pronouncements about colonial madness, European settlers represented a significant proportion of patients confined in the new hospitals. At Manouba, Europeans constituted some three-quarters of the female patient population and nearly a quarter of the male population. Blida documented a similar pattern, with Europeans comprising over a third of patients, but less than a tenth of the general population. While Muslims constituted two-thirds of male patients, there was a "slight majority of European women" in the female population.[18] At Berrechid, nearly two-thirds of new patients in 1937 were European, despite the fact that settlers only amounted to 200,000 in a total Moroccan population of five million.[19] Yet European patients' relatively successful treatment accounts in large part for the illusion of fluid movement in colonial hospitals. Despite extensive rhetoric about the "civilizing" prospects of modern psychiatry in colonial terrains, in actual practice in the 1930s the hospitals served far higher proportions of Europeans than North Africans, and apparently served them more effectively. Although more Europeans were admitted, more were also released in short order, while Moroccans experienced substantially longer hospitalizations.[20] This scenario raises important questions, including, chiefly: Why did the European patient population turn over more quickly than the Muslim population? Did Europeans receive preferential treatment or merely more effective treatment? Were some of the same behaviors considered normal in European patients but aberrant in Muslims? What social effects and practices informed these hospitalization patterns and generated divergent outcomes?

Abandonment, rather than a failure of treatment, offers one explanation for these disparities. In some ways, the hospitals were victims of their own success. The opening of the hospitals suggested a new space for the transfer of the unwanted by family, community, and state. Ambiguous claims about a subject's potential and public danger rendered hospitalization a useful mechanism for managing criminal, deviant, or disturbed subjects at the protectorate's expense. A 1936 circular from the Tunisian public health directorate noted the extent to which Tunisian Muslims in particular had taken advantage of the new hospitals. The minister indicated that many patients at Manouba and the Tékia were "currently cured and may be, without risk, released to their families." Yet he also noted that "the latter have not responded to notices" announcing the imminent release of their relatives. Abandonment to colonial authorities amounted to a mechanism of repudiation, an absolution of responsibility for the patient, that dated to the tradition of the *maristans* and continued to plague North African hospitals through the postcolonial era. As a consequence, Manouba found itself in the mid-1930s "encumbered by healthy persons and obliged to refuse care to numerous patients due to a lack of space."[21]

Patterns of internment indicate that not all of these "healthy" patients were terribly sick from the outset. Among the most widely shared attributes of patients who found themselves involuntarily confined in North African hospitals were poverty and delinquency, a factor reinforcing the impression of psychiatry's ambivalent position on the cusp between medicine and penology. In the hope of ridding their communities of recidivist criminals, addicts, and the insane, police, *caïds* (Muslim authorities who served as intermediaries between the colonial state and local subjects), and other colonial administrators repeatedly emphasized their subjects' absolute lack of resources and especially their danger to public safety in demands for internment. Even in cases of minor disturbance, requests uniformly suggest the dangers posed by the mentally ill, indicating the requestor's hopes of transferring responsibility from village and community to the state. Such was the case of one patient who suffered, according to police files, from a "mania for stealing bicycles in the absence of their owners"; police implored higher authorities "to take the required actions so that in the future he cannot resume [these] misdeeds."[22]

Many, if not most, patients in colonial hospitals suffered from a range of addictions. These cases presented important ambiguities, with implications for epidemiology, confinement patterns, and the politics of colonial medicine. Psychiatrists pointed to forms of substance abuse that were specific to North Africa, such as "teaism" and "coffeeism" in addition to the more familiar "hashishism," heroin addiction, and alcoholism. Authorities interned most of these patients not because of their addictions per se, but rather because of antisocial behavior and public endangerment that followed from intoxication. In Algeria, a Kabyle who had murdered his wife offers a typical case: according to Charles Bardenat, an intern at Blida, chronic overconsumption of coffee and tea had provoked the patient's reaction.[23]

Despite Islamic prohibitions, alcoholism also played a significant role in shaping patient populations. Heavy drinkers "whose consumption generally surpasses two liters of wine and several apéritifs per day" constituted a quarter of the patients at Blida in May 1941. More significantly, they constituted 40 percent of Blida's criminally insane population and included as many Muslims as Europeans. Maurice Porot, Antoine Porot's son, student, and colleague, who had written his 1938 medical thesis on alcohol poisoning, concluded from these figures that "alcohol in all its forms and in any quantity is a danger at least as serious for the Muslim as for the European."[24] Responding to this danger, a law passed in October 1941 prohibited the sale of alcoholic beverages to indigenous Algerians.[25] The Berrechid psychiatrist André Donnadieu noted that "despite the Prophet and despite the *dahirs* [the sultan's proclamations], alcoholism is beginning to bring to Morocco ravages as serious as those in European countries." Berrechid's population comprised a "considerable" number of alcoholics, of whom half presented symptoms of maniacal excitation. Alcoholism was predominant in soldiers, but was also found in diverse urban occupations: "drivers, café workers, cooks, and manual laborers" proved the most widely affected populations. Even some Muslim women—"nearly exclusively in the categories of prostitutes or domestic servants"—presented alcoholic symptoms. Few alcoholics came from the liberal professions, perhaps because "intoxication is slower there and due to this factor violent reactions are rarer." These "violent reactions" precipitated confinement: "Due to his excitation, the indigenous alcoholic arrives in the ward sometimes through administrative means for agitation, scandalous public behavior, vagabondage; sometimes through judiciary means for violent crimes, murders."[26]

Heroin abuse constituted a major scourge among indigenous patients in the interwar period, especially in Tunisia. Nearly a fourth of the male Tunisian patients who entered Manouba between 1935 and 1937 were heroin addicts, and French newspapers in the protectorate predicted that 80 percent of the youth in Tunis used the drug. Heroin addiction cut across the social spectrum, but concentrations in urban Muslim youth gave rise to the suspicion among nationalists that "the French government fostered the dispersion of the drug in Arab intellectual circles in order to annihilate the movement."[27] The lack of police action and the "complacency" of customs officials favored this interpretation, but Pierre Maréschal, the director of Manouba after 1936, ascribed this sentiment to paranoia rather than evidence.[28] Maréschal argued instead that "the Tunisian Arab has always been prone to addiction," and the introduction of heroin into Tunisia provided "the poison he needed [and] . . . dethroned other intoxicants." Drug addiction suited the Arab personality, according to Maréschal:

> the penchant for dreaming and inaction; the contempt for the notion of
> time; the relative importance given to the truth; this conception . . . that

to purchase by credit is to purchase for free; that to be convicted with
a suspended sentence is to be acquitted; and finally, this "small-time"
lifestyle [*façon de vivre "à la petite semaine"*] seem to be common traits in
the Arab and the drug addict.

Addiction treatment offers important clues to the appearance of movement in the patient population. Although addictions remained difficult to
cure, detoxification enabled psychiatric hospitals to turn beds quickly. As
resident-general Marcel Peyrouton noted in 1935, "I think that Manouba
will have many clients, which will be a rather pleasant life: intoxicate yourself for a month, detoxify for fifteen days at State expense."[29] Psychiatric hospitals came increasingly to serve as refuges for chronic patients, a
problem compounded by the abandonment of the healthy at their doors,
and psychiatrists found themselves besieged. This was a nearly universal
problem in the 1930s. Long-term patients overwhelmed hospitals and asylums in Europe and the United States during this period, resulting in the
phenomenon that the historian Jack Pressman called "silting up," in which
chronic patients clogged hospitals. A result of the rapid urbanization and
industrialization of Europe and the United States, population growth in
cities led to an expansion of populations at risk for diseases and disorders with long-term psychiatric consequences, such as syphilis and schizophrenia. The added stresses of the Depression and a resulting inability to
provide care through private means left more of these cases than usual in
public hands. As Pressman argued, regardless of a hospital's efficiency,
"even a low retention rate will retire enough beds that an institution's ability to process the large number of patients pressing at the entrance will be
significantly impaired."[30]

By contrast, the short-term detoxification of drug-addicted patients
represented an important means of facilitating releases. Including detoxification patients in the hospital's aggregate population generated an illusion of flow because of the procedure's capacity to empty beds quickly. As
the medical anthropologist Lorna Rhodes has argued about an American
psychiatric unit in similar circumstances, colonial psychiatric networks
"advertised treatment while offering movement."[31] The release of detox
patients after fifteen days preserved the statistical illusion that the modernization Manouba brought to confinement proved effective at the level of
treatment. Balancing admissions and discharges, the figures show an institution in equilibrium and demonstrate the efficacy of the modern technologies it employed. This was particularly important in a colony such as Tunisia, in which Maréschal presided over a virtual monopoly on psychiatric
expertise. Although this position invested him with significant authority,

it also meant that physicians unacquainted with psychiatric diagnostics ordered the internments of most patients from the interior. Inexpert medical judgments resulted in the confinement of chronic patients who might have been treated more effectively in nursing homes than in an acute care facility. In contrast with the encumbrance problem chronic patients posed for Manouba, heroin addicts constituted an attractive patient base: supervising detoxification presented few problems to the overwhelmed Maréschal, who was free to devote his attention to more demanding patients.

These cases call attention to the close relationship between psychiatry and criminology. In French law since the Napoleonic era, Article 64 of the penal code had specified that proof of mental impairment in the culprit absolved the criminal of any wrongdoing; indeed, such proof meant that no crime had taken place at all. This element of the code was applied in colonial settings in various ways and created close links between psychiatric expertise and the judicial process. In the Tunisian case, Article 38 of the code followed the French model in declaring that infractions committed by children under the age of seven and those "in a state of dementia at the time of the action" were "not punishable": these cases reflected an "absence of criminality."[32] Yet in contrast with French law—which explicitly removed authority over confinement from the judiciary to the administrative branch by assigning that power to the prefecture—in Tunisia the decision over a defendant's mental state rested with the judge. Lay witnesses, including arresting officers and victims, might influence the court's ruling, but psychiatrists retained the most significant influence over decisions for internment. In one case where a police officer and a second witness "testified that the accused did not appear to enjoy his full mental faculties at the moment of the crime" and "random witnesses confirmed these two testimonies," the magistrate followed the opinion of a psychiatrist who examined the culprit six months after the fact and contradicted the others, concluding that he was responsible for the crime.[33] Yet other cases likely to have been treated in a penal setting in other contexts—the punishment of alcoholism and heroin use in the United States in the same period is one example—often brought patients into psychiatric rather than judicial disciplinary settings.[34]

Psychiatric rather than penal confinement often pertained where more traditionally "medical" diagnoses might apply. In a number of cases, physiological and neurological disorders that entailed criminal behavior resulted in judgments of irresponsibility and orders for psychiatric confinement. Encephalitis caused Ben Alied S., a twenty-year-old Algerian at Blida in the mid-1930s, to hurl a child into a well. The disease, according to the treating psychiatrist, freed the patient's deepest murderous instincts. Once at Blida, he turned these instincts on himself, banging his head against a cell wall and wounding himself repeatedly. Epilepsy was also imagined to provoke criminal episodes in North African patients. Epileptics such as Moussa S., who stabbed his mistress and mutilated the corpse, and Mohamed B., who killed his mother-in-law, found their way to Blida, where doctors treated them with heavy barbiturates.[35] These organic manifestations, like chronic intoxication, provided strong evidence for the "state of dementia" required for a verdict of criminal irresponsibility and psychiatric rather than penal confinement in Algeria. Other cases were murkier. Psychiatrists often assigned diagnoses of paranoid psychosis and persecution delirium to cases where jealousy provided a strong motive. The courts confined Ahmed D., an Algerian man, at Blida after he attempted to slit his neighbor's throat after the neighbor made advances toward Ahmed's wife. The patient's three-year history of jealous outrages and his attempt to kill his wife with an ax upon his release—which may have indicated premeditation in other circumstances—indicated paranoia to psychiatric experts at his trial.[36] Psychiatrists also diagnosed a number of criminal patients with a general "acute psychosis," as in the case of Em. Ben F., an Algerian interned at Blida after claiming that voices told him to kill a romantic "rival." Although Em. still heard voices after three years in the hospital, his physicians released him as "cured" after he learned to resist the voices' demands.[37]

These examples highlight the general mechanisms of confinement in the French colonies. In most cases, violent or disruptive behavior led authorities to question an individual's mental state. Evidence uncovered during the judicial process located the deep-seated roots of antisocial behavior in mental disorders of organic or chemical origin; psychiatric expert witnesses at trial found confinement the most appropriate response and the likeliest pathway to rehabilitation. Yet they point only obliquely to factors that complicated the process. With the exception of abandonment by relatives, they tell very little about the intersection of cultures that marked psychiatric diagnosis and treatment and the ways in which cultural assumptions informed what "normal" responses to psychiatric disorder should be. In a colonial setting, judgments about illnesses and treatments were subject to intense and ongoing negotiation, a process that greatly exacerbated the already loaded dialogue between psychiatrist and patient.

Patterns of Treatment

The installation of colonial psychiatric hospitals coincided historically with one of the most prolific phases in the development of psychiatric technologies in the twentieth century. The late 1930s witnessed the introduction of a wide range of new therapies that aimed at the social and medical re-organization of the psychiatric discipline and exacerbated tensions between local healing practices and European ideas about psychopathology. The colonial setting offered an ideal laboratory for experimentation with new techniques that alternately aimed either at the body or at a pathological social fabric as the principal locus of insanity, efforts that merged closely with efforts at the medical and social engineering of colonial space.

Two important trends marked Western psychiatry in the 1930s and 1940s. Social and medical forms of intervention that were developed in this period widened the scope of psychiatric treatment considerably. Since its inception psychiatry had occupied a unique position between social and medical science: Pinel and Esquirol aimed simultaneously at social renewal and the elevation of psychiatry to a medical science. But the in-terwar period introduced new means for facilitating psychiatry's applica-tion at both its social and its medical poles through a range of "soft" and "hard" treatments. The conjunction of this period of professional renewal and the development of psychiatric hospitals in the Maghreb means that from the outset new technologies in mental health care complemented the "modern" architectural and legal frameworks with which psychiatrists had endowed the assistance networks anchored at Blida, Berrechid, and Ma-nouba. This intersection provides an important location for exploring the ethical implications of psychiatric innovation, on the one hand, while un-derscoring the clash of medical cultures in French North Africa between the 1930s and 1950s, on the other.

...

Although Paul F. had acted strangely for years, his real trouble began in 1938. Early one January morning he burst into a neighbor's apartment in a working-class section of Algiers and began firing a revolver. Under subse-quent observation, he claimed that the neighbor had persecuted his family relentlessly. At this point he revealed an extraordinary family history. Paul suffered from paranoid delusions, a brother was confined in an asylum with schizophrenia, and a younger sister had suffered a "complete mental breakdown" a decade earlier. Two of Paul's other sisters and his parents demonstrated an even more interesting trend. Once Paul's delirium ap-peared, they all manifested nearly identical symptoms, absorbing his delu-sional paranoia and lashing out violently at the family's perceived enemies. This case of *folie à quatre* prompted the treating psychiatrist, Jean Sutter, a die-hard organicist who had long considered neuropathology the origin of madness, to rethink the relationship between heredity and psychological disturbance.[38] The extent of pathology in the family upheld standard paradigms about biological predispositions to deviance. Yet the epidemiological pattern hinted at a strong social element in this case of what appeared to be contagious madness. The root of the delirium may have been biological, but its simultaneous explosion in a number of family members suggested that a social intervention might have proven just as effective as a medical one in halting transmission.[39]

Cases such as these suggested to psychiatrists and social workers that all was not well in Algeria's European community. Modern psychiatric medicine, physicians argued, had the potential to alleviate the social burden of epidemic insanity. Yet efforts to improve the mental health of European settlers also entailed an important component of social engineering. For psychiatrists in Algeria, madness was as much a social as a medical problem and therefore demanded both social and medical solutions. As Sutter noted about cases like Paul F.'s, "The coexistence of a number of cases of mental illness in the same family can at times be explained by a 'social' mechanism, contact with psychopaths being able to create conditions in the individual that are favorable for the formation of mental disorders."[40] Mental health experts in the colony espoused a gendered division of labor—between the almost always male psychiatrist, who treated patients in hospital settings, and the female social worker, who sought to reshape the "social order" of mental illness—as an ideal means of staving off pathology as well as the scandal that attended European deviance in Algeria.[41]

First-line services dramatically extended psychiatric outreach into North Africa's European and Muslim communities by streamlining the admissions process. Yet the mental hygiene units and social services programs that Porot and others had so strenuously advocated reached a far more limited community than did psychiatric confinement in general. Although intended to improve the operation of the colonies' relatively small facilities for long-term confinement—designed to house hundreds of patients, in contrast with the thousands held at their metropolitan counterparts—in practice, they appeared most suitable for coping with mental illness and social disruption in North Africa's settler community. This was particularly the case in settler enclaves such as Algiers, where the relatively large and well-staffed social services unit at the Mustapha hospital engaged in a defense of European sanity and respectability on the front lines of empire.

The trope of European madness in the colonies is a familiar one. Literature teems with references to the colonies as spaces of moral and emotional danger in which Europeans took their psychological lives in their hands; Conrad's Kurtz is only the most prominent example.[42] The medical literature in which these anxieties found expression reveals how threatening signs of social and biological weakness could be in a colonial environment. In Algeria, with its vast European population, aberrance within the settler community threatened to undermine European prestige and self-confidence.[43] Since the late nineteenth century, social theorists had considered Algeria and its settler population to be a critical environment for the rejuvenation of French civilization.[44] Yet mental weakness threatened to betray this goal and the illusion of superiority on which it was based. Medical theorists had long recognized the problem of mental pathology in Algeria. Some critics even found settlers to be self-selected for breakdown, as the lure of easy financial gain and the capacity to rapidly climb the social ladder drew members of the purportedly "dangerous" working classes—in which psychopathology was believed to take a disproportionate toll—to the colonies in droves, rendering the settler community a "refuge for the unbalanced."[45] Yet it was only with a major restructuring of the Algerian public health system in the 1930s that colonial officials devised a broad framework for dealing with the problem. Authorities dedicated significant sums to the development of programs for educating the population about the constant menace of madness and death that plagued the urban poor, pointing out the "pathways to death" that threatened the "constantly growing European population," as a poster produced by the Office of Preventive Medicine and Hygiene reflects (see figure 9).[46]

In Algeria, as Eliane Demassieux documented in her 1941 thesis, the social and biological sciences combined to produce a truly comprehensive program for preventing, treating, and managing mental illness. A crucial dimension of this program was a social welfare system housed in mental hygiene dispensaries, which aimed both at the prevention of mental illness and at "reducing the consequences of illness in the individual, familial, and social order to a minimum" (see figure 10). These interventions represented an essential complement to the physicians' bolder approach. Although medical treatment could ameliorate the patient's condition, discharging that patient to a sick environment could undo medicine's achievement. The social worker could ensure effective social recuperation as a means of providing the best prognosis for released patients ("SSP," 19, 44). Yet this was only one of the social worker's duties. She also sought prospective cases through surveys of the urban landscape, determined which individuals merited early treatment, corresponded with patients' families, and found employment for released patients. Perhaps most important, the social worker tried to implement the least invasive solution possible, attempting to avoid the expense and legal difficulties of hospitalization at all costs.

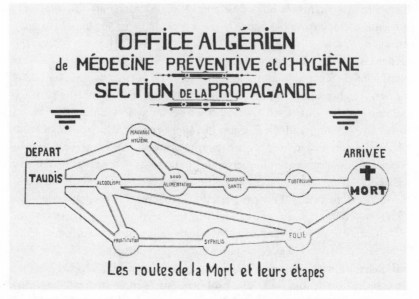

Figure 9. Office Algérien de Médecine Préventive et d'Hygiène, "Pathways to Death," 1934. From "Compte Rendu des cinq années d'action de l'OAMPH," Algérie, GGA 9 X 184, Centre des Archives d'Outre-Mer, Aix-en-Provence.

If social outreach thus represented the core of mental hygiene, according to Demassieux, the social worker was the "very heart" of this service itself ("SSP," 20, 38). And although the medical profession was dominated by men, this "heart" of mental hygiene was an explicitly feminine one. Only a woman could conduct effective social work, Demassieux argued, as "her very nature" rendered her "better adapted to this type of activity." The position required a woman's tact and diplomacy. According to one authority, "The feminine sex possesses psychological attributes that recommend her for these functions." These attributes included "a readier affection, a greater compassion, an easier and more sympathetic intuition for . . . the suffering of others." A woman's "biological constitution" predisposed her to "devotion," to providing that "'gift of oneself' that is so precious for the perfect exercise of this eminently feminine activity" ("SSP," 38).

The tasks that required this tact, intuition, and devotion frequently entailed intervention in domestic entanglements and the regulation of private affairs that threatened to explode into public crises. A case might be "an inveterate drunk, [who] menaces and insults his wife, beats his children, but refuses to come to the hospital." Or a case could be an "unbalanced" teenager who "doesn't recognize that he is sick and protests . . . hospitalization." One could never read these cases at face value. Families might

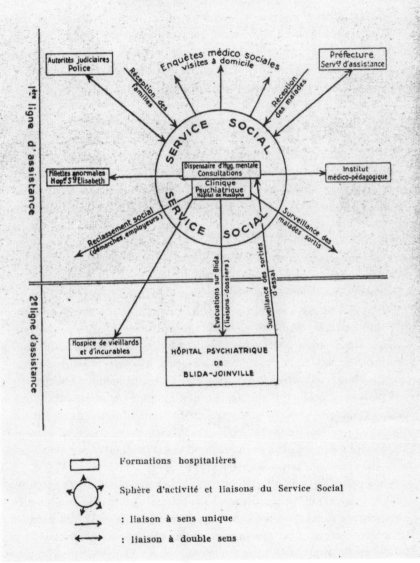

Figure 10. Organizational schema for the mental hygiene dispensary at the Mustaphà Psychiatric Clinic, Algiers, 1941. From Eliane Demassieux, "Le service social en psychiatrie: Son application à la Clinique Psychiâtrique de l'Université d'Alger" (med. thesis, Algiers, 1941). Reprinted by permission of Bibliothèque nationale de France.

wish to rid themselves of a burdensome elderly relative and exaggerate his senile dementia. Others might downplay a patient's symptoms: a sentimental family, or a "terrified woman" who feared reprisal from an abusive husband. In any of these cases, "only a delicate and able woman" had the requisite "tact and diplomacy," and "even in a charged situation, she will succeed where one would have shown the physician to the door, or hostilely received the police." The social worker not only dissolved social tension, but also "greatly facilitated" the doctor's healing role by convincing patients to enter care willingly ("SSP," 42–43).

These hypothetical examples depict the social worker as a representative of the state, an official running reconnaissance for other agencies. But the case histories Demassieux cites suggest a far more active role in reshaping the social landscape as a means of fostering mental health. Standard procedure in any investigation involved close scrutiny of a number of apparently extramedical factors in the patient's life. The social worker explored finances, "family and social relations, habits, vices, [and] interaction with neighbors" as a means of "better understanding the situation." The case of an unemployed mechanic with a history of depression revealed how these factors connected to the patient's condition. In the autumn of 1940, his joblessness and financial anxieties overwhelmed him. He began drinking and stayed inside the house. The social worker failed to convince him to try hospitalization, so she resorted to another tactic. She told the patient that a prospective employer awaited him in the street; when he stepped outside, three orderlies seized him and took him to the clinic. Although an unwilling patient, he proved responsive, and after two months of shock therapy, the social worker eased his release by securing him a position. In this case, the disorder and the social condition informed one another. The patient complained chiefly of his uselessness, that his duties as a husband and father required him to be productive. Treatment was necessary for his underlying depression, but his social condition also mandated employment to establish the best possible chances for recovery ("SSP," obs. I).

This patient's outcome suggests the important relationship between gender and mental hygiene. Regardless of the nature or origin of his disorder, a reconfiguration of his social position that enabled him to meet what he considered to be appropriate standards of masculine productivity proved essential to maintaining his mental health. Many cases in Demassieux's analysis indicate a similar pattern, whereby social workers deemed proper environments crucial for the regulation of a healthy population. This social regulation project focused principally on women, who constituted on average two-thirds of the European patients who entered psychiatric care in Algeria.[47] In one example, a woman presented as a paranoid schizophrenic: she shouted at neighbors and accused them of trying to steal her husband. Yet the social worker discovered community discord that compounded her disorder. An investigation revealed that certain neighbors had left dead flowers, rotting food, and garbage on her doorstep, and that one neighbor had ordered her son to follow the patient in an attempt to incite the woman to violence so that they might bring a complaint against her. While the patient may have been sick, problems in the social environment at the very least exacerbated her illness. Relocating cases such as these individuals and their families to new neighborhoods avoided hospitalization but still facilitated peacemaking in Algiers' settler districts by removing the patients from hostile surroundings ("SSP," obs. VII; also obs. VI).

Social workers in Algiers also emphasized the prophylactic effects of domestic harmony. Happy marriages represented an ideal standard, but social workers recognized that for some couples this was impossible. Demassieux noted a case in which one woman hospitalized for a nervous breakdown was a victim of domestic abuse. Once in the hospital—and away from her husband—she recovered quickly, but upon release she faced the danger of a fractious home, where her husband abused her physically, sexually, and emotionally. The social worker took her into protective custody and helped her to win separation and custody of her children while also finding her suitable employment. An act of social protection, this also constituted a "consolidation of the cure" without which she would likely have suffered further breakdowns ("SSP," obs. II).

Yet in most cases, the social worker considered the presence of a husband and a commitment to domestic labor as a woman's major defenses against mental illness. Demassieux referred to two women who had become manic-depressive after their husbands departed for the front early in the Second World War. Both of the women were skilled workers—one a dressmaker, the other a bookkeeper—but both felt isolated. The dressmaker lost contact with her family and found herself alone, despondent, and panicked in the settler community. The bookkeeper vacillated between bizarre hallucinations and devastating depression, all the while preoccupied with her husband. For these women, consultation with the social worker amounted to companionship, a sole human contact binding these women with their communities in their husbands' absence ("SSP," obs. VIII and IX). In another case, a widow's depression had driven her to attempt suicide. In her consultations, the widow pleaded with the social worker to help her find employment, preferably through domestic service. The social worker placed her with two priests in Oran, where she found sufficient fulfillment to transform her outlook on life. In a letter to the social worker, the patient emphasized her happiness with her new position and expressed her gratitude to a psychiatric system that healed her illness by alleviating social pressures and providing an outlet for expressing her talents: "Here, life is calm and reclusive, and I do everything I can to satisfy these gentlemen. Mademoiselle, I thank you for your kindnesses on my behalf" ("SSP," obs. XI).

Scholars such as Elizabeth Lunbeck and Regina Kunzel have shown that social workers' interventions are often about more than patients' health alone, frequently reaching into broad social engineering programs.[48] There are strong similarities between mental hygiene programs in French Algeria and the efforts of social workers in much of Europe and the United States, where the activities of a range of private and public agencies lay at the heart of an interventionist welfare state. In the French case, particularly, scholars since Foucault have highlighted the state's normative and governmental-ist approaches to the family, considered a barometer that reflected social tension in the population.[49] Yet the Algerian case merits close attention for a number of reasons. The mental hygiene programs of public psychiatric clinics represented only one of dozens of efforts at social intervention in twentieth-century Algeria that targeted the settler community in particu-lar, indicating the state's profound interest in preserving the social order of the European community.[50] More particularly, the emphasis these mental hygiene programs placed on settlers highlights an important discrepancy in the operation of colonial medicine. While many social development pro-grams also aimed at Muslims, the success stories highlighted by Demas-sieux all concern European patients. This suggests that colonial psychiatry achieved greater efficacy when it could treat patients within their cultural idiom. If healing mental illness necessitated the renegotiation of the pa-tient's social role, doing so across as few cultural barriers as possible could only have helped the process.

...

In 1939 Dr. André Donnadieu reported proudly that the Berrechid hos-pital in Morocco had accelerated its "medical" activities after installing a laboratory two years earlier. The lab enabled "every admission" to undergo "a blood test and a lumbar puncture," which permitted the detection of syphilis and spinal meningitis in the patient population. When patients tested positive for syphilis, he noted, cocktails of mercury, arsenic, cy-anide, and bismuth promised to curtail spirochetic reproduction in the body.[51] Pronouncements such as these were widespread during this period. According to one observer, such "daring treatments as paludotherapy, in-sulin comas, and cardiazol have revolutionized therapy and have given

these institutions more and more of a 'hospital' character." Case histories
from throughout the 1930s and 1940s also reflect the increasing importance of somatic treatment to psychiatry as practitioners developed new
drugs and therapies. Psychiatrists' papers emphasize a range of invasive
and radical procedures, including lumbar punctures, cardiazol injections,
malaria therapy, sedation by barbiturates, and the use of volatile chemi-
cals such as Antabuse (disulfiram) with their alcoholic patients.[52] As Porot
was eager to report in 1943, "therapeutic activity" at Blida was "very extensive," with "4510 insulin shocks, 2483 cardiazolic shocks, 383 lumbar
punctures, [and] 5805 laboratory examinations" in 1940 alone.[53]

The privileging of medical therapies over social interventions—at least
where Muslim patients were concerned—reflects an increasing faith in
the physical and chemical makeup of mental illness and in the capacity of
scientific means to treat mental disorders. As with the use of these treatments in Europe and the United States, widespread experimentation with
somatic therapies for mental illnesses in colonial hospitals demonstrates a
need among psychiatrists to find a physical pathology at the root of mental
illness in the hope of bringing their field into parity with other medical
specializations.[54] Yet such practice in the colonies also points to the ways in
which psychiatrists saw the Maghreb as an experimental terrain for testing
the safety and efficacy of new healing technologies, as well as the uses of
these treatments for establishing the colonial clinic as a theater of biomedical prowess.

Medical, technological, and somatic interventions in psychiatry predated the development of hospitals in the Maghreb by at least a century.
Rudimentary shock therapies such as the "circulating swing" and stabiliz-
ing devices such as chairs equipped with manacles—designed alternately
to shock the mind into tranquility or to relax the mind by calming the
body—date to the late eighteenth and early nineteenth centuries, while the
administration of calming and stimulating nostrums and compounds dates
to the Hippocratic era and earlier. Yet the twentieth century was particularly prolific in the development of promising, if audacious, new therapies
that appeared to work, at least for certain conditions. Paludotherapy—the
deliberate infection of a tertiary-syphilitic patient with malaria so that the
ensuing fever would kill spirochetes, a treatment developed by the Vien-
nese psychiatrist Julius von Wagner Jauregg in 1917—introduced a new era
of development through which psychiatrists pursued a range of possibilities for healing the mind by acting on the body.

In the early 1930s somatic therapies marked the leading edge of psychiatric practice. Ladislaz Meduna's cardiazol injections promised to counter
schizophrenia by inducing seizures, conforming to the belief that epilepsy

and schizophrenia were incompatible.[55] Manfred Sakel's insulin therapy sent the patient into hypoglycemic coma for up to two hours, five to six times per week, in an effort to rupture "functional synergies" between mind and body.[56] But significant complications offset their promise—cardiazol produced uncontrollable convulsions that often broke patients' bones in addition to producing a "vivid anxiety" between injection and onset, while insulin shock frequently entailed cardiac arrest, pulmonary edema, and irreversible coma as unfortunate complications.[57] Electroconvulsive therapy or ECT, developed by the Italian psychiatrist Ugo Cerletti after he learned of the uses of electric shock to stun pigs in a Roman slaughterhouse, promised to be a "simpler, non toxic" alternative to these methods.[58] Since the First World War psychiatrists had experimented with the therapeutic application of electric currents: German and British physicians found electric shock especially useful for intimidating psychopathic simulators back into service.[59] But Cerletti and his colleague Lucio Bini redirected ECT as an alternative to cardiazol rather than a neurostimulant procedure. After human trials ameliorated the condition of a schizophrenic patient, they presented their findings at the Medical Academy in Rome in 1938. "Very likely," Cerletti later noted, "except for this fortuitous and fortunate circumstance of pigs' pseudo-electrical butchery, electroshock would not yet have been born."[60]

The implementation of such treatments in France and North Africa exposes a general pattern of metropolitan caution and intense experimentation on the periphery. ECT presents the clearest example of this phenomenon. Early French publications approach the topic with interest, but also obvious trepidation. At Neuilly-sur-Marne, two doctors, Lapipe and Rondepierre, began the first, rather restrained, human trials of ECT in France in 1941, consisting of 250 sessions on fifteen patients.[61] At the same time, *L'encéphale*, a leading psychiatric journal, urged caution concerning all of the "so-called shock treatments." The physician Henri Baruk, the journal's editor and a longtime arbiter of the French psychiatric profession, argued that "a fearsome cloud of the unknown hovers over these otherwise brutal, blind, and inhumane methods." Trials on rhesus macaques showed serious consequences for brain circulation, and Baruk implored his colleagues to seek "rational, safe, and truly humane" alternatives. His conclusion pleaded for the return of an approach that characterized his discipline a century earlier: Baruk implored his colleagues to forsake such radical inventions for "the very important and too often forgotten moral treatment" for mental illness.[62]

Colonial psychiatrists, by contrast, were quick to boast about the innovative and scientific character of their therapeutic activity. While French doctors pursued animal tests—and some small-scale human trials—electroshock immediately became a bedrock of therapy in the Maghreb. For R.-P. Poitrot, the director of the Berrechid hospital, this "new method of convulsive therapy" was attractive because it "presented certain advantages over the chemical methods" that his hospital had employed since the late 1930s, with over a thousand treatments delivered between November 1942 and June 1944.[63]

In 1941—the same year in which Lapipe and Rondepierre were still conducting trials on rabbits—Maréschal revealed his zealous experimentalism as he told a French psychiatric congress at Montpellier that he and his colleagues administered ECT "regularly and systematically to all patients capable of tolerating it."[64] Even a pregnant twenty-five-year-old woman who presented a "frenzied confusional agitation" received the treatment. A first session produced uterine contractions; nonetheless, they administered a second treatment three days later, this time inducing labor and producing "a viable infant, one month before term."[65] According to one nurse's observations, use of ECT at Manouba was indiscriminate:

> Therapeutic methods? In 1943, it was an assembly line of electroshock [*électrochoc en série*]. . . . All patients, even epileptics, passed through electroshock as if we were dumping sacks in a factory, one after another. An electroshock for everyone. Families said nothing. *What did one expect them to say?* They had a madman, they were happy some took care of him.[66]

Results appeared promising. In Morocco, ECT seemed to reduce transfers to chronic confinement by a third, and in Algeria by half.[67] Yet sources suggest an abusive approach to ECT. A psychiatrist in Rabat, for example, told of using ECT on a recalcitrant Moroccan patient to obtain "a confession about his sexual life and his social . . . conduct," presaging the horrifying uses of electricity during the Algerian war.[68] Doctors in Algeria also employed ECT as a diagnostic tool to intimidate those who feigned mental illness in order to avoid military service. But aside from these clear abuses, the explicitly medical usage of ECT indicates a broader pattern of experimentation in North Africa that persisted for the next two decades. New machines allowed physicians to control convulsions to an unprecedented degree, and the use of anesthetics and paralytic agents eliminated some of ECT's least desirable complications, most important among them broken bones resulting from severe convulsions. By 1952 Maurice Porot, in his capacity as director of the Mustapha psychiatric clinic in Algiers, had personally administered nearly eight thousand of these treatments.[69] He also tested the limits of the therapy, experimenting widely on tubercular patients—despite the frequent complication of lung abscesses—and also with pregnant women and cardiac patients to determine the feasibility of application even where ECT was strongly contraindicated. Concerning his trials with tubercular patients in Algeria during the Second World War, he subsequently boasted that even in this era before streptomycin, and with a severely malnourished patient base suffering from wartime deprivation, out of forty-one cases, only nine deaths could be connected directly to treatment; this 22 percent mortality rate was promising enough to merit further study.[70]

Among psychiatry's therapeutic practices, the more radical proved the most polarizing for Muslim patients. As chapter 5 notes in some detail, for the Algerian author Kateb Yacine, whose mother, Yasmina, was confined at Blida in the mid-1940s, ECT was a powerful signal of psychiatry's punitive dimensions. Likewise, psychiatrists at Berrechid in the 1940s noted that patients demonstrated such a palpable fear of electroshock that the procedure had to be carried out "away from any potential witnesses."[71] Others, however, accepted the treatment readily. Of ninety-four patients enrolled in an ECT trial at Manouba, for example, fourteen asked to discontinue treatment before the trial's end. But most startling is that eighty of them continued with the treatment—in an era before paralytic agents and general anesthesia rendered the treatment relatively benign.[72] Although some North Africans found psychiatry to be a brutal discipline and an extension of the colonial social order into the domain of the mind, others, like these outpatients, accepted harsh side effects as a necessary cost for receiving what they saw as the benefits of Western medicine.

Maurice Porot's papers on psychosurgery indicate that he took this experimentalist attitude into more invasive domains in the late 1940s and early 1950s. French psychiatrists on both sides of the Mediterranean were slower to deploy the Portuguese psychosurgeon Egas Moniz's Nobel Prize–winning techniques than were their British or American colleagues. But once the therapy became a common component in the Francophone repertoire, Algerian practitioners again embraced the cutting edge. Porot published the first major paper on lobotomy for a French audience in 1947, for example, peppering a synthesis of foreign works with his own observations. In the next seven years, Porot performed psychosurgeries on over two hundred patients, a number that matched that of American state hospitals in the same period, whose patient populations were double and triple those of Algeria.[73] For Porot, psychosurgery was a "blind method," whose technical function "remain[ed] obscure" and which risked "a possibly definitive reduction" in "psychological and motor functions" in addition to its relatively high mortality rate of 3 percent. But Porot also found these chances "worth taking": according to statistics obtained in Britain, the United States, France, and Algeria, "today the prefrontal leucotomy [a lobotomy technique] is no longer a careless experiment with damaging risks, and it has the right to take its place among modern psychiatric therapies."[74]

The particular circumstances that psychiatrists faced throughout the world in the 1940s and early 1950s greatly favored this optimism. As in the United States and Europe, psychiatric hospitals in North Africa had "silted up" in the postwar era. If the "internable residue" of chronic patients had encumbered North African hospitals in the mid-1930s, the problem absolutely crippled facilities a decade later. By 1954, Berrechid held a surplus of five hundred patients, with no possibility of further expansion. In Tunisia the situation was more acute. Already besieged by the late 1930s, a decade later the hospital was forced to refuse all new admissions, and administrators began exploring the possibility of transferring patients to metropolitan asylums.[75] Conditions had utterly decayed by the early 1940s. As the nurse who described Manouba's "assembly line of electroshock" noted, the hospital "was overloaded with a huge number of patients. . . . The patients wore simple gowns, [and went] barefoot, [and] the incontinent were often nude . . . no mattresses, there were horsehair mats for most, [which were] always soaked."[76] In their defense, hospital administrators argued that "*over-encumbrance* is indeed the plague of psychiatric hospitals" despite the application of "the most diverse modern psychiatric treatments." Treatments such as "electroshock, insulin therapy, sleeping cures, and also the re-education of the patient through work and occupational therapy have brought numerous cures," yet "each day five or six patients are turned away because of a lack of space."[77]

Although Algeria possessed far more psychiatric beds than its neighbors, its greater population and more efficient state apparatus left the system greatly overburdened by the mid-1950s. A 1955 article in the journal *Information psychiatrique* by a team of physicians from Blida (including Frantz Fanon) pointed to Algeria's "need for several thousand" more beds for "mental patients who require emergency treatment." Blida surpassed its capacity by over a thousand patients and maintained a waiting list of nearly another thousand. The burden of patients undermined the "luxury" that observers had celebrated a decade earlier. "Nearly all the refectories [and] the bathrooms have been transformed into dormitories," the chapel now housed an occupational therapy workshop and a nursing classroom, and the mosque held two other workshops. With no dayroom, patients spent their days wandering the courtyard in Algeria's "brutal summer sun."[78] Oran's overcrowded departmental hospital was forced to house nearly five hundred patients in a makeshift "canvas psychiatric camp," where patients lived and ate in tents and "prefabricated wooden buildings" that provided less than a square meter per patient. The hospital's director lamented that the utopian idealism of the open service had "become a tentacular ward . . . a malignant tumor that infiltrates neighboring areas, but also metastasizes further out in the city and the department." The ward was "no longer anything but a police service."[79]

This crisis in psychiatric welfare motivated efforts to rid hospitals of the "incurables" who clogged wards and hindered movement. Psychosurgical techniques presented useful tools for this purpose. Since 1947 Maurice Porot had performed psychosurgeries on over two hundred patients—roughly 10 percent of Algeria's patient population—and had experimented widely with new techniques.[80] To critics who argued that these interventions "transformed the personality," Porot countered that "when one speaks of the 'transformation of the personality,' we must first remember that it is a *diseased personality* that we are operating on"; any defect in the lobotomized patient was generally "due much more to the prior illness than to the intervention." Supporting this view, Porot cited the case of a law student who spent several years at Blida: "after a lobotomy, he spontaneously resumed his studies, finished them, registered with the bar, and currently litigates successfully." If psychosurgery killed human subjectivity, the procedure killed the sick subject, allowing the healthy one to reemerge. "The essential problem is to answer the following question: will the patient benefit personally from the intervention? If one can answer 'yes' without hesitation, the intervention is legitimate."[81] Yet Porot also argued that patients themselves and even their families were in no position to offer consent to the procedure. In these situations, Porot argued, "the treating physician" was best able to consent to the procedure. "In the opinion of the majority of authors, it is with the psychiatrist . . . that the decision should remain." Sound therapeutic choices resulted from the "conjunction of confidence—that of the patient—with a conscience—that of the physician."[82]

Such arguments raise important considerations in a moment marked by the "silting up" of wards. Overcrowding provided psychiatrists with strong motives for experimenting with means that held the promise of releasing chronic patients, either to family care or to their own devices. Tunisian and Moroccan physicians explored the possibilities of radical technologies such as ECT and insulin coma to push patients out of their wards. More important, such techniques were applied unevenly: psychiatrists were quicker to test their limits on Muslim than on settler patients. In Algeria lobotomy added a powerful weapon to the psychiatrist's arsenal. The advent of these techniques combined with a passion for experimentation that undergirded the practice of psychiatry on the colonial periphery and a desire to remake the psychiatric profession by establishing a new scientific center in colonial space. In a moment when the liberatory psychiatric utopia envisioned by Antoine Porot had failed to materialize, somatic treatments signaled the advent of another psychiatric modernity. These techniques promised to smooth the operation of a malfunctioning system. Yet, combined with the biomedical logic on which they were founded, somatic therapies also transformed the Maghreb's institutions of madness into theaters of colonial conflict.

Contesting Diagnosis, Negotiating Treatment

In November 1952 a man complained to authorities in Algiers about his son, Chokri Smiri, who had been suffering from mental disorder for nearly a month. In that period, Chokri had become so unmanageable that he was kept "constantly chained." The father was unable even to approach his son, "who constantly menaced [him], as well as his mother and brothers and people" from his village of Tamazirt. Unable to care for Chokri, the father demonstrated a clear understanding of Algeria's bureaucracy of madness. He brought in a physician, who confirmed Chokri's condition and established a dossier of internment ordering his extended observation at the Mustapha hospital's psychiatric ward in Algiers. When rebuffed, the father implored authorities to take his son into confinement. After byzantine negotiations involving a number of patient transfers between Blida and the regional hospital at Tizi-Ouzou, departmental officials secured a place for Chokri at Blida.[83]

Algeria's police files from the 1940s and 1950s teem with similar cases. 'Iadh Moussaoui of Algiers and his family begged police daily to find some means of taking his daughter-in-law Leila, a "furious madwoman" whom the family kept locked in a room in their apartment, into confinement. The family of Zorah Beneghadi in Kabylie designated her "as dangerous to those around her" and actively sought her confinement at Blida-Joinville. Hassan Amir pleaded with the both the prefect of Algiers and his representative in the Assemblée Algerienne to intern his grandson. Along with countless other Algerian, Tunisian, and Moroccan Muslims, these parents, grandparents, husbands, and wives saw French authorities as a potential source of aid and comfort in their efforts to cope with their insane relatives. This sentiment is echoed throughout the 1940s and 1950s, when Muslims seeking to hospitalize sick relatives and neighbors collided with overcrowding that made admission into Blida, Manouba, and Berrechid nearly impossible.[84]

Cases such as these complicate one of Frantz Fanon's central arguments in a famous essay, "Medicine and Colonialism." Written at the peak of hostilities during the Algerian war, the essay outlines one of the clearest formulations of the fractious nature of colonial medicine. For Fanon, it was

> a good thing that a technically advanced country benefits from its knowledge and the discoveries of its scientists. . . . But the colonial situation is precisely such that it drives the colonized to appraise all the colonizer's contributions in a pejorative and absolute way. The colonized perceives the doctor, the schoolteacher, the policeman through the haze of an almost organic confusion.[85]

The colonial physician provoked strong ambivalence in the colonized. Not "socially defined by the exercise of his profession alone," the doctor represented the vanguard of an occupying force (*DC*, 135). According to Fanon, the patient was an object of derision for colonial physicians, a being who is "told that [he is] a savage because" of his medical customs and his noncompliance. Patients thus understood their doctors' instructions as "a manifestation of the conqueror's arrogance and desire to humiliate" (*DC*, 125–26). For their part, doctors found their patients superstitious and stubborn, presenting with diffuse complaints rather than clearly defined ailments and unable to translate their experience of illness into a comprehensible symptomatology. Where the colonial physician saw recalcitrance, Fanon saw active disruption of an oppressive regime. Where the physician saw superstition, Fanon saw the native "getting even with" the colonizer. "Colonial domination," Fanon argued, "gives rise to . . . a whole complex of resentful behavior and of refusal on the part of the colonized" (*DC*, 130–31). For Fanon, Algerians rejected colonial medicine because they could: it was a means of resistance under a totalitarian state.

Fanon's arguments reflect the moment of their creation. When the war broke out in 1954, French authorities weaponized medicine, prohibiting the sale of nearly all medical supplies to Algerians, including bandages, alcohol, antibiotics, and surgical instruments. Physicians had violated their claims to neutrality by participating in acts of war and defending colonial interests above their Hippocratic commitments. Fanon's model thus throws a fascinating light on the clinic as a theater of anticolonial war, but it also flattens the complexities of colonial medicine as a site for competing medical epistemologies. The fragmentary histories of patients' experiences with the colonial psychiatric regime that remain preserved in psychiatrists' case notes provide critical insight into the ways in which patients contested their diagnoses and protested what they saw as an inappropriate philosophy of healing. Patients clung to traditional beliefs in defiance of classification and treatment within European paradigms. But they did so not merely because the clinic—as opposed to the police station—was a site of possible resistance. Instead, psychiatrists and patients engaged in a protracted argument about incompatible approaches to illness. Psychiatric diagnosis exposed a deep rift between colonizer and colonized, and the doctor-patient relationship in this setting often took shape as a contest for hegemony.

Medical anthropologists and historians of medicine have argued that the understanding of disease or disorder demands a social as well as a biological interpretation.[86] For example, where the physician sees a herniated vertebra, the patient may not only feel back pain, but may also suffer from an inability to work and its social sequelae: a crisis in masculinity (in male patients), perhaps, owing to an inability to provide for a family or to participate as a productive member of society. Where the doctor sees HIV, a retrovirus with devastating effects on T4 helper cells and macrophages, the patient experiences the syndrome of AIDS: not merely weight loss and Kaposi's sarcoma lesions, but also the stigma of carrying a modern plague. Where the psychiatrist sees schizophrenia and suspects problems with neurotransmitters such as dopamine and norepinephrine, the patient suffers from delusions and the side effects of haloperidol. He or she sees pedestrians cross the street to avoid him or her and faces a daily submission to a regime of dangerous medication. Merely by taking the drug, the patient must admit illness, a premise in which he or she may very well not believe. Healing—restoring the patient's health—thus entails not only alleviating symptoms, but also helping the patient to come to terms with this burden—one that is always shaped by the cultural world in which the patient resides.

This distinction is a useful one for framing patients' experience of confinement and treatment as reflected in colonial case histories. These are problematic sources. Case histories reflect the official history of madness through the doctor's perception: the unequal power of the clinical relationship refracts them. Moreover, given the marginalized social position of most of those who entered the care of colonial psychiatrists, these patients tended to leave few if any other written traces with which to compare case notes. Yet far from the physician's "monologue" about madness that Foucault proposed as a critical element of the birth of modern psychiatry, psychiatric case histories emerge through a dialogue between physician, patient, nurse, orderly, and family.[87] As Jonathan Sadowsky has argued, they are "polyphonous," showing traces of the myriad voices that assist in the production of a narrative about madness.[88] They contain glimpses of patients' protests that reveal how doctors and patients advocated for entrenched and contradictory beliefs about sickness, health, and healing, rendering each case assessment as much a cultural battle as an attempt to cure.

Although Fanon's visceral opposition to French colonial medicine was not necessarily the rule, help-seeking through official channels rarely entailed an admission of the superiority of French medicine. Instead, patients and their families often sought hospitalization as a last resort. The case of Fatma K. demonstrates how some North African patients negotiated their illnesses across cultural contexts and signals the particularities of psychiatric practice in the Maghreb. A fifty-five-year-old Algerian woman, Fatma suffered from severe headaches and visions. Instead of presenting herself to colonial physicians, she originally sought treatment by visiting a *zaouia*, or meeting-lodge of a Sufi brotherhood, seeking a cure for her illness through trance therapy. Having failed on this front, Fatma visited several *marabouts* (in this context, folk healers), hoping that the *baraka* or spiritual power surrounding these men and places might facilitate a divine intervention to cure her misery. Fatma's condition had meanwhile worsened, and her suicidal leanings brought her to official attention. Fatma passed through the psychiatric service at Mustapha and then entered Blida in 1937.[89]

The *marabouts* whose help Fatma sought are central figures in the medical history of the modern Maghreb. Both colonial and contemporary anthropologists have researched them extensively. Writing in 1908, the ethnographer Edmond Doutté provided an early elaboration of maraboutism conceived as an Islamicized form of magical thought throughout the Maghreb. On the basis of fieldwork in Algeria, Doutté argued that in classical Arab thought "the physician is nothing but a counter-sorcerer." North African Muslims ascribed their illnesses to possession by *j'nun* (sing. *jinn*), which originated in a transgression against a given *jinn* or in a spell cast by a *marabout*. The Arab doctor was for Doutté as much an exorcist (or *taleb*) as a healer, and the best among them claimed to be *chérifs* (direct descendants of the prophet Muhammad).[90] Doutté claimed that *marabouts* operated as transitional figures in the Islamicization of superstitious practices. These Islamic saints' *baraka*—the powerful blessing or divine favor they carried with them—endowed their burial places with curative powers and passed through their lineage so that not only saints but also their descendants could claim maraboutic status. Standard treatments included most prominently the prescription of talismans, usually curative verses from the Qur'an inscribed on paper, which they believed would expel the offending *jinn* and protect against future possession.

More recently, Vincent Crapanzano has interpreted maraboutic therapies as an elaborate set of protocols for the social recuperation of an individual in crisis.[91] Responding to individual conditions, therapies such as what Crapanzano calls the Hamadsha complex seek either to restore patients to their former roles or to provide them with new social roles, and offer explanations for both psychological illness and its cure. Religious treatments—including musical or trance therapy, pilgrimages, and the prescription of talismans—introduce an order to the chaos of psychopathology according to cultural norms. Possession by *j'nun* does not occur arbitrarily, but instead relates to transgressions committed against them that often coincide with violations of social conventions. In one example, Crapanzano relates the case of a woman whose infant became ill as a result of the woman's failure to fulfill a promise of an animal sacrifice to a *marabout*. When the daughter became feverish shortly before her second birthday, both parents and neighbors assumed that this failure had angered 'Aïsha Qandisha, one of the most powerful of all female *j'nun*, who struck the child ill. The parents then undertook a pilgrimage in order to offer restitution to the *jinn* and to Allah. When they returned home the child was cured.[92]

The concept of demonic responsibility for illness offers an explanation where none can be found and therefore plays a significant role in psychological disorders. The *j'nun* operate at the level of common sense, a given within North African Islam. Like witchcraft beliefs in other cultures, theories of spirit possession serve "as an elaboration and defense of the truth claims of colloquial reason": if one has offended the *j'nun* by violating a social obligation, then their intervention naturally follows.[93] The identification of the attacking *jinn* poses an important challenge to the practitioner, because a diagnosis and appropriate therapy follows. The *taleb* often serves in this capacity, identifying the *jinn* "by oracular or mechanical means," such as reading patterns in scattered stones. Once the *jinn* is identified, its demands must be determined. The patient must then meet these demands, often through a pilgrimage to a saint's tomb or a *hadra* (an extended musical performance in which the patient enters a trance and renegotiates his or her relationship to both the community and the attacking *jinn*). The saint's *baraka* places the patient in a "potential state of health," and the following of a strict regime dictated by the *jinn* effects a cure.[94]

The Hamadsha complex is specific to one Sufi order in Morocco, but variants on the formulae of pilgrimages, exorcisms, and negotiation with *j'nun* are pervasive throughout the Maghreb.[95] The British traveler Norman Douglas scathingly describes a *hadra* as performed by the Aïssawa, an active and widespread brotherhood, in his 1912 account of a tour through

Tunisia's oases, which reads as an indictment of Maghrebian Islam. Douglas's portrayal of this "weirdly fascinating" *hadra* at Gafsa is rich with
Orientalist fantasy:

> There were wild strains of music and song; a wave of disquietude, clearly,
> was passing over the beholders. These performances, at such a time, may
> originally have taken place for purposes of nuptial excitement or stimula-
> tion; but it requires rather an exotic mentality to be stimulated, other-
> wise than unpleasantly, by the spectacle of little boys writhing on the
> ground in simulated agony with a long iron skewer thrust through their
> cheeks. . . . Mixed with them are a certain proportion of unbalanced,
> half-crazy individuals, who really work themselves into a frenzy and give
> the semblance of veracity to the entertainment.[96]

As with contemporary French descriptions of the *maristans*, Douglas
compared the *zaouias* to "our own medieval convents . . . mere menageries
of deformed minds and bodies" and argued that *marabouts* "pander to all
the worst qualities of Arabs": "In a land where no one reads or writes or
thinks or reasons, where dirt and insanity are regarded as marks of divine
favour, how easy it is to acquire a reputation for holiness."[97] Some Muslims have corroborated Douglas's disparaging picture. Antagonism toward
maraboutism originates in two different Islamic camps. Many orthodox
Muslims consider maraboutic groups, with their traditions of saint worship, to be little better than idolatrous corrupters of Islam.[98] And many
Islamic intellectual nationalists attacked maraboutic traditions as barbaric,
superstitious, and ignorant in the initial post-independence period.[99] Yet
maraboutism has historically been entwined with a range of social practices in the Maghreb, including Qur'anic education and jurisprudence.[100]

For many colonial physicians, belief in *j'nun* and their actions constituted a sign of pathological difference that played a central role in shaping
mental illness. When patients claimed they had been victims of sorcery,
for example, psychiatrists argued that this was evidence of a paranoid temperament, indicating schizophrenia as a root disorder. Yet case notes also
highlight a sense of betrayal among colonial patients. They had entered
French hospitals with specific expectations about the nature of proper care
for disordered minds, and those expectations had been violated by con-
flicting medical belief systems. Cases documented during the late 1930s by
one psychiatric intern at Blida, Suzanne Taïeb, offer rich insight into this
phenomenon.[101] Unique in the psychiatric canon of the colonial Maghreb,
Taïeb was nearly the only woman among her colleagues and spoke fluent
Arabic. She also worked extensively with female patients and sought to

understand the nature and meaning of her patients' hallucinations and delusions. During her internship at Blida between 1936 and 1939, she drew on her experiences growing up in Tunisia, where she had sat among local women in the *hammams* and learned to glean rich ethnographic details from her conversations that eventually informed her interpretations of patients' medical histories.[102] Although Taïeb's intention was to document the social factors that shaped the content of patients' delusions, her attention to detail provides insight into patients' experiences of confinement and cultural conflict.

Zohra Y., for example, made a pragmatic distinction between European and traditional medicine when she sought treatment for psychological disturbances. Hospitalization through the colonial state was free, and she could not afford to pay a *marabout* for care. Yet Zohra was astonished at her treatment by colonial psychiatrists. When doctors performed a lumbar puncture to detect neurosyphilis or meningitis, Zohra protested furiously that *j'nun*, not microbes, caused her torment. Her beauty had doubtless inspired the envy of a neighbor, whose spell in turn brought on her mental debilitation. Her case required the specialized talents of a *marabout* to relieve her from the *'ayn*, after which "she would certainly have been cured" (Taïeb, obs. 18).

An insistence that the interference of *j'nun* lay behind a broad range of physical and mental disorders fostered considerable misunderstanding between patients and their doctors. In one of the most tragic cases, an Algerian woman seeking dental work was sent into long-term psychiatric confinement. Understanding her ailment in local terms—she argued that possessing spirits caused pain in her teeth—she presented as paranoid to physicians in the Mustapha hospital, who ordered her internment at Blida (Taïeb, obs. 36). Other patients echoed Zohra's disbelief at the nature of French psychiatric medicine, insisting on maraboutic treatment inside the hospital. One woman, who had entered Blida at age fifteen with a diagnosis of schizophrenia, insisted even after five years of confinement that *j'nun* caused her illness, and she begged her physicians to exorcise them (Taïeb, obs. 13). Another patient at Blida refused treatment altogether: she insisted that she suffered from an "Arab disease" that French physicians could not cure (Taïeb, obs. 4).

These patients complained about receiving treatment that was nothing of the kind. Some argued that their treatment was incongruous with their illnesses; others denied that they were sick at all. A thirty-year-old schizophrenic male, for example, acknowledged that *j'nun* told him to attack the hospital staff, but also wrote of his fear that the hospital itself was pathogenic: "If [my confinement] continues, I might lose my sanity or die from this" (Taïeb, obs. 24). Others complained of serious illness that doctors ignored, even exacerbated. A thirty-four year-old woman diagnosed with chronic delirium claimed she was neglected, and screamed for medical attention: "I am very sick, and you are letting me die!" (Taïeb, obs. 39). Such complaints may attest to the trauma surrounding confinement, but evidence suggests that neglect was a serious problem in colonial hospitals, with patients often waiting months between consultations.[103]

Resistances to confinement and protestations of neglect call our attention to what Jonathan Sadowsky has called the "content" of colonial case histories.[104] In many cases, the colonial environment shaped both the experience of madness and psychiatrists' notations as insanity liberated the subject from the normal constraints of political domination. Yamina B.'s hallucinations, for example, exposed her fear and envy of European women. She saw a persecuting female *jinn* who appeared before her with a young blonde woman and signaled to her that the blonde would "take her place" (Taïeb, obs. 38). At times delusions of grandeur allowed the patient to usurp the colonizer's power, as in the case of a twenty-nine-year-old male syphilitic patient who told the doctor that he was a billionaire and that France had defaulted on his loan (Taïeb, obs. 42). More frequently, patients' delusions expressed their everyday experiences of exploitation and domination. Mohamed B., a patient in his early twenties, saw *j'nun* "dressed as European soldiers" who ordered him about: "take this road, sit down, don't eat couscous" (Taïeb, obs. 8). Others complained that the French wished them harm, that doctors wanted to poison them, that *j'nun* betrayed them to authorities, and, in the case of one elderly domestic servant, that a "white" *jinn* ordered her to do his laundry (Taïeb, obs. 6, 14, 43).

Most of all, patients protested the trappings of hospitalization. Hospitalization constituted the most pervasive emblem of colonial psychiatry's abuse of power. In some cases, family members who had eagerly sought to admit their relatives to care wrote authorities and hospital directors pleading for their release after years of confinement.[105] The complaints of patients and their families regarding endless confinement are highly suggestive. Few of these actors denied the existence of mental illness. Instead, they protested the function of hospitalization, which led in their view to neglect as the underlying illness went untreated. Hospitalization opened an unbridgeable gap between local and European knowledge about madness. Sick Muslims who sought maraboutic treatment received constant attention to their suffering; in the rare cases when a *marabout* "hospitalized" a patient in a *zaouia*, confinement lasted for several weeks, rather than several years, and the *marabout* attended the patient constantly. Interaction between healer and patient consisted of an untiring effort to restitute the patient to himself or herself, in terms the patient understood. By contrast, an overcrowded colonial hospital often shocked patients who anticipated quite different responses to their illnesses than the long-term confinement and aggressive treatments they received at the hands of colonial physicians.

French psychiatric hospitals in Algeria, Tunisia, and Morocco were foreign institutions for Maghrebian patients. Few of their practitioners spoke Arabic, and patients found themselves subjected to new and ever more invasive treatments they did not understand. These treatments might have relieved symptoms, but they took no account of the social world in which these illnesses had emerged. Patients' resistance to French psychiatry contains multiple meanings. While Fanon may be correct that many rejected confinement as a sacrifice of control to colonizing authority, we must recognize that many also rejected their treatment as ill-informed. By calling on doctors to expel their *j'nun*, by referring to them as *marabouts*, by protesting the inefficacy of somatic care, patients were not refuting their psychiatric status so much as contesting diagnoses they found inaccurate from the outset.

Taïeb, who treated many of the patients described here, cited their cases to argue that "primitivism on the one hand, and mental defects on the other, explain the great frequency, poverty, and systematic weakness" of ideas about the origins of "native psychopathology."[106] In contrast, I suggest that behind North African Muslim conceptions of the origins of madness lay an elaborate theoretical framework that was tightly bound to religion and culture in the Maghreb. By disregarding Muslim attitudes to mental illness as merely another sign of primitivism, French psychiatrists revealed a prejudice that rendered the effective treatment of patients' illnesses impossible. Far from recalcitrance or ignorance, patients' comments and protests to their physicians constituted a means of expressing concern about a healing system they regarded as inadequate to their needs. Patients' voices in these accounts, though mediated, point to the ways in which institutions exacerbated the cultural conflict at the heart of the colonial predicament even as their architects hoped they might cement bonds between Europeans and Muslims. The very nature of mental illness means that its practitioners and its patients can only speak about psychopathology in a halting conversation.[107] In a location where profound cultural and linguistic difference deepened the normal rift between doctor and patient, this barrier became practically insuperable.

...

Critics of colonial psychiatry have charged that the discipline operated purely as a scientific system in the defense of settlers' interests. Close scrutiny, however, reveals a more complex story in the field's development in North Africa. The historical contexts for the development of psychiatry in the colonies are crucial for understanding the Algiers School's development and its concern with innovation. By French medical standards, no psychiatric system existed in North Africa at the moment of French conquest. Moreover, the looser regulation of the psychiatric discipline itself in the colonies also paved the way for somatic experimentation in the mid-twentieth century. French psychiatrists in the Maghreb operated under their own authority, as opposed to their metropolitan colleagues, who were forced to work at the behest of the prefectures. For the physicians, this environment offered both a crucible for scientific inquiry and an incitement to scientific practice. Colonial medicine and psychiatry held the potential to conquer new domains through the deployment of a scientific arsenal. The papers of the Algiers School reflect this imperative at every turn. Congress meetings in Rabat in 1933 and Algiers in 1938 displayed the new institutions to an international audience as a symbol of the combined achievements of French colonialism and psychiatry, and witnesses extolled "the civilizing work of benevolent France in its expansion." Such institutions could "develop the manifestations of modern life, above all from the hygienic point of view" in a desolate region.[108]

Practice in colonial terrains and the charge to care for both settler and Muslim patients shaped fascinating and troubling patterns through which this innovation unfolded. The experimental work of psychiatrists practicing in the Maghreb met the accepted gold standard of European psychiatry in the first half of the twentieth century. By the early 1950s, colonial psychiatry had achieved recognition in France, marking the Maghreb as a new center for scientific inquiry. Although significant mental hygiene programs were simultaneously implemented on the European continent and in the United States, in Algeria mental hygiene and social work represented the anchors of the entire psychiatric system—the "very heart" of social welfare. The mental health care available there embraced a biosocial approach that was attempted in France on a major scale only after the Second World War. Although this correlates with a reading of the colonies as experimental spaces for scientific innovation, it also corresponds to a growing literature on the continuing influence of social factors in much of colonial medicine even as biomedical approaches dramatically reshaped medicine and public health in Europe. In a political context that repeatedly emphasized the role of "civilization" in marking racial difference in health matters as well as all others, conforming to the mandates of civilized society—that is, adhering to a strict regimen of social hygiene—was as

important as avoiding microbes in maintaining mental and bodily sound-
ness.[109]

Psychiatrists and social workers envisioned a society directed by science, but their focus on European patients also suggests a preoccupation
with facilitating social coherence as a means of preserving white respectability. Historians exploring the significance of gender and sexuality in
European empires have outlined a number of ways in which colonialism
was essential to the production of whiteness, concluding that modern
bourgeois society and its emphasis on domestic respectability was as much
a product of colonial expansion as it was a precursor to colonial ideology.[110]
Psychiatrists and social workers who engaged in mental hygiene projects
were key participants in this task. Working at the intersection of science
and society, they attempted to restructure social interaction in the interest
of producing a model settler community. Settlers stood as representatives
of European civilization in constant contact with indigenous populations.
Efforts to curtail deviance served the interest of protecting French prestige
on the front lines of empire and ensuring the position of settler culture as
a legitimate branch of French society.

Yet colonial practice also reveals problematic patterns of innovation
linked to ethnic difference. Although the biocratic dimensions of mental
hygienism expanded the "soft" interventions of modern psychiatry into the
lives of European settlers through social interventions, "harder" programs
for testing the safety and efficacy of radical somatic therapies applied dis-
proportionately to Muslim patients. As much as these trials were geared toward advancing the psychiatric profession, they also constituted weapons
in an effort to conquer resistant mentalities. As one psychiatrist asserted
in 1933, "It is indispensable . . . that the [colonized] population feels in
its physical and psychological health the benefits that today's medicine is
capable of bringing to the sick in mind."[111] Colonial psychiatrists occupied
the front lines in a struggle between Western biomedicine and what they
considered to be superstitious tradition. According to their view, Muslims'
understandings of illness were pathogenic in their own right, constituting
a rejection of the "advantages that French civilization has procured for"
the colonized. Psychiatric hospitals, dramatic and invasive therapies, and
publications in leading journals were weapons designed to facilitate the re-
lentless march of science across the obstacle of indigenous madness and local knowledge systems. For North African Muslims, *j'nun* caused convulsions, hallucinations, and maniacal outbursts. For the French psychiatrist,
epilepsy, delirium, and schizophrenia offered better explanatory labels for
these symptoms. For North Africans, mental illnesses were phenomena;

for the French, they were manifestations. Yet although patients were often materially powerless at the hands of their physicians, their utterances demonstrate that they refused to recognize the authority of their captors. Even as they submitted to confinement and to treatment, they did not concede the power to heal.

Between Clinical and Useful Knowledge
Race, Ethnicity, and the Conquest of the "Primitive"

Mohamed S. had a particularly trying year in 1937. A nineteen-year-old Moroccan student at a French colonial lycée, Mohamed faced the daunting prospect of the *baccalauréat*, an examination he had failed twice before. He also began showing new signs of psychological disorders that had plagued him four years earlier, and on the evening of 16 May he attempted suicide with a friend. In the moment, his friend found he could not take his own life, and implored Mohamed to kill him. After murdering his friend, Mohamed survived his suicide attempt and was admitted by Dr. André Donnadieu to the French psychiatric hospital at Berrechid for observation. But perhaps the lowest point for Mohamed was the factor that may have precipitated his suicide attempt. His immersion in French culture in preparation for the *bac* led him to realize that as a "poor Moroccan," life held nothing for him: he could never be truly French. As a result, his life became "nothing but an eternal torture." Mohamed argued, "We are pulled in two directions. France has made us see the light, she has illuminated our souls, we young Moroccans. But when our souls want to fly toward this horizon, we find ourselves rooted by our bodies, our customs, our traditions." This obstacle in the path of civilization proved insuperable for Mohamed, who concluded that Moroccans' cultural predicament was incompatible with modern progress.[1]

Over months of observation at Berrechid, Mohamed S. fascinated Donnadieu. The psychiatrist dwelt on the novelties of the case: his patients were rarely anxious, as the Muslim "lives day to day, without concern for tomorrows." Suicidal manifestations were also exceptional among North African Muslims, and Donnadieu noted that this double suicide was most likely the first of its kind in Morocco. And finally, the "polymorphism of ideas enunciated by the patient was equally remarkable": the patient's philosophical bent was incongruous with the psychiatrist's conception of a Muslim mentality.[2] The case thus pointed to potential similarities in the psychical makeup of Europeans and North Africans. Although atypical for a Muslim patient, tendencies toward anxiety, depression, suicidal ideation, and philosophizing were common among well-educated European patients, suggesting the possibility of an underlying universality to the human psyche that transcended racial, ethnic, and cultural boundaries.

Yet Donnadieu concluded that Mohamed's problems resulted from an ineradicable psychological difference that prevented his adaptation to French culture. Mohamed spent every day living as a French student, enjoying the freedoms that accompanied civilization, and returned home every evening to "plunge back into Muslim life." Mohamed left Donnadieu with "the impression of . . . an insufficient assimilation," a double entendre that captured both the patient's ineffective use of knowledge and the persistence of his cultural background. Rather than elevating the patient out of misery, "civilization" *produced* the patient's psychopathic anxiety and depression. The case presented Donnadieu with an important lesson. A population rooted in primitivism at the level of its "bodies, customs, and traditions" could not be "civilized" overnight. The best means of avoiding future cases like these, Donnadieu concluded, lay in significantly limiting France's efforts to bring its colonies into a European modernity, chiefly by restricting education to only a tiny fraction of the colonized.

Mohamed's case history highlights salient aspects of psychiatric theory and colonial practice in the French empire for much of the twentieth century. Like many European intellectuals, psychiatrists in the colonies became fascinated by the relationship between psychology and culture. Many thinkers found in the so-called primitive mentalities of colonized populations elements of a primordial, universal human subjectivity with prevalent instantiations in the modern European psyche and used these observations to demonstrate an essential human psychic continuity. Yet by the outbreak of the Second World War, the practitioners of the Algiers School of French psychiatry insisted that an overdetermined difference—based in bodies, customs, and traditions—separated "civilized" Europeans from "primitive" North Africans. This difference, they argued, exacerbated the inherently conflictual nature of the colonial encounter, a scenario in which the Muslim's lot in a modernizing environment was one of displacement, alienation, and incongruity, each of which entailed potentially dangerous outcomes for the subject and his surroundings. In some ways, their work drew on the legacy of the psychological anthropologists, physicians, and racial biologists who, as historians beginning with William Cohen in 1980 have argued, guided France's approach to sub-Saharan Africans from the eighteenth century to the early Third Republic.[3] Yet the psychiatrists of the Algiers School also introduced a range of novel elements to the study of the relationship between race and difference. Just as the implementation of new institutional designs in colonial hospitals pointed toward a pathway for metropolitan reform, locally produced knowledge promised to make the colonies and their institutions critical sites for the development of the new science of colonial psychiatry. Its architects positioned this new subfield as pragmatic in its applications and advocated changes to judicial, social, and military policies in France and its colonies based on their findings.

This chapter explores colonial psychiatric discourse in French North Africa by considering the practical implications of medical ideas. Historians have argued that since the nineteenth century, French psychiatrists have marked the North African Muslim as inferior to the civilized European by documenting the Maghrebian's temperamental violence, fatalism, superstitions, and mental debilitation.[4] But although these authors offer accurate readings of the psychiatric literature on North Africans, they fail to situate this literature in a larger medical and political context. From its origins colonial psychiatry was a military organism. Beginning during the First World War, its practitioners articulated their mission in the language of battle, detailing a daily struggle against the North African's recalcitrant alterity. Psychiatrists such as Antoine Porot construed this project as a matter of domination over not only indigenous madness, but also the personality and character of the North African Muslim. The deployment of psychiatric knowledge in the service of colonial power is most explicit in the French army's psychological warfare programs, developed during the Algerian struggle for liberation. Yet it also appears in psychiatrists' efforts to shape debates over law enforcement and immigration and indicates the ways in which settlers could speak of "civilizing" a colony while engaging its population in overt conflict. From its origins in the early twentieth century to the end of the Algerian independence struggle, the historical development of the Algiers School presents a crucial example of colonialism's discordant logic in practice, where a nuanced, detailed, responsive, and even progressive scientific circle with utopian ambitions was simultaneously an uncomprehending, violent entity driven by militant racism.

Of Climate and Character: Mentality and Environment in the Nineteenth Century

The concept of the North African's psychological difference is most familiar from Frantz Fanon's *The Wretched of the Earth*. Fanon argues that under Antoine Porot's direction, the Algiers School of French psychiatry educated its students to understand that North Africans were irremediably primitive, mentally deficient, and criminal by nature.[5] Yet medical and scientific discourse about race and ethnicity long precedes the foundation of the Algiers School in 1925. Psychiatrists had speculated about the relationship between race, climate, and madness since the origins of the profession. Early modern theories about the effects of climate on bodily equilibrium extended to mental balance as well and remained influential for much of the nineteenth century. Excessive heat and light were deemed to pose significant dangers for European minds, best suited for temperate climes. In addition to these environmental approaches, French psychiatrists tended to privilege the place of "culture" and "civilization" in their assessments of the epidemiology of insanity. Following the Rousseauist notion that insanity marched in step with modern progress, they proposed that madness was the price Europeans paid for living in civilization; psychological well-being, by contrast, appeared to be the privilege of so-called primitive populations.[6]

Although such ideas were based more on philosophical precepts than on actual fieldwork, early medical expeditions refined rather than corrected this logic. The work of Jacques-Joseph Moreau (de Tours) offers a key example. Having toured North Africa and the eastern Mediterranean, Moreau published a major study on insanity among Muslim populations in the first number of France's most prestigious psychiatric journal, the *Annales médico-psychologiques*, in 1843.[7] Within his psychiatric paradigm, an absence of enlightened civilization meant that North Africans should suffer from a lower degree of mental alienation than Europeans. Yet he proposed several caveats to this theory. He considered "Islamic fatalism" to engender a lack of will, and the intense heat and sun of the North African climate to render the population utterly torpid. He also stressed that madness meant not merely alienation from one's self, but also from one's social environment, Moreau argued that insanity was therefore technically infrequent in North Africa. Few Muslims were "abnormal"—that is, psychologically distinct from other Muslims—yet Muslim North Africans as a people were essentially abnormal in their normal psychological state.

The relationship between climate, culture, and madness articulated by Moreau and others meant that the naturally degraded nervous systems of colonial subjects could easily collapse under certain circumstances. But such a process could affect Europeans just as it affected natives: the stifling heat, combined with a general state of poor health, led quickly to mental breakdown. A permissive and exotic space, the colonial realm served as a site for the exploration of forbidden human passions; those Europeans whose temperament could not withstand the intense pressures of heavy drinking, drug use, colonial violence, boredom, and intense heat served as symbols of the psychological menace of colonial space. By the turn of the twentieth century, however, the idea that psychological difference was a function of climate and culture had fallen out of favor among practitioners in the colonies.[8] Increasing European settlement in tropical climes was not the least of the reasons for this change in perspective: the notion of climatic pathogenicity was certain to fall out of favor in a moment when European nations encouraged dramatic expansion into the colonies. This was especially the case for French Algeria, where a significant increase in the settler population after 1870 constituted a demographic backdrop for the development of new ideas about native psychopathology.

An 1884 thesis by the Lyonnais physician Adolphe Kocher on crime among Algeria's Arab population marks this shift. For Kocher, climate played a significant role in shaping behavior: "It seems that as one approaches the equator bloody crimes become more frequent." Yet violence among Arabs was chiefly "a matter of race" and of culture rather than a function of climate. Presenting statistics that suggested that Arabs committed the vast majority of violent crimes in Algeria, he argued that this was "nothing surprising, knowing the mores of these people": "Vengeance is necessary for them: to leave an injury unpunished would be to pass for a coward."[9] Moreover, Arab violence was a sexual and inhuman violence. "Like all Oriental peoples, the Arab is a *sodomite*," and "bestiality is observed at times among Arabs. They have relations with goats, sheep, even mares": as the "native has the animal's instincts, he also takes on its habits."[10]

Kocher's argument rested on a cursory reading of crime statistics gleaned from the Algiers Cour d'Assises, in which Algerian Arabs constituted nearly 90 percent of those convicted for violent crimes.[11] The conclusions are problematic: among the study's flaws is Kocher's failure to consider qualitative factors that might have influenced both a higher conviction rate for Arabs than for European settlers in a colonial court and the discriminatory policing of colonial urban space. Instead, these figures suggested to Kocher a clear propensity for violent sexual assault that constituted strong evidence of a constitutional difference between Arabs and Europeans. Subsequent commentators agreed with Kocher's claims as biological descriptions of race and psychology became more elaborate.

Abel-Joseph Meilhon, the director of the Aix asylum in 1896 charged with the care of the institution's Arab wards, insisted that "the issue of race dominates all psychopathology for the Algerian native." Meilhon asserted that "an asylum composed exclusively of [Algerians] would show us how madmen were in the age of barbarism."[12] The key "sign of a state of native cerebral inferiority," Meilhon noted, was the Arab's "instinctive" nature (which in Europeans was "only found . . . among the most inferior degenerates"). The Arab's "depravation of instinct, already frequent in the healthy man, will be found in the madman with the exactitude that madness imprints on all exaggerations of the human passions"—a problem so acute that "a young Arab child . . . should be observed in an entirely special manner to shield him from the lubricious appetites of his coreligionaries."[13]

Changing social patterns in the colonies and new scientific ideas contributed to psychiatrists' increasing conviction that biology, rather than culture, shaped mentality. Extensive French settlement in the late nineteenth century provided the financial resources essential for building a modern medical infrastructure in Algeria.[14] But a concomitant turn away from assimilationism opened a logical space for settlers to consider colonized populations inherently different while maintaining their defense of colonialism as a civilizing influence. New ideas that marked a larger trend in European human sciences at the *fin de siècle* lent intellectual weight to psychiatry's increasingly biological associationism. Ideas and anxieties about evolution, development, degeneration, and modernity shaped aesthetic, political, social, and psychological discourses in a range of contexts, but also contributed to a simultaneously emerging intellectual concern with comparative psychology. Commentators drew on the existing ethnographic literature and at times engaged in fieldwork as a means of developing new theories about race and mind. Although practitioners in this new discipline focused primarily on distinguishing diverse ethnicities according to mentality, as good social Darwinists and physicalists they concentrated especially on demarcating boundaries between civilized and primitive groups.

Figures such as Bénédict-Augustin Morel, Valentin Magnan, Cesare Lombroso, and Gustave Le Bon had long signaled the merits of evolutionary approaches to psychology. But the psychiatrist Auguste Marie's work offers perhaps the clearest indication of how evolutionary biology informed comparative psychology at the turn of the twentieth century. In a seminar series at the École d'Anthropologie in Paris, an institution founded by Paul Broca in the mid-nineteenth century dedicated to physical anthropology, Marie drew on Lamarck, Haeckel, and Darwin to argue that physiological and evolutionary factors accounted for psychological differences among populations.[15] Cerebral topography and emotional complexity separated higher from lower orders in the animal kingdom, but even human beings passed through stages from absolute simplicity to the greatest complexity.[16] This evolutionary pattern provided humans with the intellectual capacity for reflection and marked a distinction between sensory and reflective capabilities. For Marie, psychiatry's greatest accomplishment was the realization that physical ailments accounted for the impairment of these capacities, revealing lesions at the origin of all pathology. "If," he argued, "having operated on a brain where you have sought lesions in the cortical centers in vain, you make a [deeper] cut, you find that lesions are sometimes here, sometimes there."[17]

Marie established a scale of mental sophistication that ranged from unicellular to complex organisms. "Contemporary man" occupied the highest rank, followed by children and then "savage" or "primitive man."[18] But all humans passed through the entire scale, "because all of us are issued from a single cell, linked later with another, and so on, through proliferation." Intellectual capacity for rational thought increased in the process. Marie thus locked "primitive man" biologically in an evolutionarily prior moment, arguing that his mentality represented an intermediate stage between the "monocellular" and the "pluricellular psyche." For Marie, "the mentality of the savage, the primitive" was also "a transitional mentality that is therefore normal for a certain period," which explained the European child's similarly "simplistic manner of considering things." In the child's physical development, which operated through a process of "cellular colonialism," an original "animistic, unrefined mentality passes to a purer conception." Marie also saw the phylogenic development of entire races as a mirror of the individual process, which culminated in the modern scientific mindset: "Thus, the individual grows more and more, as Humanity has grown to superior ideas: it passes from fetishism to polytheism, from polytheism to monotheism, then to a metaphysical state and to the positivist period." Yet the "savage's mentality" remained "fetishistic" and "unrefined." Marie therefore characterized psychological development as "evolutions of mentality graphed onto organic evolutions." The individual followed a developmental evolution that corresponded to "the cycle that humanity has followed," and therefore "little by little he arrives at a mentality that is more adequate for the realities which surround him." [19]

This psychological model had two important consequences. First, organic factors accounted for mental pathology: lesions or regression to an earlier stage of development represented the principal origins of madness. Second, the brain's developmental level accounted for the social environment, and not the reverse. European children evolved from unicellular to civilized stages of mental development in a process that rendered their psyches well suited for the modern world's social environment. Marie's conclusions contrasted with early-nineteenth-century Rousseauist ideas about mental development. For Marie, civilization did not cause madness; in the new model, it merely did not tolerate madness. Instead, biology held the key. As Marie argued to a psychiatric congress in Vienna in 1909, "The question of races is the order of the day." His studies in the Middle East and North Africa revealed that "accentuated anatomical character-istics are accompanied by psychological characteristics [that are] no less typical." The apparent explosion in mental illness in nineteenth-century Europe had little to do with modernity's overstimulation of the senses. Instead, the environment had changed. Lunatics who could have merged seamlessly with village life in a peasant society now stood out, deracinated and displaced in a less tolerant urban world, much like the colonial student who could not navigate the divide between European "civilization" and the Muslim life in which he was rooted.[20] In the colonial world, then, "ethnic and comparative psychopathology could clarify the problem of normal psychology as powerfully as general pathology clarifies normal physiol-ogy."[21]

Not all doctors agreed with Marie. Victor Trenga, a French doctor in Al-geria, argued in 1913 that culture—especially Islam—defined race in what he called the "Arabo-Berber" context.[22] Yet his argument is as scathing as those of his organicist colleagues. Muslims thought and acted differently from Europeans, but because the "brain of Arabo-Berbers is well made, constituted from a cerebral substance of good quality," cultural factors must account for fatalism, indifference about the future, and "contempt and haughty indifference" in this "deceitful" population.[23] These observa-tions led Trenga to specific conclusions regarding the French role in usher-ing the Muslim world into modernity. The French, he argued, must teach Muslims to drop their "blissful torpor" and embrace the French qualities of "clarity of thought and conception, frankness and decisiveness in the smallest actions."[24]

Despite its emphasis on culture, Trenga's work also points to a criti-cal shift in perspective that emerged alongside the increasingly biological model of ethnic psychological difference. Although he was careful to dis-tinguish European settlers from Jews and Muslims, he never distinguished among Muslims themselves. This indicates psychiatry's significant de-parture from its contemporary scientific counterparts. For much of the late nineteenth and early twentieth centuries, divide-and-conquer policies encouraged fine distinctions among North African populations—divided into Arabs, Berbers, M'zabites, and Jews in addition to national divisions between Algerians, Moroccans, and Tunisians. As Patricia Lorcin has ably demonstrated, the distinction between Arabs and Berbers in nineteenth-century Algeria was particularly pronounced in selective policies that promoted French cooperation with the "good Kabyle" and not with the "bad Arab." A similar logic undergirded distinctions that colonial officials often made between so-called aggressive Algerians and their more docile Tunisian neighbors.[25] Such important distinctions persisted but retained less significance at the turn of the century, when increasing settlement favored a hardening of racial boundaries between Europeans and North Africans as a group.[26] With a few significant exceptions, early psychiatric commentators dedicated little attention to distinctions among populations, arguing instead that the critical difference was that between Europeans and Muslims.[27] This collapsing of difference—one psychiatrist used the terms "Arabs," "Algerians," "Muslims," and "North Africans" interchangeably—set an important precedent for the Algiers School, whose members across the Maghreb employed an ambiguous shorthand that deepened the rift between *l'homme civilisé* and *l'homme primitif*.

Overdetermining Difference: The Algiers School and the Remaking of the Primitive

The outbreak of war in 1914 marked an important transition in psychiatry's approach to race. Although wartime budgets eviscerated social spending in the colonies, the war itself created unprecedented opportunities for studying colonized populations under stress. Psychiatrists were conscripted en masse alongside other practitioners as the intense psychological pressure of the trench experience initiated a great demand for mental health expertise. The presence of significant numbers of colonial subjects in the French infantry provided a critical data set for the study of racial and cultural influences on psychopathology. For Antoine Porot, service at the Maillot military hospital in Algiers presented the opportunity both to study comparative psychology in a controlled setting and to redirect the relationship of psychiatry to the colonial state.

North Africa presented an ideal setting for launching a major study in psychiatry and ethnicity. To Porot and his colleague Angelo Hesnard, a naval psychiatrist and later a founding member of the Parisian Psychoanalytic Society, the Maghreb was "a crossroads where very different racial elements and conditions meet." For the duration of the war, the two psychiatrists' caseload included many Algerian Muslims, whom they described as "the most thwarted beings, the closest to nature," alongside "the most defective products of civilization"—poor whites drawn from settler populations. The two volumes they produced after four years of study, *L'expertise mentale militaire* (Military Mental Expertise) and *Psychiatrie de guerre* (Wartime Psychiatry), present a range of ideas about how informed psychiatric opinions might determine recruits' psychological aptitude for military service and how psychiatry could facilitate the understanding of psychological trauma suffered in the course of service. Yet ideas about race are also central to the texts, and along with Porot's subsequent works, the volumes mark an important turning point in the history of colonial psychiatry and the development of the Algiers School.

The texts are adamant in their effort to establish a racial hierarchy of suitability for military service. Owing to "anomalies in intelligence or character," the authors argued, "each *race* has its own *mental level* and its own particular complexion." Echoing the growing literature on *mise en valeur* and the suitability of different colonial populations for labor, Porot and Hesnard claimed that these phenomena informed a soldier's capacity to serve effectively. In some cases, cultural phenomena shaped capability. For example, colonial soldiers often exhibited pathologies that also plagued Europeans, but with greater prevalence. This was especially the case with breakdowns that stemmed from nostalgia: "*syndromes of stupor and inhibition*" that appeared as a result of the homesickness experienced by all soldiers on the front were more common among the Algerian "'fellahs' [peasants] uprooted from the archaic life of their 'douars' [villages]." Other characteristics of North African soldiers, however, presented what Porot and Hesnard saw as racially specific pathologies: "It has so happened that on several occasions we have received . . . natives labeled 'mentally debilitated' who were not, however, inferior to the mean of their race." Instead, their "passivity, inertia, nonchalance, [and] a certain degree of superfluous pithiatism had been misrecognized in their exact and ethnic significance."[28]

North Africans exhibited other traits that had serious implications for military service. Muslim recruits showed "violent episodes of angry mania": their worst attribute was "the violence and brutality of their hysterical episodes." Although this same characteristic supposedly rendered West African soldiers such as the infamous Senegalese riflemen highly suitable for some military duties—French commanders praised the *tirailleurs'* allegedly "innate" capacity for brutality—in North Africans "these episodes often signify an impulsive disposition . . . and necessitate a definitive discharge from the army." Language and cultural barriers rendered psychiatric intervention "very difficult"—these "hysterics" possessed a "tenacity and a force of perseverance" that obstructed "all efforts" to heal.[29] For Porot and Hesnard, the psychological character of North African Muslims rendered them more impulsive and less controllable than other colonial soldiers. Just as Muslims proved recalcitrant when shown the purported benefits of French civilization, the authors intimated, so they also resisted military service by virtue of their inherent psychology rather than through force of will.

Psychological character at the front resulted from biological difference rather than a geography of race. Of all soldiers from the North African colonies, only Muslims posed significant psychological problems. Colonial soldiers of "French stock" proved "remarkable in their moral robustness and tonicity." Members of "this energetic race" flouted the "shocks and privations" of war, and "their 'drive' . . . inspired the admiration of all those who saw them in action." European settlers with Italian and Spanish roots were more prone to breakdown, as were Algerian Jews. Officially members of the "French family" since 1870, Jews were hypersensitive and showed depressive and nervous tendencies when pressed into service. Still, they proved capable of "springing back" to mental health after psychotherapy and presented few unmanageable chronic problems.[30]

The situation was different for Muslims. In both *Psychiatrie de guerre* and his 1918 "Notes on Muslim Psychiatry," Porot argued that before the war the few North African men who joined the French army tended to be like the "legendary" Turkish warrior: "engaged, fond of the uniform and adventure," "brave" and "fierce."[31] The Great War's unprecedented conscription confronted military officials with an "indigenous mass, a formless bloc of primitives, profoundly ignorant and gullible for the most part, greatly distanced from our mentality and our reactions." The war thus revealed the *nature* of that "ignorance" and "gullibility" as increasing numbers of Algerians, Moroccans, and Tunisians passed through psychiatric clinics. Conscription drew North African men away from their "free, peaceful, and archaic lives" and "threw them into a life where the most scientific and infernal inventions loomed before their eyes, which had only known the calm serenity of infinite horizons."[32]

This "indigenous mass," this "formless bloc of primitives": the language is familiar, although it belongs as much to *fin-de-siècle* psychological discourse as it does to colonialism. Like Le Bon and the crowd, Porot describes Muslim recruits as a suggestible throng that defied civilizing progress.[33] The psychiatrists linked Muslims' failure to perform at the front to a general resistance to civilized modernity. In contrast to the vigorous settler who struggled in an arduous climate and rendered an unforgiving land fertile, the hapless native merely clung to his "miserable earth." Likewise, the colonial conscript rejected the purportedly civilizing influences of the front, with its emphasis on a technological order and military discipline.

These soldiers broke down as a function of their material incongruity with the new environment of war: they were "thrown" from the "hypnosis of brilliant sunlight" into an "infernal" but also "scientific" cataclysm. As Porot argued, "Suddenly, we were able to measure the entire moral resistance of simple souls, the powerful force of certain primitive instincts as well as the misery of certain mental deprivations and the deviations imprinted through credulity and suggestibility." The war therefore put indigenous mentality to a test that it failed miserably. The plucky settler proved resistant to the horror of the trenches; the North African merely revealed his homesickness, fatalism, suggestibility, and mental childishness.[34] Whereas exemplary military service proved Jews' capacity for assimilation into French culture, French psychiatrists argued that North Africans' psychological composition prevented them from serving France as effective soldiers, despite their dying in droves in the trenches.[35]

Historians have noted that Porot described North Africans as "psychically entirely other," "fixed . . . in an irremediable alterity."[36] Yet scholars have overlooked the political and practical consequences of the Great War studies. Racial stereotyping proceeded beyond the establishment of insurmountable mental boundaries between Europeans and North Africans and marked colonial psychiatrists' transition from professional to political advocacy. More than an effort to expand psychiatric knowledge of the Other, Porot and Hesnard's works are user's manuals for the clarification of indigenous mentalities. These guides—which base conclusions about "normal" mentalities on the observation of psychiatric patients—are rooted in medical and colonial prejudices but at the same time are mired in the historical context of the war as well as the interwar reconceptualization of civilization and primitivism.

As Michael Adas has shown, the savage brutality of the trench experience prompted reassessments of the basis of European superiority. Measuring human worth according to standards of industrial progress had proven morally bankrupt in the wake of technologically driven destruction.[37] In a climate that interrogated the very basis of civilization, an ethnologically driven psychology offered a useful outlet for a new intellectual fascination with primitivism.[38] The philosopher Lucien Lévy-Bruhl had explored this problem in his 1910 *Fonctions mentales dans les sociétés inférieures* (Mental Functions in Primitive Societies), but it was only with the explosion of interest in primitivism in postwar France that he achieved widespread recognition.[39] Based on the author's interpretations of others' observations—Lévy-Bruhl never undertook fieldwork—*Primitive Mentality* (1923) pointed to an essential difference between "primitive" and "modern" thought patterns: whereas Europeans enjoyed a logical, scientific consciousness, "the primitive's mentality is essentially mystic," displaying a "decided distaste for . . . the 'discursive operations' of thought."[40] Scholars have rightly castigated Lévy-Bruhl for his essentialist assumptions about "primitives"—a term he used to describe alternately sub-Saharan Africans, Native Americans, and Australians—but he was careful to note that the primitive's "indifference" to "reasoning and reflection" reflected "neither incapacity nor inaptitude." Lévy-Bruhl insisted that those who explained the behavioral, psychological, and intellectual differences of "primitives" by referring to "the feebleness and torpidity of their minds" failed to "take the facts sufficiently into account." Rather than any evolutionary or biological defect, Lévy-Bruhl asserted, "group-ideas" and "collective representations" of primitive societies—cultural and environmental factors—accounted for the "prelogical and mystical" nature of primitive mentality.[41]

Reactions to Lévy-Bruhl's work reflected a profound divide between the metropolitan and the colonial. Military and colonial physicians seized on his claims that "modern" and "primitive" mentalities displayed fundamental differences, while others followed Lévy-Bruhl's argument that cultural rather than biological factors accounted for this difference. Military and colonial physicians also were quick to accept Lévy-Bruhl's ideas of the practical difficulties that arose from "the primitive mentality." For example, two military doctors, René Jude and Victor Augagneur, argued at the 1925 Congress of French Alienists that the French military's increasing dependence on colonial troops mandated officers' understanding of "prelogical and mystical" mentalities. They found that

> the native, in general, has an innate, profound sense of elementary, simple justice, and . . . an unjustified action or reprimand, for a minimal infraction, that appears to us to have no importance, will appear to his mind to be an injustice of the greatest seriousness. In the brain of the primitive or the most evolved native, the reaction will be swift and violent and will manifest itself immediately through actions that appear to us to be disproportionate to their initial cause. By contrast, such actions, gestures, spoken orders that appear to us to be of capital importance will scarcely hold his attention.[42]

A "thorough knowledge of the mentality of natives" was a prerequisite for the fulfillment of France's civilizing mission. Institutions such as the École d'Application du Service de Santé des Troupes Coloniales in Marseille thus organized programs of "psychological and psychiatric instruction" for colonial officials.[43] According to one instructor at the

École, understanding native mentalities was critical for civilians as well as military personnel: "No European succeeds with natives" without being "quite familiar with their mentality, their character, their modes of reaction." Effective administration relied on sound knowledge: "To act usefully on populations, to obtain what one desires from them, to make them accept the advantages of what we are bringing them, it is indispensable to understand them and to know how to make them understand you. Your influence can only be civilizing under this express condition."[44] E.-L. Peyre, head physician of the French colonial forces in the early 1930s, agreed that as overseas settlement rose, increased contact between European and colonial populations rendered ethnological knowledge about mind and behavior essential for the continuation of the civilizing mission. For colonized populations, increasing settlement entailed the "upheaval of all their old ancestral notions," a rapid "evolution" that strained intellectual development with profound consequences for mental hygiene; for settlers, cross-cultural contact heightened the suspicion that mental illness was more frequent in natives.[45] Psychiatric understandings of "native" mentalities, Peyre argued, could bridge these gaps.

In contrast with these practical exhortations, Lévy-Bruhl's work encouraged the romanticization of primitivism in some circles. In the context of a postwar assault on reason among European intellectuals, surrealists such as the former psychiatrist André Breton were receptive to alternatives to "Western civilization," many of which they found on the margins of European society. Children not yet corrupted by education's moral straitjacket, hysterical women, and madmen reflected the kernel of unconscious brutality hidden within all subjects. But "the primitive" offered an antithesis to European modernity. Unlike the cubists, who explored only the formal possibilities of a primitive aesthetic, in the postwar era the surrealists interrogated what they believed to be the meaning of primitive art and ritual.[46] At the same time, the foundation of the Institut d'Ethnologie, which functioned largely for the training of colonial officers, by Lévy-Bruhl, Marcel Mauss, and Paul Rivet signified the emergence of a new scientific fascination concomitant with the primitivist revolution in aesthetics.[47] Some medical practitioners also denied the existence of such hard-and-fast distinctions between mentalities. The psychoanalyst Pierre Rubenovitch, for example, wrote in 1934 that "in every society" there existed "two categories of individuals": in contrast with "a small minority" who could drive evolutionary progress forward, "the vast majority of men" were incapable of acting with historical consequence. "In this sense," Rubenovitch declared, "the majority of men possess a mentality that is no different from primitive mentality." The "civilized" masses existed in an evolved milieu "with the same absence of critical spirit . . . as the primitive."[48]

These arguments signaled a redemption of the primitive that paralleled developments in other psychological communities but that remained absent from most colonial circles. As early as 1913, Freud argued in *Totem and Taboo* that the psychological processes of Europeans represented a vestigial primitivism in the modern psyche with powerful links to the "mental lives of savages." Drawing on the work of Frazer, Mauss, and Robertson Smith, Freud argued that far from a psychical other, the modern primitive was functionally equivalent to a European without a repressive mechanism.[49] By the 1930s the Hungarian psychoanalyst Géza Roheim had begun to test Freud's claims through fieldwork among Australian aboriginal populations near Alice Springs. Although Roheim noted that such populations demonstrated markedly different behaviors from Europeans—especially concerning sexuality, violence, and family organization—he concluded that these phenomena resulted chiefly from the absence of a superego in aboriginal society rather than from an essential racial or biological difference between "primitive" and "modern" man.[50]

Psychoanalysis served as a critical organizing tool for those who considered "primitivism" to constitute the heart of the modern ego. So-called primitives proved useful to psychoanalysis by demonstrating the existence of an unconscious as a fundamental human condition. If the incest taboo, ambivalence toward the father, and the tension between the indulgence and repression of violent instincts or drives operated at the level of the contemporary "primitive" in Australia, Melanesia, New Guinea, or sub-Saharan Africa, psychoanalysis could point to the universality of its central tenets. The field's concern with revealing the underlying irrationality of the modern, autonomous ego encouraged a fascination with primitivism among its practitioners as well as psychoanalytically oriented ethnographers and critics, who saw in the violence of everyday civilization an atavistic return of a savage mindset that lay in the unconscious. This concern with the psychological continuities that linked the family of man undergirded the works of a range of scholars and analysts in the interwar period, from the renegade surrealists Georges Bataille and Michel Leiris, to the ethnographer and curator of the Musée de l'Homme Paul Rivet, to the analyst Rubenovitch.

A similar dynamic operated within Parisian psychiatric circles. Although noted for their early hostility to psychoanalysis, psychiatrists in metropolitan France reveal a powerful Freudian influence in their writings on primitivism in the interwar period.[51] By the 1930s they had begun to consider parallels between "primitives" and mentally disordered Europeans, noting especially the connections between paranoia and primitive mentality. Some considered "paranoid" aspects of primitive mentality—such as the belief in sorcery—to be evidence of psychological underdevelopment: one medical student compared such beliefs to medieval European psychoses.[52] Another psychiatrist described a "striking" congruity between "the paranoid mentality and the primitive mentality," but also noted a crucial difference: primitivism was a social phenomenon, where paranoia was an individual affliction. A change of environment could thus initiate a transformation of a primitive mentality as the subject adapted to a new social milieu by transforming thought and behavior, while the European paranoiac could only follow the "psychobiological laws of his thoughts."[53] The psychiatrist Jean Lévy-Valensi echoed this idea. Like the paranoiac, the primitive suffered from deliria of persecution and ambition; and just as paranoiacs were "hallucinatory," Lévy-Valensi argued that "the savage is so in his normal state."[54] But for Lévy-Valensi, the primitive—as opposed to the paranoiac or the schizophrenic—retained the possibility of adaptation. Lévy-Valensi's student Pinkus-Jacques Bursztyn pushed the analogy further. In almost Lacanian terms, Bursztyn argued in his 1935 thesis, "Schizophrenia and Primitive Mentality," that for these subjects the symbolic order is not fixed. "The patient and the primitive lack consciousness of the unity of the self," which is "fragmented into elements . . . that are often projected outward and personified."[55] In this magical conception of the world, the self was easily dissipated into forces or qualities that inhabited various objects. But whereas "the primitive's representations" concerned "the ambient world"—and were therefore subject to "the action of the real"—"the schizophrenic's representations were drawn from outside the real." For Bursztyn, as for many of his colleagues, while "the mentality of the primitive is normal, that of the schizophrenic is pathological."[56]

As formerly impermeable boundaries between reason and madness dissolved after the First World War, paranoia and schizophrenia fascinated the French mental health community precisely because they destabilized these categories. For psychologists and psychoanalysts, these diagnoses signaled the "psychopathology of everyday life," while psychiatrists insisted that paranoia resulted from constitutional defects in the personality.[57] For all disciplines, however, the study of primitive mentality's analogies to paranoia and schizophrenia promised insight into the nature of these pathologies—especially because practitioners such as Jacques Lacan noted a strong correlation between paranoid symptoms and violent criminal behavior.[58]

The explosion of interest in primitive mentality in the interwar period indicated that an ethnological sub-specialty was gaining steam within the

French psychiatric profession. Yet like Lévy-Bruhl, psychiatrists such as Dumas, Lévy-Valensi, and Bursztyn had no direct experience working with colonial populations, and they based their comparisons of primitivism, paranoia, and schizophrenia on a reconciliation of psychiatric theories and ethnographic data collected by others. And for all their emphasis on practical experience in the colonies, many military and colonial physicians tended to treat colonized populations interchangeably. Gustave Martin of the École d'Application in Marseille, for example, considered Indochinese, Maghrebian, and West African populations to be basically identical when he argued that these "primitive societies immutably conserve the same traditions."[59] Such pronouncements, critics argued, only encouraged widespread romanticism of a vaguely defined "primitivism" by eliding differences among colonial populations.

Targeted studies of specific populations—defined by ethnicity or region of origin—offered a pathway out of such generalization. In contrast with their metropolitan colleagues, who considered primitive mentality more of an intellectual curiosity than a practical exigency,[60] psychiatrists practicing in North Africa insisted that close contact with colonial patients revealed the practical and political importance of specific ethnopsychiatric knowledge. As the psychiatric luminary Henri Claude noted in 1933, colonial research could bring to light "many curious details concerning a pathological psychology that is unfamiliar to us."[61] By documenting patients who had remained unexamined by Western medicine, colonial psychiatry brought to the profession "an incomparable education in psychology, the psychology of peoples, [and] a great lesson in human culture." Colonial practice presented new opportunities for the advancement of the profession. "The colonial contribution to pathology in general has been considerable," Porot argued in 1935, and it promised to add "several new chapters to neuropsychiatry."[62] In the same way that the study of tropical diseases had transformed understandings of the mechanism of infection and contagion, so the diagnosis and treatment of thousands of patients drawn into a new network of care offered a new pool of subjects for the development of psychiatric knowledge.

As early as 1909 Auguste Marie contended that meaningful ethnopsychological research necessitated a proper colonial institutional setting. "Such study," he insisted, "is only possible with a scientific field of observation in the entirely special milieu of the lunatic asylum."[63] By the 1930s, the Maghreb presented ideal conditions for this research to unfold. Porot had assumed a chair in psychiatry at the Faculté in 1925 and had begun training students immediately, for which the patient populations of psychiatric institutions in Algeria, Tunisia, and Morocco offered a vast research subject pool. As Porot's colleague Henri Aubin noted, psychiatry had found increasing practical applications since the First World War: it had become "a precious instrument of research in the hands of psychologists" as well as "an indispensable guide for the judge and the criminologist" and "the inseparable companion of the pedagogue." The sub-field of "ethno-psycho-pathology" offered new opportunities for psychiatrists to enhance their profession's applicability, and Aubin concluded that in the ethnopsychiatric field, the "University of Algiers, a natural link between the Metropole and its global Empire, appear[ed] especially qualified" to seek the practical uses of knowledge.[64]

Algeria's importance as a site of contestation over settlement and assimilation made the colony a logical site for the development of this knowledge. As Algerian settlers increasingly distanced themselves from French metropolitan attitudes and policies, so colonial psychiatric doctrines departed significantly from the works of metropolitan theorists. Their work reflected the hardening of racial lines that characterized Algeria in the interwar years as a distinct mentality emerged among the so-called *pieds-noirs*, or French Algerian settlers.[65] An insistence on the biological nature of psychological constitution that had shaped approaches to difference in the colonies since the turn of the century lent itself easily to explicit political advocacy, while the establishment of the Algiers School as a new scientific research center invested such statements with institutional clout.

The school's first formal product—a 1925 thesis by Porot's student Don Côme Arrii—reflects a clear effort to use science as a tool for shaping policy. Arrii's study, "The Criminal Impulsivity of the Indigenous Algerian," presented the Algerian mind as a threat to public safety. The origins of "impulsivity," a constitutional pathology in which the subject responded to stimuli with unmitigated, explosive reactions, lay in a "deficiency" or "imbalance in the superior functions of the ego" that weakened the functions of "judgment and voluntary control."[66] Although pathological impulsiveness was found occasionally in European patients, Arrii argued that psychiatrists found such manifestations as a matter of course in indigenous North Africans. Like earlier theorists, Arrii collapsed categories such as Kabyles, Arabs, and Moors into the figure of "the *indigène*." Yet Arrii focused his argument on Arabs, whose constitutions, temperaments, and traditions, he noted, invariably blazed a path toward criminally impulsive behavior. The "childish" Arab was a "monster of amorality" who remained "arrested in the progressive march toward knowledge, fixed by his indolence and his fatalism, to no good." Islam encouraged such mental characteristics in Arabs, who depended on the will of Allah rather than their own initiative.

Islam also exacerbated innate tendencies toward closed-mindedness and stubbornness, which in turn enhanced "brutality and savagery."[67]

This appalling characterization of "the" indigenous Algerian contains a number of conflations that mark most of the Algiers School's psychiatric discourse. First, although based on observations of Algerian psychopaths, these manifestations are described by Arrii as the Arab's normal mental state.[68] Second, Arrii slips from a description of all North Africans to a description of Arabs, using terms such as *indigène*, *Arabe*, *musulman*, and *Algérien* interchangeably. Third, Arrii readily vacillates between ascribing pathology to religious and "racial" factors by linking Muslim cultural tendencies to heredity in a Lamarckian fashion. The Algerian's "mental debilitation" was tied to "his numerous hereditary defects," which in turn pertained to all Muslims, and especially to Muslim men. Islamic customs favored impulsive behavior from their origins, and Muslims naturally inherited their ancestors' character attributes. For example, Muslim men "too frequently" murdered their wives "like one does with a useless animal, an unproductive beast."

> But we cannot really attribute complete responsibility for these brutal repercussions to debilitated subjects of a violent nature. Indeed, holy principles govern marriage. The husband purchases his wife, who becomes his property. The law forces him, moreover, to marry a virgin, and the *indigène* sees in this prescription an invitation to take exclusively young girls. Didn't Mohammed set the example himself by taking Aïcha as his fiancée at the age of six, and consummating the marriage with her as soon as she reached her ninth birthday?

Where Muslims understood Muhammad as their foundational prophet, Arrii saw him as a foundational criminal. North African men naturally followed the prophet's lead. A society that considered statutory rape to be a sexual norm inured its population to violent crime. The "legal conception of rape in marriage" led "naturally to . . . indecent assaults or plain rape." More important, "murder impulsively follows rape, to overcome resistance or to conceal the screams of the victim." North African men therefore murdered "in full sexual excitation," for "erotic intoxication is an extra contribution to impulsion and to aggravation, to the unleashing of this homicidal furor."[69]

As David Macey has noted, Arrii based his work on an extremely small and limited sample.[70] By studying twenty cases heard in French-Algerian courts, he concluded that a flawed mindset predisposed Algerians to vio-

lent conflict. Despite its methodological weaknesses, Arrii's thesis offered
a persuasive logic for the interpretation of an apparent incompatibility between settler and Muslim populations in the Maghreb. If Muslim culture
and its pathological heritage were as immutable as biological heredity, leading by a chain of events from legally sanctioned rape to "homicidal furor,"
the Arab remained impossible to assimilate. A revised version of the thesis
published by Porot and Arrii in the *Annales* in 1932 advocated a stronger
police presence in colonial cities. Whether motivated by "social protection" or "the educational value of punishment," the authors concluded,
"justice should follow its course" in cases of constitutional impulsivity.
French North Africa required intense policing, as "it is above all through
. . . sanctions that we teach these thwarted and overly instinctive beings
that human life must be respected . . . a thankless, but necessary task in the
general work of civilization."[71]

It is difficult to determine whether real rates of violent crime were in fact
rising during this period. Yet it is clear that crime was on the rise in the interwar imagination. In both metropolitan France and the colonies, steadily
expanding literacy promoted the development of a sensationalist press that
popularized random violence through the mechanism of the *fait divers*.
The *faits divers* were and remain unique to the French press. Brief, usually
anonymous stories located alongside serialized novels, theater listings, and
puzzles, they provided capsule narratives of violent crimes for a consum-
ing readership eager for distraction.[72] Yet like stories of Jack the Ripper and
the "Maiden Tribute of Modern Babylon" in turn-of-the-century London,
the *faits divers* created an atmosphere of mediated chaos in which violent
crime could strike anywhere and at any time in the urban environment.[73]
The sensationalist press was equally pervasive in Algeria, where the *faits
divers* highlighted crimes committed by Muslims in the colony's major
cities. In the interwar period, the consolidation of land holdings by large
agricultural concerns exacerbated patterns of land expropriation initiated
in the nineteenth century and forced destitute and unemployed Algerian
peasants into the cities in a pattern of push migration.[74] The rapid expansion of poor and poorly assimilated Muslims in the *bidonvilles* of periurban
Algeria, Morocco, and Tunisia intensified colonial anxieties about crime
and conflict, while psychiatric theories provided a useful explanatory logic
for the defense of settler interests.

By the 1920s anxieties over migration had touched metropolitan France
as well. Although most commentators in interwar France focused on the
economic and cultural threats posed by immigration from Eastern Europe, large numbers of Muslims began arriving in France in the same period as North African men sought employment. Arrii argued that Mus-

lim impulsivity thus "no longer remained only an Algerian medicolegal problem." According to metropolitan police, "the crimes of these 'Sidis'" demonstrated that "the Muslim native, who mingles more and more with our national life, brings the psychopathological heritage of his race to our civilization."[75] More than resisting France's civilizing entreaties, the Muslim's predisposition to violent criminal madness threatened to undermine civilization's very foundations. Immigration compounded the problem in a number of ways: beyond bringing unpredictable madness to the metropole, in France the absence of Islamic social pressures to abstain from alcohol meant that immigrants were even more likely to indulge their criminal impulses than those who remained in North Africa.

The criminal stigma that psychiatrists in Algiers attached to North Africans' normal psychology provided a strong counterbalance to those who attempted to romanticize primitive mentality after the First World War. Because of the so-called endemic criminality of North African Muslim culture, civilization could be accomplished only through punishment and confinement—by building institutions that could constrain native impulses. Further theses and papers by psychiatrists in Algiers, Blida, Manouba, and Berrechid built on Arrii's claims by elaborating his theories about the origins of Muslim criminality. In Tunisia, Pierre Maréschal linked crime and deviant tendencies to heroin addiction, while in Algeria, Porot's student Jean Sutter argued that epileptic seizures opened a pathway to the Algerian's natural "extraordinary violence and savage furor."[76] But the paper most relevant to questions about primitive mentality and ethnopsychiatry was Jean Sutter and Antoine Porot's 1939 article on "the primitivism of North African natives" and its "manifestations in mental pathology."[77] Elaborating on Arrii's work, the paper reflects the efforts of colonial psychiatrists to position themselves as France's foremost experts in the practical applications of ethnopsychiatric research by virtue of their empirical study of the problem.

Porot and Sutter began by lamenting psychiatrists' and psychologists' widespread misunderstanding of the concept of "primitive mentality." Whereas most theorists considered primitive mentality to be "an ensemble of dispositions of the mind found constantly among the least evolved groups and peoples," Porot and Sutter found that their clinical practice made possible a "much more specific idea of primitive mentality." Strictly speaking, they acknowledged that North Africans were not primitives. This "would be a manifest exaggeration," because North African Muslims were "collectively much more evolved than the Negroes of Central Africa or Polynesian tribes who have served as models" of the primitive. Yet at levels of psychological structure, psychiatric symptomatology, and patients' "practical

activity and comportment," "a fragmentary and partial" primitive mentality "imprint[ed] a specific character on [the North African's] mental pathology." Patients were "fatalistic" and "monotonous," never showing the
great variations in symptomatology found in more sophisticated mentally
ill Europeans. Their intelligence was "not only poorly developed, but even
generally fragile," marked by an absence of the logic, "critical spirit," and
"powers of reflection" that marked European character.

The authors placed their strongest emphasis on their patients' behavior. Primitive tendencies shaped patients' "external action phases," violent
outbursts that frequently led to "assault, laceration, degradation, and often murder" in male subjects—women, held in "quasi-servitude," experienced too little freedom to engage in such actions.[78] Explosive criminality
constituted the strongest evidence of a basic difference between civilized
and primitive mentalities: "While the evolved individual always remains
. . . under the domination of superior faculties of control, the primitive
reacts . . . through a complete liberation of his automatist instincts, and
here we find the law of all or nothing: in his madness the native knows no
restraint." This phenomenon meant that "in our modern psychiatric hospitals, we have had to multiply the isolation chambers, which have proved
still insufficient for containing the astonishing number of 'violent natives'
that we have to confine." Such tendencies resulted not from a "lack of
maturity" or "arrested development," but instead stemmed from a dangerous intersection of biology and culture. Fatalism, superstition, and other
psychological characteristics of the North African "primitive" originated
in Islamic traditions, but primitivism also had "much deeper roots" in the
"'dynamic' hierarchization of the nervous centers" of the North African's
brain. "A certain weakness of cortical integration" gave "free reign to the
predominance of diencephalic functions." Specific descriptions of physical pathology went beyond the article's clinical purview. Instead, Porot and
Sutter merely demonstrated that the primitive nature of "the North African mind" was overdetermined: while cultural factors shaped character,
a deviant brain structure meant that civilizing endeavors were doomed to
failure.[79]

Critics and historians since Fanon have dwelt on this inflammatory
article, but none has situated this crucial piece effectively in the context
of interwar debates over primitive mentality and colonial politics.[80] The
paper appears almost as a response to the Blum-Viollette law of 1936. A
cornerstone of the Popular Front's colonial policy, the law, proposed by
Léon Blum and the former Algerian governor-general Maurice Viollette,
promised the gradual and progressive enfranchisement of Algeria's male
Muslims, who could attain French citizenship while retaining Muslim civil

status in Algeria. The project's authors intended the law as a wedge that would eventually promote social, political, and economic equality for the Muslim population while tabling the issue of independence. It was vehemently opposed by settlers, as well as by a substantial minority of Popular Front deputies.[81] Porot and Sutter's paper on primitivism marshaled a trove of evidence that demonstrated the impossibility of such a program's success. The North African as a clinical subject presented difficulties to psychiatrists that were unclear to colonial administrators, who considered the North African only as a theoretical citizen. The authors moved debates about primitive mentality out of the ivory tower by noting the real consequences of primitive mental structures. For the Algiers School, a rigorous, ethnologically specific clinical psychiatry was a critical tool of colonial administration. As ethnographers and aesthetes romanticized the difference between Europeans and Africans and as critics of colonial policy proposed greater efforts toward assimilation, colonial psychiatrists underscored the recalcitrant difference between colonizer and colonized and emphasized their discipline's indispensability to effective governance.

Yet there is a crucial irony in the notion that the danger of North African Muslims lay not in their difference from Europeans, but in their similarity to them. Even Porot and Sutter acknowledged that North Africans were among the least "primitive" of France's colonial subjects and were at least superficially far more assimilable and far more intelligent than other colonial populations. But North Africans who succeeded in the lycée and demonstrated a capacity for assimilation threatened the colonial project in myriad ways. They undermined the notion of difference that validated French rule. And yet, colonial subjects who effectively mimicked the trappings of French culture remained inherently different. As postcolonial literary critics have argued about other contexts, North Africans' inherent differences made any successful assimilation a mockery of French civilization, rather than a success of the civilizing mission.[82] The assertion of physical difference in brain structure therefore represented a strategy of dominance on two levels: on the one hand, the dominance of Europeans in the colonial environment; on the other hand, the dominance of the Algiers School's authority over discussions of primitive mentality.

André Donnadieu's case history of Mohamed S., the Moroccan student who attempted suicide in 1937, appeared as the Algiers School's discourse about native difference had crystallized. With the First World War, observations of North African mental patients en masse led to discussions about their incapability of living in French culture. By the Second World War, clinical observations undertaken in new institutions raised this discourse to more sophisticated levels. The Algiers School introduced few new themes: psychiatrists had discussed North Africans' fatalism, deviant sexuality, and excessive violence since the mid-nineteenth century. But Porot and his students established the overdetermined origins of these tendencies. Whereas earlier writers had argued that climate, culture, or biology accounted for the native's violence, sexuality, and "lack of a critical spirit," the Algiers School maintained that multiple factors determined Arab mentality: they were "rooted by their bodies, their customs, their traditions." As Bardenat, at the Mustapha hospital in Algiers, argued, even the educated colonial subject only "borrows the exterior forms of Western civilization," which were undermined by the constant "flow" of the "crude substance of his deep instincts."[83] Initiatives that sought to assimilate North Africans only encouraged an ill-advised hybridization. As with Mohamed S., efforts at assimilation produced "civilization psychosis," not intelligence, because they ignored the multiple barriers between civilized and primitive mentalities. For the Algiers School, the essential structures for civilizing North Africans were therefore penal rather than educational, medical rather than cultural.

...

That these arguments emerged from the colonial setting is unsurprising. Similar theories about sub-Saharan Africans, Indians, and Southeast Asians emerged from British and Dutch colonial contexts, and French travelers since the early nineteenth century had considered the Muslim world a repository of lurid sexuality, savage violence, and uncontrollable madness. But such ideas were also generally limited in their reach. With a few notable exceptions, historians of colonial psychiatry have often depicted its practitioners—usually those with no formal psychiatric training—as physicians who operated at the margins of their profession in the peripheral space of empire.[84] Besides providing a strong counterbalance to novelists, artists, and armchair ethnologists who romanticized "the Orient," the works of Porot and of his colleagues also noticeably informed psychiatric and lay thought about the practical realities of civilizations in conflict. Just as the experimental services and treatments of the Maghreb had driven psychiatric innovation in the Francophone world, so the Algiers School's research shaped ideas about the relationship between race, madness, and crime.

Porot and his students were able to promote their authority effectively because they disseminated their views widely in both medical and popular circles. Journals such as *Algérie médicale* and *Tunisie médicale* (which Porot had founded in 1911) provided a venue for communicating colonial research to other practitioners in the empire. Such media also enhanced the growing authority of the University of Algiers as a new center for inquiry into ethnicity and insanity. The school's members published in major metropolitan journals such as the *Annales, Information psychiatrique,* and *La presse médicale* as well. But even though important pieces such as Porot and Sutter's article on primitivism sometimes appeared in obscure journals, reviews of these articles in major journals assured a wider audience and reinforced the importance of local knowledge about race and psychiatry. The *Annales'* prominent review of the "primitivism" article, for example, summarized Porot and Sutter's central arguments. The review indicated that the key elements of North Africans' primitivism were "their fatalism, indolence, the conception of a nature that is entirely charged with affective potential," their "inaptitude for precision, abstraction, generalization," and their "belief in spirits, omens, witchcraft." The *Annales* noted that "such a milieu fetters the psychological development of the individual" and identified the "frequency of fear, jealousy, anger, that is, instinctive reactions" among North Africans. Highlighting "external action phases of extreme violence" as one of the "most common psychopathic forms" in these patients, the *Annales* also included Porot and Sutter's slip from psychopathology to the North African Muslim's normal psychology:

> This penetrating analysis of the mentality of the indigenous African [*sic*], observed in his mother country, should be familiar to those who observe him transplanted into the Metropole, where he becomes one of the most picturesque forms of mental dislocation [*anatopisme mental*]: that of the "sidi" of the large cities.[85]

Even readers with no access to *Le sud médical* could thus extract the key principles of North African primitivism from the review. Observation "in his mother country" revealed knowledge that merited the attention of French practitioners as "sidis" increasingly traveled to work in French cities. Between 1932 and 1950, reviews such as these appeared in every issue of the *Annales* and other prestigious journals, exposing the pioneering work of psychiatrists in Algeria to the French psychiatric community and legitimating their ideas as cutting-edge research. Written by prominent French psychiatrists, these reviews constantly reiterated familiar notions. North Africans—especially men—were uncivilized and superstitious alcoholics, and when educated they became neurotic.[86] They were dangerous drug addicts: "chronic hashish intoxication [is] very widespread in North Africa."[87] They were frequently epileptic, and when epileptic they were killers.[88] They were vengeful, pathological liars.[89] Publications and reviews after the Second World War affirmed the conclusions of 1918: Al-

gerians were incapable of military service.[90] Even Algerian children were
not exempt from psychiatric vitriol. A review of a 1950 article by Antoine
Porot's son Maurice ascribed the greater frequency of delinquency among
Muslim children than Europeans to congenital cultural attributes of the
Muslim family, especially the sexual segregation of the family, alcoholism,
and amorality.[91]

A critical component of the group's increasing influence was its cultiva-
tion of a general psychiatric expertise alongside its ethnological special-
ization. In contrast with colonial psychiatrists such as J. C. Carothers of
the Mathari Hospital in British East Africa, practitioners in the Maghreb
published extensively on a wide range of psychiatric topics that had ostensibly nothing to do with practice in the colonial field. Between the 1940s
and the early 1960s members of the Algiers School produced substantial
research on the somatic treatment of mental illness and the uses of early
social intervention for treating acute cases (see chapter 3), but also generated volumes on medicolegal psychiatry and a psychiatric textbook for use
in the general medical curriculum. These works also provided an outlet for
reiterating the central claims of the group's ethnopsychiatric research. By
seamlessly integrating claims about race and mentality into these general
works, the school found a much wider distribution for its specific expertise
than would otherwise have been the case.

In 1952 the Presses Universitaires de France published the *Manuel alphabétique de psychiatrie clinique, thérapeutique et médico-légale*, written by
Porot and nine colleagues, eight of whom practiced in Algeria. The authors
aimed this practical guide at the widest possible audience. In "forty years
of practice and twenty of teaching," Porot had been aware of students' constant misunderstanding of psychiatry's confusing and often "hermetic"
language. He and his colleagues therefore intended that the manual rectify
this problem for psychiatrists, students, and general practitioners by sta-
bilizing the language, illustrating the origin of terminology, and offering
specific clarification of the psychiatric lexicon. The volume was a précis of
contemporary psychiatric knowledge designed to bring the essence of the
discipline to anyone's fingertips.

Alongside articles on electroconvulsive therapy, psychosurgery, and
open services were other pieces that reinforced the place of ethnological
knowledge in modern psychiatry. Specific entries included Henri Aubin's
article "North African Natives (Psychopathology of)," in which he argued for the importance of understanding "primitive mentality." In these
patients, one could expect "an explosion of furor, analogous to the one we
see in Blacks, and also nearly murderous, especially if intoxicants (alcohol
or hashish) have impregnated the nervous centers (even in small doses),

or if basic instincts (of conservation or sexual: frequency of jealousy, homicide) enter the game."[92] But more casual references to North Africans
throughout the volume are more scathing. An entry describes bestiality as
"rather rare," except "among North Africa's *indigènes*" (52–53). The entry
on homicide notes that hashish, a widely used intoxicant among North African populations, could incite "murderous reactions" and that "decapita-
tion is rather in favor among certain peoples (Africans, among others), as
is the use of the dagger" (189–90). Antoine Porot wrote that murderous
"impulsivity" was more prevalent among "certain racial categories" than
among others, citing the "external action phases and criminal impulsivity of North African natives" as evidence (211–12). Other, more subtle
references abound: the entry on jealousy dwells on the case of Othello, the
Western canon's most famous Moor, as a specific example of that affliction's murderous consequences. And the authors were careful to situate
North Africans in the school's racial hierarchy as well, as in Porot's classification of drug abuse:

> on the racial scale, each people tends toward the intoxicant that corre-
> sponds to its temperament: opium, favorable to the contemplative isola-
> tion of the Chinese; hashish, proper to the reverie of the Oriental; alcohol
> corresponding to the dynamic temperament of Westerners. (425)

The French medical establishment responded enthusiastically to the
manual's publication. "This original presentation of psychiatry in the form
of an alphabetical manual," wrote *La presse médicale*'s critic, "will be particularly appreciated by the student and the physician." The book would
become "the indispensable instrument of labor for more or less all who are
interested in psychiatry" and "the daily workbook for the student or the
young physician."[93] The *Annales* praised the volume even more effusively,
claiming that "we cannot laud Professor Porot enough for having conceived
the idea of producing a psychiatric lexicon." More than a dictionary, this
project was psychiatry itself in six hundred entries. The volume promised
to "render the greatest services to any student," who could merely "open to
the term sought in order to find immediately all the desired information."
Porot's "long and far-reaching clinical experience" and the contributions
of collaborators "educated by him" meant that this text would "complete
and advance" the work of "the great treatises of psychiatry."[94]

Soon after publishing the volume Porot entered into a new collaboration
with one of the project's co-authors, Charles Bardenat, an expert in fo-
rensic psychiatry, to produce two volumes on medicolegal psychiatry. Addressed primarily to psychiatric specialists, the volumes outlined the major

issues surrounding psychiatric expertise in the courts, the fine points of civil law, and the protocols court psychiatrists should follow in determining criminal responsibility or irresponsibility, illustrating basic concepts with case studies.[95] As with the manual, the supporting details teem with references to North African criminality, fatalism, and impulsivity. The discussion of sexual deviancy is salient. Porot and Bardenat argued that impotent North African men often murdered their wives, suspecting that they had stolen the men's virility. In a deft analysis Porot and Bardenat thus linked murderous impulses to sexual violence while simultaneously raising questions about North Africans' masculinity.[96]

Although the psychiatric press endorsed Porot and Bardenat's ideas, some practitioners contested them. Many psychiatrists who worked with immigrant patients, for example, attributed their high prevalence of mental disorders to nostalgia and the trauma of dislocation rather than to a constitutional defect.[97] The Marseille psychiatrists Joseph Alliez and Henri Descombes acknowledged in 1952 that many patterns they saw in their immigrant patients "corroborate the observations already made in North Africa."[98] Yet to Alliez and Descombes the political economy of metropolitan racism and the stresses of immigration and isolation, rather than some inherent primitivism, appeared to be the principal causes. These patients "were uprooted, their way of life was abruptly modified, and they find a more materially evolved society around them, whose complexity disconcerts them and forces them to face their status of inferiority and inadaptability[;] . . . as far as real psychoses are concerned, we do not believe that an ethnic factor is involved."'A team of researchers at the Sainte-Anne hospital in Paris led by Georges Daumezon largely agreed. Immigration had dramatically increased the proportion of North Africans in the Sainte-Anne hospital's population, which the authors attributed only partly to "antisocial character" of the North African's "pathological mental reactions." More significant were the stresses of poor job security and poverty.[99]

Yet the outbreak of the Algerian war in 1954 helped the Algiers School's ideas to achieve a higher degree of medical currency. Daumezon and his team, for example, shifted their views radically between their initial studies of Sainte-Anne's population and a revised publication of 1957. In a monograph commissioned by the Institut National d'Hygiène, Daumezon and his colleagues addressed "one of the foremost demographic problems" in France and its impact on the mental health system. Admission of North African psychopaths to Sainte-Anne alone had increased more than tenfold, from twenty-seven in 1945 to over three hundred in 1955. Now citing Porot's and his students' works extensively, the authors asserted that "above all else" this constituted a problem of "mental hygiene," because "an intense movement of North African Muslim immigration into the metropole has entailed the formation of a Muslim new wave of population in metropolitan psychiatric hospitals." The root of this "Muslim new wave" was the "liberalism" of immigration regulations between France and North Africa, which precluded "the application of health protection measures (especially concerning mental health)" and resulted in "a series of problems" for mental health practitioners faced with the "marked originality of this population."[100]

The idea of an unstable immigrant population also drew the attention of police authorities. Charles-A. Hirsch, a commissioner at the Paris Préfecture de Police, found in the Algiers School's works the keys to understanding an apparent immigrant crime wave that unfolded in the late 1950s. Like "Puerto Ricans in New York" and "*wet backs* in Texas," North African immigrants presented Parisian authorities with an endless "source of conflicts."[101] North Africans were "masses of poorly adapted and displaced humans" whose "mental evolution has remained quite retarded" despite the fact that life in France immersed them "in the beginnings of the Atomic Age" ("CNA," 129). North Africans had "to learn in several weeks what the European man has learned in several generations": the evolution from "tribal life" in "the Islamic pre–Middle Ages" to life as citizens in a democracy. Crime rates had risen sharply as a result of the tension between civilization's demands and primitive culture: North African men constituted only 7 percent of total convictions in Paris in 1946, but by 1954 this figure had more than doubled, exceeding the immigration rate. Worse, "violence" marked North African crimes: typical offenses included "murder, possession of arms, attacks, sexual violations." Worse still, with the outbreak of the decolonization struggle, Hirsch argued that "a climate of civil and racial war" supplanted the petty crime of "small and medium delinquencies" ("CNA," 131–32).

For Hirsch, the Muslim immigrant was destined to a partial and dangerous assimilation. Religion played a powerful role in limiting the immigrant's acculturation: "the bewitching that the Islamic religion exercises" is something from which "Mohamed is never completely liberated." But a fundamental difference in personality constituted assimilation's major stumbling block. An innately criminal nature limited the possibility of education, for example. Although Muslims were able to "acquire sufficient understanding for operating complex machines," they tended to be drawn to technology's dark side: thus the North African "prefers the firearm to knives when he settles his accounts [and] for bombarding Blida with mortar attacks, alas! the rebels of the FLN have acquired the means"

("CNA," 137). Even the so-called evolved North African—the partially assimilated student—was psychologically predisposed to violence. "Like psychiatrists," Hirsch argued, "detectives are familiar with this great phase of emotional discharge that brings a wise and reserved boy before the Cour d'Assises" ("CNA," 135). A "characteristic aggression and violence" was imprinted on the North African "brutalities" and "rebellion against authority": close correlates of Algerian anticolonialism's desperate acts of terrorism. For this criminologist, a fundamental rift between French and North African psychology explained why "the comportment of the delinquent Arab or Berber had not changed in more than a century" ("CNA," 133).

Gabriel Alapetite, the resident general of Tunisia, had remarked in 1919 that the North African "brain does not reason like ours."[102] By the mid-1950s, the Algiers School's constant reiteration of North Africans' primitive difference brought scientific corroboration to this prejudice. Far from neutral, this knowledge encouraged discrimination on a number of levels. According to judicial observers, the idea of criminal impulsivity in North Africans brought severe condemnation from the bench in cases where Europeans would have found leniency.[103] It provided a justification for the disparities of the Code de l'Indigénat, for the limiting of educational opportunities, and for the banning of Muslims from medical practice. But although the Algiers School's ethnopsychiatric knowledge had often found a ready audience in the French medical and criminological establishment, with the outbreak of the decolonization struggle in the 1950s it caught the attention of a new group: the French army's newly founded Fifth Bureau—the architects of psychological operations during the Algerian war.

Psychiatry at War: *Action psychologique* and the Conquest of Alterity

It is early 1957 in Algiers. The Front de Libération Nationale (FLN) has called a general strike to demonstrate the Algerian people's solidarity with the revolution. Paratroopers have stormed the Casbah, abducting men from their homes and forcing them into work details. A loudspeaker transmits a series of messages in French: "The FLN wants to keep you mired in misery. Revolt against the orders of the FLN. People of the Casbah, France is your country." Days later, the strike continues. A helicopter circles overhead. The voice over the loudspeaker announces the names of prominent revolutionaries killed or in custody. "People of the Casbah, the FLN has already lost the battle. Join us in rising up against those who would oppress you." Armed paratroopers patrol the rooftops, searching for concealed terrorists. They force their way into homes, examining all possible hiding places. At the police station, at the El Biar prison, in hospitals, they brutally interrogate those suspected of harboring any information about the FLN's cells in Algiers. They drown their charges, bind them, beat them, burn them with blowtorches, electrocute them. Meanwhile an ambulance speeds through the city, dropping a body from its rear doors. Pedestrians rush to the body, shocked to discover that the victim is a doctor. The ambulance's passenger begins firing randomly into crowds on the street; moments later, the ambulance careens into a group waiting at a bus stop in a suicide attack.

These scenes from Gillo Pontecorvo's 1965 film *The Battle of Algiers* capture the paradoxes of the Algerian war. It is perhaps these incongruities that account for the conflict's ongoing emotional charge. The war brought to a head the central contradictions that marked the French colonial enterprise in the Maghreb. It witnessed torture in the name of republican civilization and terror in the name of liberation. It enfranchised a population that colonialism had dehumanized for over a century. It was bitterly fought to defend an integral part of France, yet it also forced the "repatriation" of a European population that had never called France its home. The French army insistently proclaimed its advocacy for the incorporation of France's Muslim brothers into the republican project, yet its actions betrayed its contempt for the colonized as irremediably other. The army's psychological warfare programs—like the obtuse loudspeaker messages of Pontecorvo's film—demonstrate a crystallization of the conflict's double edge. Embracing tenderness and brutality at once, the announcement offered promises of assimilation (France is your country!) while the violence of the paratroopers signaled that France would carry out its civilizing mission at the point of a gun.

The war also brought colonial medicine's most incongruous elements to light, revealing its helping hand to be a crushing fist. Colonial medicine and psychiatry were strong instruments of persuasion that balanced the stick of the legionnaire's rifle with the carrot of medical relief. By exploiting the vulnerabilities of a miserable population, the doctor was at the vanguard of colonial expansion. Yet the war laid bare the coercive elements of medicine and psychiatry. As Frantz Fanon argued compellingly in his famous essay on medicine and colonialism, written at the height of the war, the French weaponized medicine during the struggle. By prohibiting the sale of medicines, bandages, alcohol, and surgical instruments to Algerians, by requiring physicians to report all wounded Algerians to the police, by employing physicians and psychiatrists as agents of torture, the colonial government gave the lie to the notion that medicine and science were objective and neutral fields. The physician had become fair game, violating claims to neutrality by participating in acts of war and defending colonial interests over Hippocratic commitments.[104]

The outbreak of hostilities provided a critical opportunity for psychiatrists to enhance their commitment to the colonial state. Psychiatry not only promised to account for the nature of the Algerian's revolutionary consciousness, but also offered its expertise as a new weapon in the struggle against an enemy mindset. Members of the Algiers School offered ready explanations for the appalling violence that marked terrorist attacks on European communities in Algeria. In 1960 Porot and Bardenat claimed that a pathological form of Arab "xenophobia" was the origin of attacks "against subjects belonging to an occupying race." Although these attacks appeared to be politically motivated, "in reality, it is always a matter of solitary [lunatics], engaged at base in the mystique of their religion, which orders them to behave hostilely to the foreigner."[105] Religious fanaticism and mental instability rather than oppression and a revolutionary program directed the Algerian's criminal impulses against European settlers. The FLN's methods also signaled a pathological mindset, especially "the emasculations and eviscerations and profanations of cadavers by terrorists and insurgents."[106] For psychiatrists, the FLN was a collective of deviant fanatics rather than a coherent political organization. Psychiatric thought explained the origins and the course of the revolution in Algeria, finding its clearest evidence in the slaughter of women and children and the bombing of settler enclaves in Algiers.

The deployment of psychiatry in the service of the state represents a key example of what one settler called "information à sens unique"—the one-way information so pervasive during the war as a "collective madness blinded all classes in society."[107] An insistence on the enemy's weakness, a constant reiteration of "chimerical hopes" of retaining *Algérie française*, a mediated emphasis on French protection of Algerians balanced against the savage brutality of pathological *fellagha:* these elements characterized the obtuse campaigns of the French-Algerian press and the army. Fanon argued that this voice "avowed its own uneasiness"—that a hysterical insistence on the permanence of *pied-noir* society marked its death throes.[108] The vehemence of French Algeria's voice may reflect colonial society's own pathology, but it also points to an operation in which psychiatric knowledge played an important supporting role: the tools of *action psychologique* (psychological warfare) deployed by the Cinquième Bureau, the French army's psychological operations unit, in an attempt to weaken the enemy and stiffen the settlers' resolve.

The army's use of psychological warfare techniques predated the 1957 creation of the Cinquième Bureau. As early as 1945 French military officials recognized that they were embroiled in a "conflict of opposing ideologies" in their struggles against the Viet Minh in Indochina. Finding it "essential to examine the psychological aspect" of the revolution in Southeast Asia, and especially the place of Marxist anticolonialism in revolutionary indoctrination, army officials initiated a small-scale intelligence operation devoted to psychological warfare on Indochinese populations that remained limited to propaganda distribution, interrogation, and the provision of support to anticommunist forces.[109] Inspired by American propaganda campaigns in the Pacific theater during the Second World War, the French also dispatched intelligence officers to the United States for advanced psychological warfare training.[110] In a 1953 report on his experiences at Fort Bragg and the Pentagon, Captain Jacques Giraud wrote that "conventional warfare will no longer exist without Psychological Warfare, this being the obligatory support of the former, in all phases of battle." As "the fruit of acquired experiences," the American system promised to help the French to "avoid the inevitable period of trial and error at the start."[111]

The program's efficacy elicited contrasting opinions from its practitioners. The battalion commander Albert Fossey-François, the program's director, considered it "a solid and coherent instrument whose efficacy was never placed in doubt": the Viet Minh's "virulent" opposition to the propaganda program reflected "the degree to which the Psychological War that we have conducted has been able to hinder our adversaries."[112] But another officer recorded a more skeptical view when he admitted that "this arm is not yet ready": although "our Psychological Warfare services have not committed significant errors," they suffered from "serious gaps in the domain of cultural anthropology, and singularly on the subject of mores, customs, social values, superstitions." French forces also possessed a "considerable handicap": their propaganda emanated "from Frenchmen" and therefore "provoke[d] skepticism despite its truth," while Viet Minh propaganda "could permit itself all excesses, because, being indigenous, it benefited from a favorable predisposition from the outset."[113]

As a mimicry of the American program in the Pacific, the Bureau de Guerre Psychologique failed utterly to compete with Ho Chi Minh's message of Marxism for the peasantry. French prisoners released from Viet Minh camps after the defeat at Dien Bien Phu testified to the unshakeable conviction of their captors, suggesting the enhanced fighting capacity of ideologically motivated revolutionaries and the essential need for counterinsurgent psychological weaponry.[114] The French program's greatest value was its "most useful" lessons for the future. It was unsuccessfully adapted to the intellectual and demographic climate of the nascent Vietnam but inspired a redoubled effort to develop an effective program for use in other settings: "In an era when our Indochinese position is shrinking away, it is suitable to direct our gaze to other horizons, drawing from this experience the 'constants' that appear likely to remain valuable, whatever the field of ulterior action."[115]

Algeria represented the clearest "field of ulterior action" for French colonial forces. In contrast with the situation in Indochina, the French possessed extensive ethnographic information on Algerian "mores, customs, social values, superstitions." Military authorities also quickly recognized the psychological implications of a struggle for the retention of French Algeria. Building on their experience in Indochina, the general staff launched a response to the FLN's propaganda campaigns. The new program distinguished carefully between what the army and the government-general considered "friendly" or "uncommitted" groups (the targets of "psychological operations") and "hostile" populations (targets of "psychological warfare"). The Bureau Psychologique, which became the Cinquième Bureau in 1957, avowed that its central mission was "to struggle against [the] diabolically clever propaganda" of the FLN—which deployed "technical procedures for organization and action borrowed from the Soviets, but corrected for the Arab temperament." Such propaganda motivated Algerians to undertake "the systematic recourse to violence" that correlated so closely to the "Arab's specific character."[116]

The French response consisted of a three-pronged assault through the diffusion of information, propaganda, and deception. The goal of the bureau's program, according to one report, was to "take from the adversary the desire to resist."[117] Psychological engagement with the FLN entailed the "systematic implementation of diverse measures and means destined to influence opinion, sentiments, attitude, and the behavior of adverse elements (authorities, armies, populations) in such a manner as to impose our will on the adversary."[118] Tactics to facilitate this goal included press censorship, loudspeaker announcements, graffiti, and the use of photographic images to convince indigenous Algerians of the benefits of the French presence and the destructiveness of the FLN. Executing these programs entailed applying *fin-de-siècle* lessons about mass psychology. According to one officer, for the proper conduct of psychological operations "it is necessary to massify the crowds, to give to men the behavior of mass men."[119] "Mass man" was excitable, suggestible, and imitative—psychological characteristics that also marked the normal North African in psychiatric discourse.

It is difficult to discern the extent to which the work of colonial psychiatrists informed psychological warfare programs. Yet from the outset, *action psychologique* shared the Algiers School's basic assumptions. Military officials not only referred to the Algerian's specifically violent temperament, but also described explicit policies that sought to enact what the Algiers School had already accomplished in the discursive field. Whereas the Cinquième Bureau hoped to create "mass man," Porot had produced this suggestible "indigenous mass," this "formless bloc of primitives," in his 1918 descriptions of conscripts. Army officials understood that the psychological "field of action" in Algeria posed important challenges. Effective *action psy* had to account for the fact that "Muslim Frenchmen"—a wartime euphemism for Algerians—"present extremely different psychological complexes from those of Metropolitans."[120] The interrogation of suspects thus sought two sorts of information: clues about the operations of the FLN, but also ethnographic data about the lives of soldiers in the resistance. A document titled "How to Obtain Information from a Prisoner of War," for example, pointed to the importance of intelligence about the psychological state of the enemy: "To know the state of the adversary's soul and the disagreements experienced inside the enemies' organization is to know the rifts that divide them." Most important, "to know their mentality and the circumstances that oblige them to become engaged in the enemy ranks is to know the enemy's conduct and politics." The efficacy of these tactics required a sound a priori understanding of the "enemy mentality," prompting the Cinquième Bureau to go to great lengths to accumulate knowledge about Muslim culture.[121]

A top-secret memorandum of 1959 indicates that the Cinquième Bureau actively sought information about North African mentalities from key members of the Algiers School. An army official argued that "researching quality information" for an "objective study of the mentality of Muslims" necessitated the input of "Drs. Porot and Sutter."[122] The study's chief goal was to "provide evidence for stereotypes" about "the most profound elements of Muslim culture." Questions about Muslim self-perception, the effects of education and personal experience on cognitive development, and the role of religion in the shaping of Muslim psychology reflect the army's deep concern with enemy psychology. Officials hoped that by answering these questions, Porot and Sutter might adapt information extracted from their patients in order to design a psychological operations program to be implemented in internment camps for Algerian prisoners of war, and then more broadly throughout the population.

More than coincidences, there were thus direct connections between the Cinquième Bureau's programs and the oeuvre of the Algiers School. Close reading of psychiatric publications informed the army's understanding of Muslim mentality and prompted solicitations for Porot's and Sutter's involvement in shaping military programs. Sources say little about the extent of their engagement in the project, but close correlations between military and medical pronouncements about Algerian mentalities indicated the significant attention the bureau paid to their works. The central goal of *action psychologique* was to "modify unfavorable attitudes" among Algerian Muslims, which included "the tendency toward religious fanaticism based on xenophobia." Ethnopsychiatric research into Muslim "character traits" helped bureau operatives to target populations with effective information, as did programs that reached beyond mere propaganda.

The Sections Administratives Spécialisées, the military organizations that one critic called "a velvet slogan and an iron fist," represent a key example.[123] Created in 1955, the SAS were small-scale outposts dispersed throughout rural Algeria with the goal of demonstrating the benefits that French civilization brought to the Maghreb. Through tried and tested means such as vaccination campaigns and rural education, the SAS worked to foster French interests in hundreds of villages. But the SAS combined these tactics with psychiatric revelations about Muslims to deploy these propaganda measures to greater effect. An SAS chart indicates how knowledge about Algerians' character traits shaped psychological operations tactics and reveals startling parallels with the terminology used by Porot and his students:

Character Traits	Consequences
—Extreme emotional sensitivity: the Muslim "thinks with his heart."	To convince him, employ arguments of a sentimental rather than a logical order.
—Being passionate, he has highs and lows.	Be patient, try to keep him calm whatever the current situation
—*He does not tolerate irony.*	Avoid mockery absolutely, and be aware of the "joke" that will not be understood and will wound deeply.
—He is extremely attached to *Muslim religion*, even if he does not follow all its practices.	Avoid all religious controversy: *this does not concern us.*
—His intelligence is oriented differently from ours. We are scientific, he is a dreamer and a mystic.	Do not be astonished if he fixes his attention on other things than those that we fixate on, if his mores are different from ours. Exploit what interests *him*, not what interests *us*.
—He lacks a critical spirit.	A great lie proffered by the enemy can be perfectly believed.[124]

This précis also outlined contrasting ideas about Europeans in Algeria. Unlike Muslims, *pieds-noirs* respected "logic": "*Explain* and *prove* if you wish to convince him." They were skeptical: "Avoid brainwashing." And they were profoundly attached to the soil: "Translate problems into hectares of cultivated land as often as possible."[125] But the emphasis of the SAS campaign—as well as psychological warfare more broadly—was to "influence opinions, passions, attitudes, and behavior" in the Muslim population "so as to assist the realization of national goals." According to this officer, although settlers were easily convinced of the benefits of a continuous French presence in Algeria, Muslims inevitably resisted such ideas. Because they were "still affected by a primitive mentality, psychological work based solely on intellectual constructions and logical demonstrations is ineffective." Instead, the "Muslim masses only understand our arguments if their heart is touched before their mind." To this end, "we need to present ourselves not with a straight face or a condescending air, but with the warmth of a friend who is engaged in a persevering struggle and who will bring the guarantee of Peace and Justice."[126]

Authorities worked on two sets of assumptions. First, they asserted that a primitive mentality governed the Muslim's psychological processes. Second, they assumed that not all Algerians were committed to the FLN's "xenophobic" and "fanatical" mission. Exploiting this tension through propaganda campaigns was the key to effective psychological warfare. The army's chief task through these campaigns was an insistence upon the civilizing presence of the French in Algeria: "If he does not see that the European brings considerable development to the country from which he indirectly profits, the Muslim may think that he is exploited by a colonial regime."[127] Whereas psychiatric assumptions about the Algerian mind governed the language of *action psychologique*, the civilizing mission guided its methods. Army officials stressed the importance of hospitals as tools for pacification: propaganda documents emphasized that "free medical assistance" had more than doubled in 1957.[128] Schools also played crucial roles in serving these interests. In 1958, after French paratroopers' savage use of torture brought the battle of Algiers to a close, the minister of national education ordered that all schools offer "a special lesson on France's work in North Africa" that would emphasize "economic, social, and human" accomplishments—including the production of a modern medical infrastructure in Algeria.[129]

Military control of information technology was crucial for maintaining psychological control of the population. As an editorial in *France outre-mer* argued in 1956, France could not leave the psychological initiative to the *fellagha*: because "the man and woman of the countryside . . . form their judgments based on the small facts of daily life," every soldier must act as a representative of French civilization.[130] Censorship of the press and the disruption of enemy radio broadcasts were essential components of the program.[131] But the military also sought psychiatrists' assistance in developing new strategies for convincing the Algerian population that their interests could be best served by a continued French presence in the Maghreb. In one test conducted in an internment camp for FLN suspects, the army's *médecin général* organized photographic displays that contrasted French contributions with the destruction wrought by the *fellagha*.[132] Banners implored viewers to choose between the *fellagha* and France, while photographs directed them toward an ineluctable decision. Images of teachers instructing Algerian children, doctors caring for the elderly, and children receiving X-rays emphasized that France "builds," "instructs," "revitalizes," and "cares"; photographs of demolished schools, of despondent, limbless children in hospitals stressed that the *fellagha* "destroys," "terrorizes," and "kills."[133] The goal was "to dis-integrate the individual" from the FLN platform by revealing that the architects of the Algerian revolution were "defective and incapable" subjects who "steal and kill" in violation of Qur'anic principles. A captive population allowed intelligence officers to determine the required length of time for "recuperating" subjects who had been "intoxicated" by revolutionary propaganda, and to calculate the primary methods for redesigning "the foundations of individual and crowd psychology . . . for Muslims."[134]

Designers of the photographic program used the technique as a sort of Rorschach test to elicit certain reactions from imprisoned revolutionaries. Critics of the program questioned the legitimacy of employing such devious techniques for attracting sympathetic populations. The insidious methods of *action psychologique* could only produce "a pseudo-conversion obtained by the most vulgar and dumbfounding forms of propaganda" rather than "a sincere and thoughtful adhesion in the Franco-Muslim community."[135] Others protested what they considered a brutal form of modern warfare. In January 1958 the Groupe d'Études de Psychologie in Paris issued a press release that took a "public stand on the use of psychology" in the military: the "use of 'Atomic weapons' is certainly dangerous," these students argued, "but that of 'Psychological weapons' is just as [dangerous], because its consequences also result in the destruction of Man."[136]

Albert Fossey-François, the director of *action psychologique* in Indochina, had argued that resistance against the program demonstrated its success: despite the campaign's losses, the vehement response to propaganda suggested the potential applications of this relatively new military technology. If resistance constitutes a reliable measure of a program's impact, *action psychologique* appears to have had a profound effect in Algeria. Journalists and students in France measured the possible successes of the program against its significant psychological costs. Prominent Algerian intellectuals also spoke out against *action psychologique*. Jean el-Mouhoub Amrouche and Ferhat Abbas, both of whom subscribed to the republican ideal in their youth, attacked the campaign as fundamentally dehumanizing for Algerians. Although they were firmly committed to Algerian independence, Amrouche and Abbas had believed in the civilizing mission until the devious techniques of psychological warfare revealed the bankruptcy of French humanism.[137]

Although *action psychologique* produced no physical casualties, these tactics sought to reshape the Algerian mind by destroying its capacity for resistance. In the same way, French colonial psychiatry—especially its incarnation in Algiers—deployed an intellectual violence that was in every sense the equal of colonialism's dehumanizing legal and social structure, a savagery concomitant with the brutality required to police Algeria's Manichaean world. The degree to which ethnopsychiatric knowledge informed settlers' opinions about native North African populations cannot be measured with any certainty; nor can the extent to which preconceived notions informed psychiatric ideas. But as the next chapter makes clear, the resistance that colonial psychiatric ideas and practices elicited attests to the degree to which contemporaries experienced the practical ramifications of these ideas. Psychiatric racism is of course the origin of Frantz Fanon's reactions against the colonial system. In addition to Fanon's diatribes against ethnopsychiatric manifestations of scientific racism, other doctors railed against medical theories that linked race and madness. Maghrebian authors detailed their experiences with sophisticated racism in their novels and memoirs as a means of contesting stereotypes. And perhaps most crucially, patients at Blida, Berrechid, and Manouba tested the limits of psychiatric knowledge about North African Muslims in myriad ways. Patients contested psychiatric authority inside asylum walls, and students such as Mohamed S. revealed the hollowness of assertions about North African primitivism through their clear intelligence.

And what about Mohamed S., this "poor Moroccan" who tried to take his own life when he realized he could never be truly French? Donnadieu's case history is so emblematic of psychiatrists' concerns about the proper means of civilizing North Africans that it becomes difficult to believe this patient ever existed—at least as Donnadieu presented him. But Donnadieu informs us that after leaving two French institutions—the lycée and the hospital—Mohamed spent most of 1938 and 1939 in blissful ignorance. Living as a gentleman farmer in the North African *bled*, Mohamed S.

never again tested his limits, having accepted his lot in life. Rooted in his body, his customs, and his traditions, Mohamed was best served, according to Donnadieu, by avoiding self-improvement. French instruction and French revitalization—the central messages of *action psychologique*—had their limitations, and for psychiatrists, the specific institutions that best accomplished the civilizing mission in the Maghreb were the hospital and the prison. *Action psychologique* sought to convince North Africans of the investment the French brought to the Maghreb. At the same time, *action psychologique* sought to preserve the division between populations by underscoring a fundamental difference between Europeans and North Africans, a difference based in bodies, customs, and traditions.

5

Violence, Resistance, and the Poetics of Suffering

Colonial Madness between Frantz Fanon and Kateb Yacine

We most often imagine medicine as a healing art, a means of alleviating pain. And yet what of a scenario in which medicine is a primary source of—or is at least coextensive with—suffering and trauma? Since Michel Foucault's critical framings of clinical knowledge and medical power, social scientists and humanists have exhaustively explored the production of biopolitical knowledge and its implications for modernity.[1] Yet concern for exposing the operation of medical power has produced fewer examinations of medicine as an explicit source of suffering. The complicity of medicine in the structural violence of the colonial situation reveals a range of iatrogenic forms of suffering and a setting in which medicine cannot be construed without also accounting for its operation as a force of oppression.

Such a perspective illuminates the overlapping of layers of violence and trauma under colonialism, a scenario in which the clinic is often a literal theater for colonial conflict. It also points to medicine as an important location for anticolonial resistance. For many, the work of the psychiatrist and anticolonial theorist Frantz Fanon best encapsulates the links between colonial medicine, violence, and resistance. His best-known works, *A Dying Colonialism* and *The Wretched of the Earth*, both published during the Algerian struggle for independence, illustrated the moral bankruptcy of the French civilizing mission and the savagery of the colonial encounter. More important, they drew on Fanon's clinical experience in Algeria to lay bare the racism of colonial psychiatrists and their complicity in colonial violence. Clearly outlining the dehumanizing structures of European colonialism in North Africa, these tracts also offered a call to action against a psychiatric tradition that labeled North African Muslims "born slackers, born liars, born robbers, and born criminals," and that thereby established a scientific armature in the interest of the colonial state.

Yet Fanon was far from a lone voice crying in a violent wilderness. A number of North African critics pointed to sickness under colonialism as an experience marked by overdetermined forms of physical, emotional, and psychological trauma. Medical papers, poetry, dramatic works, novels, and essays by Muslim authors explored the clinic and medical knowledge as spaces of colonial violence, and they conceived of their writings as a tool of resistance against both imperialism and the sickness it generated. Their works also demonstrate a wide range of experiences. For some, a scientifically rooted prejudice resulted in professional and social disenfranchisement. For others—especially the Algerian author Kateb Yacine—multiple orders of marginalization and the violence of everyday life under colonialism rendered them far more vulnerable to far more serious dangers. Madness was for many of these authors the paradigmatic sickness of colonialism, while psychiatry operated as a biopolitical machine for the regulation of colonial order. Psychiatric knowledge, colonial power, and the madness their intersection generated were a crucible of suffering and trauma, linked to an acute anguish both born and productive of colonial violence.

The works of these doctors, political figures, and poets are sources of the key meanings of violence and suffering at the heart of madness and medicine in the colonial Maghreb. I read these texts not through the eyes of a literary critic attuned to the subtleties of form and representation, but instead through those of a social historian of medicine with an interest in how they interrogate the ambiguous position of colonial medicine and how they illuminate the intellectual and political contexts of twentieth-century anticolonial resistance. Colonial violence took many forms—epistemological, structural, and physical. The works of the writers considered here, and especially those of Kateb, point to the ways in which colonial medicine and psychiatry were complicit with these forms of brutality. By reading these works alongside Fanon's more familiar critique of violence and pathology in Algeria, we can see the development of an intellectual culture of resistance that took medicine and psychiatry as its object. This frame not only contextualizes Fanon's work, but also highlights the range of experiences with colonial forms of knowledge that shaped local imaginings of political circumstance and suffering.

Fanon, Biography, and History: Mythmaking and the Violence of Everyday Life

Frantz Fanon is a complicated figure for historians. His advocacy for the Algerian *lumpenproletariat*, the marginalized and illiterate rural population ignored by French colonialists and the FLN alike, brings him the admiration of many in the academic Left. Fanon's work on the experience of race as a critical factor in the formation of the modern subject also grants him a foundational position in the field of postcolonial studies, as does his effort to identify the political and economic sources of the pathology of the colonial situation. Yet his advocacy for violence as the only legitimate means of throwing off the yoke of colonial power and creating a new postcolonial subjectivity is troubling for many and remains especially problematic in light of the ongoing bloodshed in contemporary Algeria.

Many of Fanon's biographers have downplayed his legacy of violence and have presented him instead as a pioneering reformer. From the biographies, the legends, and at times his own words, the story is familiar: Fanon's legacy rests with his revolutionary criticism, his exposés of medical racism in the colonies, and the liberatory reforms he brought to his patients in Algeria and Tunisia. Biographers have argued that Fanon took a heroic stand against the insuperable obstacles of institutional psychiatry and the French colonial regime. Fanon, these authors claim, was a colonial Pinel: a reformer whose initial move upon taking charge of the Algerian Hôpital Psychiatrique de Blida-Joinville in 1953 was to remove chains from his patients,[2] and whose writings represented the first critique of the Algiers School's racism.[3] The comparison to Pinel is insistent: Fanon's liberation of North African patients from colonial chains in the heady atmosphere of the freedom struggle echoes Pinel's utopian unchaining of the lunatics at Bicêtre in the context of the French Revolution. Likewise, Fanon's attempts to introduce culturally sensitive therapeutics at Blida revolutionized treatment at this "backward, medieval" hospital. A daring revolutionary, Fanon survived several assassination attempts in his tireless efforts to aid the embryonic Algerian nation and to discredit obsolete scientific prejudices that supported colonial racism.[4] In these assessments, Fanon's radical engagement with the entrenched forces of the psychiatric establishment in Algeria meant that this doctor was "ahead of his time."[5]

Born in Martinique in 1925, Fanon fought for the French Free Forces during the Second World War and studied medicine at Lyon in the 1940s and early 1950s. Race is paramount for Fanon beginning with his earliest publications. *Black Skin, White Masks* of 1952, originally submitted (and rejected) as Fanon's medical thesis, relates the author's attempts to transcend racial boundaries as a colonial subject bound by European assumptions and in so doing outlines the psychological pressures of racism on the formation of the black subject.[6] Although *Black Skin* treats the impact of racism on experience and identity, his 1952 article "The North African Syndrome" launches his first indictment of the racism of the French medical establishment.[7] Physicians working in Lyon's North African immigrant community often described an unlocalized illness in their patients, which they attributed to imagination and malingering. Fanon revealed that this so-called North African Syndrome was instead a widespread psychosomatic phenomenon with roots in the patients' experiences as immigrant laborers in a hostile social environment.

A year after publishing these works, Fanon applied for and received a post as a ward director in Algeria's psychiatric hospital at Blida. The beleaguered hospital was immensely overcrowded upon his arrival, and practices bore the stamp of the Algiers School's racialized psychiatry. After the outbreak of the Algerian war Fanon sided with the revolutionary Front de Libération Nationale and eventually resigned both his post at Blida and his French citizenship. Fanon then moved to newly independent Tunisia where he continued both his psychiatric work and his political activities on behalf of the FLN. Here Fanon was somewhat freer to participate in his political activities as well as his attempts at psychiatric reform than he was in Algeria. Based on his medical and political experiences, Fanon published a series of coauthored articles that criticized the inadequacies of contemporary therapy, prepared *A Dying Colonialism* and *The Wretched of the Earth* for publication, and offered university courses in psychiatry. In 1961, after fighting leukemia for several years, he died in a hospital in Washington, D.C.

Fanon's experience at Blida is crucial for understanding his criticism of colonialism and contemporary psychiatry. Although any psychiatric hospital might have shown similar problems of overcrowding and abusive treatment of patients, at Blida Fanon confronted the attitudes of European settlers in North Africa as well as the particular brand of ethnopsychiatry practiced by members of the Algiers School. Fanon responded with a scathing criticism of both colonial logic and its basis in psychiatric science. He denounced the colonial "Manichean world" that policed, oppressed, and dehumanized the colonized population in the interests of European exploitation, and argued that psychiatry operated as a regulatory arm of state power. Colonial psychiatric theories about the inherent and overdetermined inferiority of the colonized precluded any claims on their part for political or cultural legitimacy and therefore bombarded North Africans with messages of their primitive nature. Fanon claimed that colonial psychiatry, with its understanding of Algerians as "born slackers, born liars, born robbers, and born criminals," brutally assaulted the very subjectivity of the colonized.[8]

To counter this attack, Fanon located the origins of Algerian violence in the mechanics of colonial society and in the psychological formation of the revolutionary subject. Popular and scientific imaginings of Algerian impulsivity justified police repression, perpetuating an endless cycle of violence. For Fanon, colonial society was a malfunctioning organism that engendered madness and savagery in the dominated population. It was the colonialist's aggression that bred concomitant behavior in the individual. Algerians *were* unnaturally violent, he conceded, but such outbursts constituted a response to pathological violence rather than a reliable measure of the Algerian's "primitive" or "criminal" nature.[9]

Fanon also insisted on violent action as a necessary step in the development of revolutionary consciousness. Such action was essential to the revolution on a number of levels. It exposed the inherent violence of colonial society through the reprisal it engendered from the settler. It committed the revolutionary: it was an articulation that he or she had reached a point of no return and had forsaken the civilizing mission. It was an appropriation of the violence of the settler, turned toward the end of liberation and the creation of new revolutionary subjects. A mind and a society shattered by violence could only find its salvation in an equal and opposite violence, one directed at the cleansing liberation of a colonial society.

Fanon's advocacy of violence has elicited fierce debate among scholarly critics. Some, such as Ranjana Khanna, have found Fanon's response to Porot to be restrained, given the virulence of the Algiers School's pronouncements.[10] Others, such as Robert Berthelier and Jock McCulloch, have argued that Fanon was merely the obverse of Porot—that his formulation of the Algerian's violence effectively embraced Porot's description but provided an account of the stimulus that inspired the inevitable response of brutal criminal passion. Yet despite valid criticisms of the mechanistic nature of Fanon's theory of Algerian violence, it is clear that colonialism for Fanon operated in a logic analogous to that recently outlined by anthropologists such as Nancy Scheper-Hughes, Arthur Kleinman, and Veena Das in their trenchant analyses of violence and subjectivity. In these accounts, the experience of the "violence of everyday life" produces specific forms of subjectivity as state and global forces distort local moral orders that normally preserve social integrity. Violence shapes identity as it becomes the subject's principal register for framing the local social world and, in turn, individual and collective action.[11] French colonialism fractured community in North Africa. When faced with the overwhelming repressive force of the colonizer, the colonized (male) subject internalized and redirected his anguish and aggression toward other Muslims as the only possible outlet. Under colonialism, as Fanon argued, "Algerian criminality takes place in a closed circle. Algerians rob each other, cut each other up, and kill each other."[12] Yet the liberation struggle offered a new channel for this violence and a means for deploying that rage in the creation of a new Maghreb and a new Muslim subjectivity.

The Tensions of the *évolué*: Psychiatry and Epistemological Violence

Fanon was far from the first to identify the oppressive components of psychiatry in the colonies. As chapter 3 shows, colonial patients themselves resisted internment in myriad ways. Yet other forms of resistance emerged simultaneously with the formation of colonial theories about the Muslim mind. When the physician Maurice Boigey published his cutting "Psychological Study of Islam" in the *Annales* in 1908, the French-trained Tunisian physician Ahmed Chérif pounced on the article's inconsistencies immediately. Boigey proposed that the Muslim's "psychological type" was "inactive," and therefore Muslims had "never produced any extraordinary work, built a capital city [or] studied any science profoundly." Islamic expansion was "an epidemic of religious madness" that "could be explained less by theology than by mental pathology." The prophet Muhammad, he argued, had "implanted in his Believers' brains a veritable *neuropathological state*." Boigey argued that any of the accomplishments of Islamic civilization had resulted from parasitism: he asserted that medieval Islam's most notable medical philosophers Averroës (Ibn Rushd) and Avicenna (Ibn Sina) were Spanish Christians who had converted to Islam under duress.[13]

Chérif saw the article as a viciously worded assortment of lies. He asked in the *Annales* a year later "how an educated man . . . dares to treat such an important topic by employing arguments that are diametrically opposed to historical truth" and offered to correct such errors "in the name of immutable truth and scientific integrity." The essay responded to assertions about Muslims' technological and scientific incapacity by illustrating how in astronomy and mathematics Muslims had been "instructors and advisors" to Europeans, then attacked the account of Muslim psychology: "I would ask M. Boigey if he has traveled extensively through the Orient and if he has spent so much time amid all these neurasthenic and obsessive Muslims." Finally, regarding Islamic "parasitism," Chérif wondered how Ibn Sina, a Persian who had never visited Spain, might have been a Spaniard who converted to Islam, and asked the same question about Ibn Rushd, whose Muslim genealogy extended back at least four generations.

In his conclusion Chérif described his "pain" in the realization that "Europeans in the twentieth century continue to write about Islam and Muslims . . . with as many errors and as much violence as an ignorant and fanatical monk of the time of the Crusades."[14]

Boigey's attack and Chérif's parry introduce two major components of the contest between colonial psychiatrists and North African intellectuals that lies at the core of Fanon's revolutionary criticism. Boigey's assertions about the existence of a Muslim mentality clothe overt racism in scientific garb backed by military power: in lieu of presenting evidence, Boigey speaks with the voice of medical and colonial authority. But the logical extension of such ideas presented even greater difficulties for colonial intellectuals. Valorized by their medical trappings, studies of Muslims' inherent psychopathology—and, by the 1930s, primitivism—marginalized North African culture as irrelevant to the modern world. Accusations of Muslims' psychological "inactivity" and inherent "pathology" provoked major anxieties in North African intellectual circles because of the facility with which such ideas forged an unbridgeable gap between European and North African cultures and societies.

The notion of this basic rift in colonial society—the Manichaean world—is one of the most controversial aspects of Fanon's thought. It is a problem both complicated and confirmed by the experience of the *évolués*, colonial students educated in French lycées and universities who occupied the uncomfortable space between colonizer and colonized. These figures represented the core of those who resisted colonial psychiatry's role in sustaining racist inequality. They also posed significant challenges to European hegemony by destabilizing the boundaries of colonial rule. Through their success in a system that placed almost insurmountable barriers in their paths, they demonstrated the hollowness of Europeans' claims to inherent racial superiority.[15] According to one sociologist writing in the early 1960s, "European psychology" depended on such clear-cut hierarchies: "the inferiority imposed on the Muslims" appeared "to the colonizer as the justification of his presence in the colony . . . and as the safeguard of the privileges attached to his social condition."[16] Given the psychological importance of maintaining the inherent difference that supported the hierarchy of colonial power, Muslims who claimed membership in French civilization inexcusably rent the thin fabric that veiled colonial hypocrisy. Yet they did so at the expense of alienation from their own cultures. As Fanon argued, the *évolués* who formed the rank and file of the nationalist bourgeoisie sought the "betterment of their particular lot" through their "barely veiled desire to assimilate," while "scorning" the backwardness of their fellow colonized.[17]

In some ways, these experiences mirror Fanon's. Fanon was an avatar of the colonial *évolué*. As a member of an elite Creole family in Martinique, he grew up conscious of being French. He was a subject of one of France's *vieilles colonies* and therefore a fully enfranchised citizen of the republic. According to his account in *Black Skin, White Masks*, it was only his arrival in France that created his awareness of the fact of his blackness as a visible sign of inequality. Fanon's education and his family's economic status had acculturated him to believe in his cultural position as one of potentially equal partnership with the French, while his reception by white French society revealed to him a permanent, unbridgeable rift between European and colonial social worlds. His status as a veteran, his education, and his medical credentials did nothing to outweigh his blackness, which became the central quality of his being in a society organized by race.

Yet there is a critical difference between Fanon's and North African Muslims' experiences. The constant presence of colonial settlers in North Africa reinforced the importance of racial difference in the Maghreb from cradle to grave. Although this situation could preclude the shock felt by Fanon in Paris, it also presented a terrible burden for the *évolué* schoolchild in the colonial lycée. A number of Fanon's North African contemporaries fixated on this problem in autobiographical novels—a key genre for exploring the psychological effects of the *évolué*'s split consciousness. In *Le passé simple* the Moroccan author Driss Chraïbi, for example, describes himself as an academic prodigy who rejects Islam and Morocco—his own "simple past"—in an attempt to assimilate into French culture. A European admonishes the protagonist: "We, the French, are in the process of civilizing you, the Arabs. Badly, in bad faith, and with no pleasure. Because, if by chance you come to be our equals, I ask you: in relation to whom or to what will *we* be civilized?"[18]

The Tunisian Jewish psychologist and author Albert Memmi provides another incisive analysis of colonial logic. *Le statue de sel* ("the pillar of salt") carries a message similar to Chraïbi's—that the lot of the *évolué* is to "never look back." In the novel Memmi describes the torment of his adolescence as his teachers discouraged him from scholarly pursuits: after he had slipped into slang during an oral report on French literature, a teacher berated him for using "the language of a janitor." Despite his efforts to "penetrate the soul of the civilization by mastering its language," he only succeeded in "acquiring a sort of appropriated wisdom" in which "nothing was spontaneous, everything became effort and calculation."[19]

Memmi's anxieties betray his fear of a phenomenon that colonial psychiatrists described as common. As one Algiers psychiatrist argued, signaling the limited possibilities for colonial assimilation, even the educated

North African, he argued, "only borrows the exterior forms of Western civilization" while "the rude substance of his deep instincts flows" within him.[20] Memmi describes the particularly colonial dimensions of this taunting in his 1957 treatise *The Colonizer and the Colonized*. This analysis of the psychology of colonization portends *The Wretched of the Earth*'s Manichaean world as Memmi theorizes his experiences. Seeking admission to French society, the *évolué* meets derisive scorn as he "apes" the colonizer: "The shrewder the ape, the better he imitates, and the more the colonizer becomes irritated." The colonizer seeks "the telltale nuance in clothing or language . . . which he always manages to discover"—like Memmi's "language of a janitor."[21] Any manifestation of alterity becomes woeful inadequacy in the colonizer's eyes, a phenomenon that Memmi tied to the nature of colonial education. Educated solely in *French* history and culture, the colonized's own "simple past" was marginalized in the lycée. The colonized was therefore "in no way a subject of history any more." Although "he carries its burden," he does so "always as an object," having "forgotten how to participate actively in history": "The colonized seems condemned to lose his memory" (*CC*, 92, 103).

These reflections signal the links between structural violence and the tensions of the *évolué* in colonial society. As the medical anthropologist Paul Farmer has framed the concept, structural violence is produced in scenarios in which overwhelming social, political, and economic forces combine to limit the subject's potential agency.[22] Such forces organize a (mostly) unidirectional flow of power down what Farmer calls "steep gradients of inequality" and structure experience for victimized populations.[23] The epistemological violence that marked colonial assessments of the *évolué* reflect the political-economic dimensions of Farmer's structural violence. The poet Jean el-Mouhoub Amrouche, an Algerian Christian who moved in France's highest literary circles, argued that the colonizing process annihilated local history and culture, provoking a crisis of identity for the colonized student. Colonial authority rested on the assumption of "the natural, absolute, inarguable, and undiscussed superiority of the Europeans," a notion upheld through "contempt for and ignorance of" the history of Muslim civilization. As these principles undergirded the colonial education system, growing up under colonialism entailed an inevitable process of simultaneous affiliation with and rejection of both his cultures: "The colonized child has no parents, no ancestors, the country where he is born has no history, no great exemplary men . . . to nourish his dreams and inspire his desire to imitate them." Soon the child's natural affection for his familiars gives way to "violent resentment" of his culture. Yet European racism thwarted the child's attempt to embrace French civilization,

because the North African invariably met rejection as a "dirty Arab." A
constant reiteration of Arabs' "imperfectibility" and their "inadaptability
to modern progress" meant that education constituted a growing awareness of the Muslim student's difference, which led him to "discover the
depths of his alienation."[24]

Amrouche fixated on questions of identity and allegiance in a context
where normality meant a profound ambivalence toward two cultures. His
torturous struggle over his identity suggests that the North African student grew up under conditions of psychological warfare, an issue Fanon
grappled with extensively. Colonialism's repetitive insistence on North
African difference and its destruction of history and culture constituted
a pathogenic environment. "An obsessional personality," Fanon argues,
"is the fruit of the 'psychological action' used in the service of colonialism in Algeria." Psychological warfare as practiced in the interrogations
of suspected revolutionary intellectuals "attack[s] from the inside those
elements which constitute national consciousness." The intellectual "is
surrounded by 'political advisers'"—including psychologists and psychiatrists—who "overthrow" the foundations of national identity: "Algeria is
not a nation; it has never been a nation; it will never be a nation. There is
no such thing as the 'Algerian people.'"[25] Amrouche's meditations reveal
that the colonized child experienced a lifelong subjection to psychological
torture in the lycée rather than the interrogation center, in which such indoctrination ensured psychological brutalization. If "every man . . . needs
social, historical, and mythological roots," then in the case of the colonized
"the entire race is stripped of its humanity": colonial discourse rendered
them "barbarians, primitives; in sum, skeletons of men."[26]

Academic psychiatry was deeply complicit in this process of marginalization. From its foundations the Algiers School's rhetoric emphasized that
"mental deficiency" represented the "mean of [the North African] race,"[27]
that the North African's natural state was one of "extraordinary violence
and savage furor."[28] The implications of these studies were not lost on
North African critics. To block North Africans' access to the European's
world, Memmi argued, "the colonizer will use all his psychological theories" (*CC*, 124): a battery of scientific knowledge was marshaled to reiter-
ate the immutability of the colonized subject. Memmi offered the example
of a French psychiatrist in Rabat who described a "North African spirit"
that was predisposed to psychopathology as a condition of the North African's essentially inhuman nature (*CC*, 75). As Memmi indicates, psychiatry was ultimately a coercive force at the rhetorical level, a discourse that
constrained the possibilities of assimilation and that served the interests of

colonial authority by outlining the limitations of North Africans' capacity for achievement and self-rule.

Yet colonial psychiatry was a physically as well as a rhetorically coercive force. In a lecture series he offered at the University of Tunis in 1959 and 1960, Fanon outlined his thesis on the psychology of colonial domination and drew explicit connections not just to the racist ideology of the Algiers School but also to the problematic nature of contemporary psychiatric practice itself. Fanon characterized the madman as a figure who was "a 'stranger' to society," and internment constituted society's principal means of "isolating" this "anarchistic element" in the interest of preserving its own safety. The psychiatrist was therefore "the auxiliary of the police, the protector of society" who patrolled the boundaries between reason and unreason in the Manichaean world of the psyche, just as colonialism safeguarded the boundaries between European and native. A modern therapy, by contrast, must emphasize the "resocialization" of patients rather than their seclusion.[29] Beginning from an indictment of psychiatric racism, Fanon then found himself at odds with the discipline's most fundamental precepts, a conviction that guided his experiments with group therapy and outpatient treatment at Manouba and the Charles Nicolle hospital.

The Tunisian psychiatrist Sleïm Ammar shared this assessment. Like Fanon and Ahmed Chérif, Ammar was the product of a French medical education. Born in 1927 in Sousse, he completed his studies at the Paris Faculté in 1954 and returned to Tunisia as an assistant physician at Manouba, where he eventually became Tunisia's most prominent psychiatrist in the postcolonial era. Ammar proposed reforms that paralleled Fanon's efforts to resocialize the patient, but whereas Fanon blamed the inefficacy of institutionalization on the sociological structure of the hospital, Ammar traced the problems of contemporary psychiatry to the discipline's historical development in Europe. A 1954 article proposed that "great historical upheavals preceding periods of human progress" witness the most "radical transformations in societies' attitudes concerning their lunatics"—a strong political message as Tunisians negotiated their independence. Thus Islamic expansion initiated a new paradigm for the treatment of the mentally ill. Arabs "prodigiously developed" medical knowledge and the Qur'an implored the faithful to "gather" the ill "and to seek their cure." By contrast, European medicine recalled a legacy of confinement and torture: "It was in France," Ammar argued, "that they burned the most 'witches.'" Historical ruptures brought reforms—Ammar cited the case of Pinel at Bicêtre, for example—but even the modern asylum "confirmed the segregation of the lunatic from society" and therefore fulfilled more of a policing than a medical function. For Ammar, European medicine's most significant achievements consisted of greater measures of confinement and control over the insane.[30]

Charges that the asylum was primarily an arm of state authority were a stock component of twentieth-century antipsychiatry, and such accusations might have been leveled at any number of European hospitals. Accounts of Nazi psychiatrists' complicity in racial hygiene and euthanasia programs had also raised suspicions about the relationship between medicine and the state by the 1940s, as had revelations about the thousands of patients who starved and froze to death in French asylums during the Vichy era. And as the use (and abuse) of radical somatic treatments such as psychosurgery and convulsive shock therapies became more widespread in the mid-twentieth century, skepticism about psychiatrists' Hippocratic commitment became the norm in intellectual circles.[31] In the colonies, however, the conditions of confinement and psychiatric abuses of power lent themselves to particularly strong anxieties about the use of the asylum for social control. North Africans were often reluctant to turn their relatives over to colonial authorities unless they had truly become unmanageable or unless the family had been ordered to do so by police. The result is that the bulk of the patients in the hospitals at Blida, Manouba, and Berrechid (in Morocco) were involuntarily confined either through authorities' intervention in the family or as vagrants who attracted police attention. Such dynamics also marked European psychiatric institutions. Yet the widespread confinement of drug and alcohol abusers and the internment of anticolonial nationalists, combined with the radical authoritarianism of colonial administration, raised suspicions about the asylum as a repository for society's unmanageable elements.

Dr. Salem ben Ahmed Esch-Chadely bore witness to these and other abuses at Tunisia's Manouba hospital in the 1930s and 1940s. Protesting the conditions of colonial psychiatry constituted the focus of his nationalist activities from 1935 to his death in 1954. Esch-Chadely, who was born in Monastir in 1896, came of age simultaneously with the Tunisian independence movement. Upon beginning medical studies at the Paris Faculté de Médecine, he formed a number of lifelong contacts with other Tunisian nationalist students, including the leader of the Parti Néo-Destourien (New Constitutional Party), Habib Bourguiba, and was monitored closely by French police.[32] For Esch-Chadely, nationalism and the decolonization of medicine soon constituted a single vocation. His 1929 medical thesis, ostensibly an account of fatigue and the physiology of neurasthenia, contains the first formal response to the Algiers School's medical racism in its condemnation of the "simultaneously fantastic and passionate pathogenic interpretation attributing the origins of psychoses in my country to race and religion."[33] In contrast with Porot and his students, Esch-Chadely argued that the "North African Muslim is neither a defective who belongs to an inferior race nor an asthenic."[34]

Despite his criticism of some of the Algiers School's central tenets, the Manouba hospital hired Esch-Chadely as a bilingual psychiatrist in the early 1930s.[35] In Tunis he continued his nationalist activities. By 1935, according to a classified report from the Tunisian Public Health director, he began "particularly violent campaigns in the nationalist press on both the operation of the Manouba hospital and regarding its medical director."[36] Esch-Chadely had communicated to *Tunis-Soir* and *Nahdha* that the hospital "had something to hide from Tunisians":[37] in violation of Tunisia's medical statutes, the hospital's director, Pierre Maréschal, had "created a paying clientele" at the hospital, despite drawing a public salary.[38] This charge appears to have stemmed from a personal vendetta, as such practices were commonplace among colonial physicians. Yet Esch-Chadely argued that Maréschal's profitable yet illegal "manner of interpreting his professional duty [was] for the least part dangerous," because the doctor "devoted his own care exclusively to paying clientele to the detriment of hospitalized patients."[39] Esch-Chadely later revealed that the authorities who confined nationalist intellectuals at Manouba also attempted to use psychiatric diagnoses to the government's advantage. After French soldiers brutally slew innocent civilians at Zeramdine in 1946, the protectorate sought to avoid public opprobrium by declaring the soldiers insane and therefore not responsible for their actions. Two years later, after his suspension from Manouba for declaring the soldiers "completely responsible," Esch-Chadely wrote the United Nations to complain of human rights abuses at the hospital. In addition to the offenses already listed, he claimed that the Nobel laureate Charles Nicolle, at the Pasteur Institute in Tunis, used Manouba's patients as unwilling test subjects in his continuing work on typhus—a report corroborated by a nurse who worked at Manouba in the same period.[40]

"The Rose of Blida": Gender, Madness, and Suffering

Colonial psychiatry's abuses of authority are crystallized in the works of the Algerian author Kateb Yacine, where they serve as a critical foil for his fierce critique of colonialism's disruption of local social worlds. Kateb Yacine was born in Constantine, Algeria, in 1929, the son of a lawyer. He received a Qur'anic education until age seven, when he entered the French colonial education system. As a student in French schools and a child of relative privilege, Kateb was a member of the paradoxical group of the *évolués*, a social position that deeply colored his experience of colonial rule. The French school brought Kateb what "the Qur'anic school could not": a passion for literature and writing.[41] Yet this came at the cost of alienation. In a frequently cited passage from *Le polygone étoilé*, one of his later novels, Kateb compares the trauma of his entry into French schools to being thrown "into the lion's den" (*dans la gueule du loup*): exposure to a harsh world of violent rejection.[42] Indeed, as many of his biographers have noted, his name itself reflects an ironic appropriation of the lycée's assault on the subjectivity of the colonized: born Yacine Kateb, the author adopted the reversed given and surnames characteristic of roll calls in French schools, reflecting the inversion of identity forced upon the *évolué*.[43] Yet beyond the ritualized dehumanization of colonial schooling, it was also as a lycéen that Kateb first experienced two interlocking and catastrophic phenomena that shaped several of the most pervasive themes in his literary works: Algerian nationalism and the failure of his mother's sanity.

At only fifteen, Kateb was directly exposed to the horrific violence of the Algerian liberation struggle. His initiation into the nationalist cause came inadvertently with his participation in the bloody uprising at Sétif on 8 May 1945, when rioting Algerian military veterans killed some one hundred Europeans. Kateb wrote that at the time, "I had no consciousness of what was happening in our country. . . . Then, I remember, there was a demonstration in the streets; and simply because there were classmates who found themselves caught up in this demonstration, as a student, I wanted to be with them, just like one wants to be with students who are horsing around."[44] The retaliation against Algerians reached well into the thousands.[45] Kateb was fortunate: imprisoned and threatened with execution, he was later freed.

Historians have long recognized Sétif as the opening salvo in the brutal struggle for Algerian independence. As it was for a number of future revolutionaries, Sétif was formative for Kateb in terms of its violence. But its significance was doubly profound for Kateb, because it also introduced him to the powerful tension between the dual sufferings of madness and psychiatric confinement, both of which he came to attribute to the inherent violence and impossibility of real subjectivity of the colonial situation. Whereas for many the experience of incarceration was the primary incitement to radicalism—writing of the Algerian revolution, the historian Alastair Horne describes French prisons as the revolutionary's "university"—Kateb dismissed it as "nothing, I was thrown in jail." For his mother, however, "it was more serious. She lost her mind."[46] Yasmina Kateb had long suffered from periodic breakdowns. Yet upon hearing rumors of the execution of her only living son (her first son, Belghith, had died at age two), she reached a crisis stage and spent the next few years in and out of hospitalization at the Dispensaire psychiatrique de Constantine. After her husband's death from tuberculosis in 1950, Yasmina's sister-in-law committed her to the Hôpital Psychiatrique de Blida-Joinville, near Algiers, where she spent at least several years.[47]

The figure of the suffering mother wracked with insanity is a recurring theme in Kateb's work and provides a framework for ordering the experience of colonial violence. "La femme sauvage" (The Wild Woman) of 1959, for example, presents a wandering and unstable yet fascinating figure who surfaces again and again in his oeuvre. "Mourning or ordinary abandonment, the nature of her illness didn't matter, since she had decided to personify in herself its indignity . . . summarized in the grotesque imagery of her mania. . . . Her gaze ran up and down the walls, then became absolutely fixed, and the shape of her mouth indicated nothing more than bitterness: a sardonic suffering deprived of its object."[48] The connection to Yasmina is more explicit in his 1963 poem, "La rose de Blida."[49] In dedicating the poem to the "memory of the one who gave me life / The black rose of the hospital," Kateb invokes both the asylum and the rose that is closely tied to the maternal figure in a number of his texts. That Blida was known colloquially as the "city of roses" adds a further level of irony to this framing. Yet the mother's beauty is offset by instability: she is a "rose that fell from its rosebush / And took flight."

The identical theme appears in his first novel and masterwork, *Nedjma*. Set in 1945 and composed between the riots at Sétif and the brutal massacres at Philippeville in 1956, *Nedjma* draws on Kateb's experiences to present the enigmatic story of four young men—Mustapha, Lakhdar, Rachid, and Mourad—who are both united and torn by their love for Nedjma. The novel orbits around omnipresent themes of violence and retribution. The character Nedjma, who appears in a number of Kateb's works, herself originated in an act of horrific violence: she was conceived during the rape of a French Jewish woman by four Algerians, including Rachid's father and another character, Si Mokhtar, an attack that also led to the former's death by an unexplained murder. Nedjma stands in for a new Algeria, forged in a crucible of brutality and seized from the colonizer.

Like Kateb's mother in "La rose," the mother of the character Mustapha (named Ouarda, or "rose") is tormented by the violence that surrounds her, manifesting her anguish in insanity. Arriving home to care for his tubercular father, the Mustapha laments, "Our courtyard is empty. No one to meet me. Mother has let the rosebush die." She is a "prone shape," a "tangle of white hair" inside the house. As he escorts his father to the hospital, Mustapha relates a song that his youngest sister is singing: "My brother's in prison, / My mother's going crazy / And my father's on his deathbed."[50] As the rose's madness and eventual death in the poem are prefigured by its uprootedness—the mad "rose that fell from its rosebush / And takes flight"—pervasive and maleficent birds in *Nedjma* reinforce the theme of flight into madness, while providing a vehicle for imagining the mother's delusions.[51] As Mustapha complains, "Mother can't talk anymore without tearing at her face, lifting her dry eyes toward the sky. She talks to the birds and curses her children" (*N*, 226). Kateb's language tracks the breakdown of her mind as he represents her in fragmented descriptions (a tangle of hair, a prone shape), impossible imaginings (a dead rose that takes flight), and oxymoron (the "black rose" that merges death and emptiness with life and beauty).

The character appears again in Kateb's play *Le cadavre encerclé*, the first installment of Kateb's 1959 cycle *Le cercle de représailles*. The play appeared first in print in *Esprit* in 1954 and was staged several times: first in Tunis in 1958, then later that year in Brussels, and eventually (but clandestinely) in Paris. *Le cadavre* includes several of the prominent characters from *Nedjma*, including Nedjma and Lakhdar, and is set explicitly during the Sétif massacres and reprisals. Like all of Kateb's works on Algeria, in lieu of a straightforward narrative the play revolves around central themes: colonial authority and resistance, imprisonment and death, love and the condition of women in Algerian society. Fatally stabbed by his stepfather, an Algerian collaborator with the French, the Lakhdar had already been driven mad through imprisonment and torture. His madness, a product of violent trauma, is mirrored in that of an escaped mental patient whom he encounters—Mustapha's mother. Stage directions specify that she appears wearing "the blue gown of psychiatric hospitals" and that the mother's "barely graying hair stands up on her head"; "Her gaze of searing intensity fixes on nothing, and neither her broken silhouette nor her gestures of distress are remotely feminine." The character speaks in verse: "And the daughters shave their heads / In memory of their demented mother / And as the birds leap, they mock / They mock me."[52]

The etiology of the mother's madness crosses textual boundaries of genre, appearing in the poem, the novel, and the play in identical forms. Her unreason stems from what Arnaud calls an "accumulation of suffering" through the imagination of her son's death—or her prescient mourning of his certain death in the nationalist cause. In "La rose," she is "the *femme sauvage* sacrificing her only son / watching him take up the knife." This presaging of death appears in other works, as in *Le cadavre* when the mother keens over the "dissipating image of her son," or in *Nedjma*, when

Mustapha complains, "For a long time she's been singing the prayer of the dead for me. Despair followed melancholy, then torpor" (*CE*, 62; *N*, 226). Yet there is also a cyclical aspect to this nexus of violence and suffering. In *Nedjma*, Mustapha, drunk with wine and rage, contemplates the murder of his father's friend, a fritter vendor. Describing his father's sickness and especially his mother's madness as a gross "injustice," he is driven to redemptive violence himself. His homicidal furor is a means of wreaking vengeance on a landscape of suffering, and the vendor is a bystander to Mustapha's misery:

> I think of my sisters, between the madwoman and their tubercular father. He might be dying at this very moment. In the back of the shop there's a razor; with a little effort, the vendor's head could be rolling at my feet. . . . Can a murder by itself assassinate injustice? Mother, I'm dehumanized, I'm turning myself into a leper-house, a slaughterhouse! What can I do with your blood, madwoman, and on whom can I avenge you? It's the idea of blood that drives me to the wine.

Through his analysis of mother-son alliances in Francophone Maghrebian writing, the Tunisian literary critic Hédi Abdel-Jaouad provides a useful starting point for interpreting Kateb's link between mourning and unmooring, between the loss of the son and the descent into madness.[53] For the Algerian Muslim woman, who faces potential repudiation by her husband at every turn, identification with the son is a strategy for physical and emotional survival. As a "custodian" of Maghrebian patriarchy, the mother's delivery of a son confers legitimacy and ensures her continued social survival. Yet in Kateb a series of reflexive turns complicates this relationship. First, there is an important narcissistic component to the mother's overwhelming suffering in Kateb's work. The mourning mother's recognition of her loss stems from a loss of recognition. As a subject dependent upon the son for her continued legitimacy as a subject, the maternal self is constituted through recognition by the son. Both Yasmina's world and her ego have become empty and meaningless. Thus, in the guise of the mother in *Le cadavre* who repeatedly calls her son's name, she clings to his image "through the medium of a hallucinatory wishful psychosis" that preserves his (and therefore her own) existence.[54] Although the relationship with the son is always ambivalent, it contains at least an implicit defense against repudiation, because her only source of subjective legitimacy rests in her perpetuation of a patriarchal lineage. The only son's death—even if merely fantasized—deals an equally mortal blow to the ego.

To push Abdel-Jaouad's analysis further, there is a second turn that complicates Kateb's relationship with the mother figure in these texts. The mother's madness resonates beyond psychoanalytic dimensions, operating as a powerful signal of the disruption of Algerian society by colonial violence. Abdel-Jaouad argues convincingly that the place of the mother in Maghrebian texts is often invoked as a defense against the onslaught of colonial modernity, a grounding of the Francophone son in the mythic past through identification with the mother as a source of "immutable" and unspoiled "authenticity."[55] Indeed, in colonial psychiatric discourse, female insanity evoked this image of immutability. As the psychiatrist Suzanne Ta-ïeb argued in her 1939 thesis, Algerian women were far less touched by the forces of "civilization" than Algerian men and thus constituted a reservoir of unmediated primitivism and superstition.[56] Yet for Kateb, this identification of the mother figure with unspoiled tradition highlights a further trauma. The son's effort to find permanence in his mother's image is foiled by her insanity, which is an insistent reminder of colonial violence. That her mourning and insanity cannot end results from the endless cycle of rebellion and reprisal that mark the modern history of Algeria. Whereas Freud sees mourning as characterized by "grave departures from the normal attitude to life," the pathologies of colonial society preclude a return to normalcy.[57]

Structural violence offers a useful frame for exploring how the colonial predicament informs the layers of suffering in Kateb's works. As Arthur and Joan Kleinman have argued, the imagery of suffering often serves as a repository for condensing social, economic, and political experience. A narrative of survival of unspeakable violence becomes rewritten as a trauma story, highlighting the horrors of victimization.[58] By this reading, Yasmina's madness serves Kateb as a source of symbolic capital: the story of her breakdown draws on a medicalized language to communicate the experience of the structural violence of colonial Algeria. In Farmer's calculus, sickness and suffering are closely linked to the operational forces of social inequality, what Farmer describes as "biological reflections of social fault lines" in which multiple forms of oppression constrain possibilities of action and shape the violent expression of communal discord.[59]

Yasmina's madness, by this reading, is a response to identifiable human actions rather than a neurological malfunction. Although it is Kateb's imagined death that appears as the primary cause of her breakdown, the son's execution—indeed, even his participation in the Sétif riots, along with the riots themselves—is a product of colonial oppression. Yasmina's madness was constituted in the field of colonial power and resistance, one that shaped all possible responses to the French colonial presence and its brutalities. As Kateb notes in his conclusion to "La rose," it is a mother's ability to witness the violence of anticolonial revolution and reprisal through the privileged lens of intuition that allows her special insight into revolution's circumstances, but that also determines her madness: "Fountain of blood, of milk, of tears, she knew from instinct how they were born, how they fell to the ground, and how they fell again, from a brutal conscience, without a parachute, burst like bombs, burned one against another, then cooled in the ashes of the birth pyre, without flame or heat, expatriated" (4).

Yasmina's breakdown is simultaneously a reflection of subjective fragmentation and an instantiation of resistance. The inherent violence of both the colonial state and patriarchal domination have inscribed Yasmina in the domain of what the philosopher Giorgio Agamben has called "bare life," a bestialized existence removed from the order of human and divine law.[60] She remains unmoored in a space of emotional discord. Menaced with potential repudiation on the grounds of her childlessness and her insanity, she faces exile to what the anthropologist João Biehl has called a "zone of social abandonment."[61] This position shapes Yasmina's field of action, limiting her possibilities of resistance to expression through emotional collapse. She is subject to multiple orders of marginalization by virtue of her social position: as Kateb perceives the situation, she is tangled in a web of power relations in which her agency is tightly constrained. "Multiaxial" forms of oppression inform her risk for breakdown. As an Algerian, the fact of difference precludes her political engagement on equal terms with the colonizer. As a woman in a rigidly patriarchal society, her self-definition through motherhood predisposes her to subjective annihilation when that which shapes her social position is taken from her—a brutal repetition of the loss of her first son in infancy, but a loss now attributable to the actions of the colonizer.

Therapeutic Violence, Resistance, and the Impossibility of Healing

Despite Yasmina/Ouarda's suffering, to seek comfort in psychiatric treatment is to perpetuate the cycle of traumatic violence. In *A Dying Colonialism* and in *The Wretched of the Earth*, Fanon presents medicine and psychiatry as ideological instruments of colonial power. Psychiatrists, by this account, see their Muslim patients as a data set for testing the limits of invasive therapies. They appear in the interrogation room, both to administer shock treatments as a tool for interrogation and to assess the validity of a torture victim's testimony, while their physician colleagues assess the body's ability to withstand pain and punishment. The doctor exploits the native's credulity—itself an invention of colonial psychiatric discourse—by selling useless medicines and performing "X-rays" with a vacuum canister. Medicine constitutes a site of colonial surveillance, and the clinic, a means of amassing useful data in the assistance of domination.[62] Even the objective truth of an accurate diagnosis is rejected by the colonized, Fanon notes, as it is always "vitiated by the lie of the colonial situation."[63]

As in Fanon, psychiatry and medicine are forces of violent social control in Kateb. *Le cadavre encerclé* provides the clearest example, as it is the presence of psychiatry itself that situates the text in the realm of madness. The cue that exposes the insanity of Mustapha's mother is her patient's gown; it is psychiatry's trappings as much as her pathological appearance that diagnose her condition for the audience. Far from comforting, the hospital is a malicious force. The patient describes herself as "the escaped madwoman," reinforcing the perception of the institution as a carceral rather than a therapeutic site. In the background a loudspeaker confirms the hospital's menacing presence: "Electroshock! Electroshock! Electroshock!" Like Oedipus, the madwoman is a social pariah who bears responsibility for her transgressions through her blindness. She is "a widow in reprieve," but at the same time a "mother in quarantine," and a chorus chants in the background, "Night falls, and our entire Universe leans out the window of nothingness! Do not throw stones at the madwoman, she has arisen to close the window, and that is why her eyes are ruined." With allusions to scripture and Greek tragedy as well as to the Algerian revolution, her escape is a form of deliverance from domination. As the patient "leaps out of the scene," the chorus seizes on her escape from Blida as a microcosm of the entrapment of Algerians in the discourses of colonial psychiatry, as well as their imprisonment in the colonial system. Linking Ouarda's escape metaphorically to the national liberation struggle, the chorus narrates her exit from the scene by calling out, "Nothing resists the exodus."[64]

In a context that perverted therapy into punition, the constant vigilance of the colonial subject constituted a form of resistance. The inscription of social experience in a medicalized language operated as a means of demystifying the power of colonial medicine and science. By decrying abuses, analyzing the mechanisms of psychological oppression, and rescuing an Islamic past buried by a colonial present, North African intellectuals such as Esch-Chadely, Memmi, and Ammar pointed to strategies for reversing the power of colonial domination and signaled pathways for liberation. For Kateb, this process went a step further, connecting the psychology of colonialism to a justification of anticolonial violence. These figures contributed to an atmosphere that linked critical analysis to a call to action, shaping a habitus of anticolonial liberation in the Maghreb that targeted medicine as a central tool of colonial domination.

Fanon's personal campaign against colonial medical racism followed a trajectory from reformism to public discontent and the production of a literature of resistance. Upon his arrival at Blida, he published a coauthored paper in the prominent journal *Information psychiatrique* that condemned the institution's egregious and overcrowded conditions.[65] Fanon reacted by introducing reforms in his ward despite tight budget confines. Here he drew on his clinical experiences as an intern at the Saint-Alban hospital in southern France. During his internship, the reformist François Tosquelles introduced him to a progressive "institutional psychiatry" that emphasized the patient's social reintegration through group work. Fanon further developed such practices at Blida, where he discovered the powerful influence of culture on therapeutic outcomes. Experiments with dressmaking, town meetings, and a hospital newspaper proved successful with European women patients, yet failed with Algerian men: only Fanon's establishment of a "Moorish café" that mimicked a Muslim homosocial environment achieved similar breakthroughs with these patients. The experiments revealed to Fanon the difficulties of conducting cross-cultural psychiatric work—especially in an environment where the manifest racism of the authorities rendered entire groups of patients highly suspicious of doctors' therapeutic intentions.[66]

These efforts were cut short with the Algerian war's outbreak. Disgusted with the manifest racism of his colleagues, he aired his grievances in a letter of resignation to the governor-general of Algeria, in which he both renounced his citizenship and argued that the practice of psychiatry in Algeria made a mockery of medicine. The response was an order for his expulsion from the country.[67] After going into exile in Tunisia, Fanon reemerged as a Pinelian figure when he removed a cage from the Manouba hospital's courtyard and introduced group and game therapy to the treatment regimen. In one former nurse's words, "with Dr. Fanon, many things changed! . . . *He* was a good doctor."[68] Fanon also experimented with an outpatient service at the Charles Nicolle hospital in Tunis, which yielded encouraging results.[69]

In Tunisia Fanon also further developed his intellectual engagement with colonial ideology. He continued his activities on behalf of the FLN, which he had begun as early as 1955,[70] and he contributed frequently to *El moudjahid*, the FLN's main propaganda vehicle. Yet he also engaged in a struggle to clarify the exact relationship between psychiatric theory and colonial domination. In *The Wretched of the Earth*, Fanon argues that his dwelling on the prejudices of colonial science is "less with the intention of showing their poverty and absurdity" than an effort "to make explicit, to de-mystify, and to harry" the dehumanizing logic of colonialism, and thereby facilitate the development of a revolutionary consciousness.[71]

These actions are characteristic of colonial intellectuals' responses to racialized medicine. Like Fanon, Salem Esch-Chadely, for example, leveled accusations against his superiors to colonial, French, and ultimately global authorities. Such remonstrations were dangerous in the context of an emerging mass nationalist movement in Tunisia, leading authorities to bury the accusations and to issue an array of spurious charges against Esch-Chadely as a means of discrediting him.[72] Memmi and Amrouche, by contrast, undertook the sort of demystification that Fanon advocated in *Wretched*. Their works reveal that any protest against the colonial system must also expose the framework that undergirded colonial discrimination: as Memmi argued in *The Colonizer and the Colonized*, the assumption of racial difference as a matter of scientific fact (*CC*, 71). In response to the characterization offered by the "Rabat psychiatrist"—who argued that "North African neuroses were due to the North African spirit"—Memmi argued that "memory [was] not purely a mental phenomenon," but instead was "the fruit of history and physiology" (*CC*, 103). But eviscerated by colonial derision and scorned by the *évolués* who mimicked their social betters, the history of the colonized lay in ruins. The destruction of a cultural framework and the insult to biology emanating from colonial science—and not biology itself—dehumanized the colonial subject. "Everything" in the colonial world—and especially science—"is mobilized so that the colonized cannot cross the doorstep, so that he understands that this path is dead and that assimilation is impossible" (*CC*, 125). Amrouche, for his part, argued that discussing colonial psychological oppression openly constituted the intellectual's only means of resistance. It was "the intellectual's duty, whether some doctors like it or not . . . not just to endure the test." Instead, "understanding"—Fanon would say "demystifying"—represented "the intellectual's own means of ensuring justice."[73]

For Ahmed Chérif and Sleïm Ammar, the process of understanding prefaced the regeneration of the lost culture of the colonized to demonstrate the legitimacy of budding nationhood. In his medical thesis, titled "The History of Arab Medicine in Tunisia" and completed at Bordeaux in 1908, Chérif's principal concern is stirring Muslims' consciousness of their own greatness and proving the inaccuracy of any notion of the Muslim's psychological "inactivity." The thesis supports the legitimacy of Tunisian nationalism by grounding Islam's rich medical and scientific heritage in medieval Tunisia. It documents the role played by Muslims in safeguarding Galenic medicine from European barbarism and concentrates specifically on the founding of a center for medical education at Kairouan in the late ninth century that persisted for nearly six hundred years.[74] Chérif's thesis performs an important rhetorical function in the context of the French seizure of medical power in Tunisia; in Fanon's words, to "remind [Arabs] of the great pages of their history is a reply to the lies told by the occupying power." As Nancy Gallagher has shown, European medicine superseded Tunisian healing when cholera epidemics struck Tunisia over the mid-to-late nineteenth century.[75] By 1908 Tunisians such as Chérif who wished to enter the medical profession were forced to do so on French terms. The experience was formative for Chérif: "impassioned by politics," according to a police report, he faded from the European psychiatric scene after 1909, but in Tunisia and later in exile in Beirut, he dedicated the rest of his life to medicine and Tunisian nationalism.[76]

Sleïm Ammar sought to rescue Islamic science not only to redeem North African culture, but also for its legacy in the postcolonial world. According to his 1954 history of mental health care, all progress could be linked to Islamic innovation in the medieval period. Emphasizing the Qur'anic injunction to humanitarianism—"Islam's message of tolerance, liberty, and progress"—Ammar also points to Arab "ingenuity" as the source of therapeutic efficacy even in the modern world. In defense of Arab medicine, Ammar cites a number of prominent innovations from medieval physicians: Er-Razi, who invented mercury treatments (a common therapy for tertiary syphilis until the 1970s) and who counseled games and abstinence from wine for melancholic patients; Ibn Sina, who recommended swinging and beating patients in depressive states ("shock treatments taken up and extended since then in the most diverse forms to wind up in our time as modern convulsive-therapy treatments"); and the scholarly work of medical pioneers such as Ibn Omran, Ibn Al Jazzar, and Ibn Rushd.[77] For Ammar, the antecedents of modern medicine were to be found in Arabic medicine: shock treatments, chemical therapies, and medical scholarship all found their origins in the Islamic past. Despite the decline of Islamic medicine since the sixteenth century, it still offered a model for a modern, humanitarian, and ultimately decolonized psychiatry to follow.

Yet it is still Kateb who reveals the closest likeness to Fanon. Indeed, Kateb's analysis of colonial madness and psychiatry—written from the perspective of the patient and the nationalist—mirrors the psychiatrist Fanon's interrogation of the same phenomena. For Kateb, the psychiatric hospital is less a technology for healing than one of powerful repression. It is a factory for the production of knowledge about the mentality of the *indigène*, manufacturing and processing clinical presentations such as the savage impulsivity of the Arab criminal and the primitive superstitions of the sequestered Muslim woman. Yet it is also a site of literal imprisonment and surveillance, a tool for the policing of deviance.

The themes of psychiatric punition and colonial pathology are pervasive in *Nedjma*. In the middle of the novel, Rachid, one of the four protagonists, arrives in Constantine and begins wandering through the city. As he stops at a smoking den, he is torn about whether or not to enter, when he spots an acquaintance: "The man holding the sachets was sitting there, an Olympian of twenty with a bulging forehead [*le front accidenté*]. Rachid had thought he was in the psychiatric hospital. 'You got away from them again, brother Abdallah!'" (*N*, 151). Through a range of cues Kateb offers a searing indictment of psychiatry as a force of imperial incomprehension. It is Abdallah's physiognomy and his occupation that brand him as an ideal Algerian clinical type. His "bulging forehead" signals his deviance, rendering him the target of an outdated psychiatric paradigm with roots in Lombroso's criminal anthropology. Far from a raving lunatic, Abdallah is merely a social reprobate, the proprietor of an illegal hash bar populated by a coterie of degenerates. After Rachid, a lycée dropout, later joins Abdallah as an employee, he "no longer left the savage collective, the Divan, the intimate reverie of the horde: ten or twenty men of all ages—silent dreamers who scarcely knew each other—dispersed along the balcony, deep in their intoxication, on the edge of the cliff. . . . He would probably die on this balcony, in a cloud of the forbidden herb." Rachid "had long known about the *fondouk* of which he had just become the master": "He knew, like every child, that the music-lovers at the *fondouk* smoked something other than tobacco—something that made them madmen, but not like drunkards." The group is Rachid's new cohort in Constantine: these "known criminals, the unemployed, the homeless, the *sans-papiers*, the *demi-fous* like this Abdallah, always just out of the asylum." For Kateb, psychiatry's function was the regulation of social deviance through the surveillance of this drug-addled "horde," this "savage collective" of "troglodytes" (*N*, 159–60).

This version of colonial psychiatry as a disciplinary force is important in *Nedjma* because the novel is also the site of a range of powerful expressions of mad violence. Here Kateb appropriates and reverses the Algiers School's stereotypes of the Algerian's impulsively violent character. Violence is omnipresent in the novel. Nedjma herself—this figure of the new Algeria—is produced in the womb of a Frenchwoman through an act of multiple rape: she is born of violence and seized from the colonizer. Other instances of violence are linked to this rape—Si Mokhtar's murder of Rachid's father, for example—or, more often, to the *pieds-noirs'* instigation. Yet such actions are specifically gendered in *Nedjma*: clear patterns dictate why Yasmina/Ouarda's experience of colonial domination drives her to insanity, while the life-worlds of the Algerian men in *Nedjma* lead to murderous outcomes. Just as the structural violence of the colonial situation shapes Yasmina's insanity, the forces of poverty, brutal labor, and the colonizer's aggression inform the possibilities of action for male Algerians. As Fanon insisted, it is these forces that "canalize" the Algerians' rage toward the colonial aggressor, a global force that deranges local social worlds.

The first of these scenes of masculine violence involves Lakhdar, one of the four young men infatuated with Nedjma; Monsieur Ernest, a French construction foreman; and Suzy, Ernest's daughter.[78] Other day laborers warn Lakhdar on his first day about Ernest's temper. "Ameziane unties the string he's using in place of a belt and shows a festering scrape on his lower back: 'There's M. Ernest's character.'" Ernest demands to know what the workers are talking about. Without waiting for an answer, he strikes Lakhdar in the head with a stick. Lakhdar watches his own blood flowing as Ernest's daughter Suzy tells her father, "He hasn't had enough, that one. . . . *He hasn't gotten what he deserves.*" Ernest moves closer to Lakhdar to continue the beating, "his daughter's heckling having raised him to the peak of heroism." But Lakhdar strikes first, knocking Ernest unconscious with a single blow (*N*, 41–46).

Ernest's violence is a pose, a ritual of the colonizer's masculinity. Driven on by his daughter, Ernest plays a role of domination. He is at center stage in a drama of colonial violence; he must act decisively or lose face in front of both his daughter and his workers. It is less Lakhdar's insubordination than the colonial situation itself that shapes this interaction: it is a scenario in which the agency of the central actors is decided in advance. Ernest's actions and Suzy's "heckling" are mandatory reiterations of domination, an ordering of the colonial world played out in microcosm. Lakhdar's preventive strike, although understood as an act of impulsive criminal violence, is a refusal of submission and a rejection of the violences of everyday colonial life: the poverty, marginalization, and coercive labor forced upon a disenfranchised population.

A second and more disturbing scene between Suzy and Mourad captures the dynamics of a bloodthirsty and "dying" colonialism lashing out in its death throes. When Mourad sees her on the street and tries to talk to her, we see how the constraints of a discourse of colonial violence inform Mourad's identity and motivate his subsequent actions. "Leave me alone," Suzy tells him.

> "And that's that," thinks Mourad, "the honeymoon's over, I'm just her father's workman again, she's going to walk back across that empty lot

... as if I'm committing a crime just by walking in the same place as she, as if we should never find ourselves in the same world, other than as a result of violence or rape. And that's that. Already she's *tutoie*-ing me, and she tells me to leave her, as if I had grabbed her shockingly and violently. . . ." Then he thought of nothing else but striking her, seeing her on the ground, maybe picking her up and throwing her down again.

Mourad's desires stem from Suzy's perceptions of him as violent and impulsive. His imaginary violation is realized on the night of Suzy's wedding to Monsieur Ricard, a contractor. Ricard is the archetypal *pied-noir*: a rough-and-tumble, hard-drinking settler with no patience for polite society. The wedding night, a travesty from the outset, degenerates into a melee as Ricard and the guests become violently drunk. As the crowd tries to force Ricard and Suzy into bed to consummate the marriage, Ricard's Algerian maid intervenes. The "orgy" of violence quickly turns on her. The guests seize the maid and force a bottle of rum down her throat. As the maid retches, Ricard begins to beat her senselessly: "The blows rained down. M. Ricard beat her with an expression of indignant stupidity . . . he knew now, in his fading drunkenness, that he couldn't stop beating her or finish off his staggering prey without turning against the partiers who squeezed around him in a circle." Like Ernest, Ricard explodes in incomprehensible violence as a means of saving face among the *pieds-noirs* who surrounded him. Yet at this point, Mourad, who has witnessed the orgy from outside, creeps into the room. "A blow from his knee doubled the contractor's body over, just when Suzy was pulling him back, and now Mourad pummeled him fiercely and unrelentingly, could not restrain his blows" (*N*, 24–25). Before the crowd is able to pull Mourad off the contractor's body, Mourad beats him to death.

Suzy rejects Mourad as a criminal, "as if we should never find ourselves in the same world, other than as a result of violence or rape." In response he becomes one: he saves the maid's life when he erupts into uncontrollable rage, killing Ricard. But Kateb reveals that Mourad's violence, like Lakhdar's, is a response to a more brutal violence, the maddening aggression of the colonizer. Kateb, like Fanon, never refutes the stereotype of the Algerian's violent impulses. Instead, he places Algerian violence in context. The revolution opens what Fanon called the "closed circle" of Algerian violence: "There are no more disputes and no longer any insignificant details which entail the death of a man. There are no longer explosive outbursts of rage because my wife's forehead or her left shoulder were seen by my neighbor."[79] In *Nedjma*, Algerian rage seeks its outlet in response to the physical and psychological violence inflicted by the settler. Ernest's beating of Lakhdar, Suzy's recognition of Mourad as nothing but a host of sexual impulses, Ricard's suspicion and brutality: each of these acts of violence merits an Algerian response. In these moments Kateb co-opts the Algiers School's portrait of the "Arab" to reveal the origins of violence in Algerians' articulation of their subjectivity. Like the "exodus" in *Le cadavre*, like the "rose's" flight from the rosebush, this appropriation is also a form of deliverance that reveals the suffering at the heart of psychiatric discourses of Algerian violence and insanity.

"This Country Is a Vast Hospital"

Colonial medicine is fascinating because of its multiple resonances. It is an efficient means of establishing control precisely because of its seductive power. The physician's exclusive knowledge grants a specific authority, one that can belittle the patient because of its monopoly status. It can amass data about the population because it can demand any form of information in exchange for its services. It can establish truth about patients because it exploits their vulnerability. It is a unique form of totalitarian power because it is one to which we willingly submit. We grant medicine's authority in domains we cannot understand; this is the bargain we accept when we seek a cure.

Yet colonial medicine, Fanon and Kateb argue, does not often meet its end of the compromise. This is the framework for Kateb's 1963 meditation on colonial medicine, "Ce pays est un grand hôpital." The sketch—only six pages long—is a fragmentary continuation of the farcical drama *La poudre d'intelligence*, the centerpiece in the cycle *Le cercle des représailles*. Jacqueline Arnaud has characterized the piece as situated "between the pamphlet and the theater," which accounts for its hyperbolic tone. Set in Morocco, the sketch explores the reciprocal relationship between clinical and colonial domination. The sultan, suffering from a fever, summons a doctor: enter Dr. Paul Chatinières, a colonial physician who assisted Lyautey's "pacification" efforts during the Moroccan conquest. The doctor's soliloquy as he enters the scene consumes most of the play. The passage is taken verbatim from Chatinières's memoirs and betrays his awareness of both the seductive force and the political uses of colonial medicine.[80] He announces that colonialism introduced doctors to "an entirely new role whose existence and utility we had not suspected." Although armed force initiated conquest, doctors used their "moral influence to consolidate French authority," becoming "agents of pacific penetration" as "France endeavored to attenuate this brutal manifestation . . . with a bit of humanity." The doctor proved useful because better than the priest, [the doctor] can lay bare the human soul with its hidden faults, its unavowed miseries. His practiced eye, which scrutinizes and which weighs heavily, quickly pierces the pride and the mistrust that opposes it: because the man who has stripped off his shirt is less hesitant to reveal his soul, and the notation of lesions and symptoms that cannot be denied forces the patient's sincerity.[81]

The sketch, a minor piece in Kateb's oeuvre, appears to have little direction outside of indicting colonial medicine as an abuse of power and pointing out the fragmentation of colonial society. When read alongside a range of Kateb's other works (as well as Fanon's), however, it becomes clear that for Kateb, colonial medicine is a political force that strips the Maghreb of its traditions as it divides the region's populations. As such it is complicit in colonial violence, serving as a means of "pacific penetration" and an agent of colonial suffering. Yet its seductive power renders it difficult to resist and to conquer. More than a form of social control, it is a factor that shapes the structural violence of the colonial situation. By insinuating itself into the deeply personal space of health and illness, through its prescriptive and proscribing powers of language and discourse, medicine is a crucial instrument in the establishment of colonial hegemony; the physician, in turn, is the architect of a colonial social and political order and a catalyst for the breakdown of local social worlds.

The historian of medicine David Arnold has argued that all medicine is at least implicitly colonial in its assertion of monopolistic control over the body and its annexation and destruction of alternative forms of healing.[82] While this may be an exaggeration, it remains clear that the extremities of colonial rule magnify the operations of power at work in the clinical space. Moreover, the invasiveness of colonial medicine was often tempered only by its negligence: as the patients' testimonies highlighted in chapter 3 attest, the inadequacy of much of colonial psychiatric practice, as well as the extreme neglect that many hospitalized patients experienced, failed to justify the coercive elements of confinement.[83] It is clear as well that this mechanism of domination was profoundly disconcerting for Kateb, Ammar, Memmi, Esch-Chadely, and others whose texts reveal the complicated intersection of medical knowledge, epistemological violence, and social suffering that were primary sites for the production of colonial marginalization. The deeply personal glimpses of madness and violence provided within Kateb's texts in particular are powerfully revelatory: as narratives of lived experience, they condense the pathological insanity of the colonial social order into the madness of the mother and the rage of young men.

The works of these authors articulate possible experiences under colonialism. They are fragments that complicate the "official" history of colonial medicine—one that often still sees biomedicine through a lens focused on its triumphs yet blind to its violences.[84] It is a tribute to Fanon's insight that his work remains emblematic of a multivalent challenge found in these writings: a contestation of the psychological effects of colonialism, a trenchant analysis of psychiatric racism's evisceration of culture and subjectivity, and exposure of an abusive medical system in desperate need of reform. These ideas were central to Fanon's critique, but they also circulated readily in the twentieth-century Maghreb.

Biographies understandably emphasize Fanon's humanitarianism and the revolutionary thought he brought to medicine as well as his politics. Yet hagiography and disregard for his antecedents do Fanon a disservice. Portraying Fanon as a lone reformer struggling against insuperable odds, a figure whose subjection to European racism hastened his death at thirty-six from leukemia, renders Fanon a mythological rather than a human figure: a Pinel for anticolonial psychiatry rather than merely a remarkable historical agent. Putting Fanon's ideas in context reveals the source of their power, their resonance within revolutionary circles. The Manichaean world of French North Africa may not be historically "accurate," but works by Fanon's contemporaries and other medical critics of colonial psychiatry reveal how this world was experienced as a historical reality.

6 Underdevelopment, Migration, and Dislocation
Postcolonial Histories of Colonial Psychiatry

Psychiatry has remained an important venue for imagining the French–North African relationship in the postcolonial era. In the idioms of medicine and public health, governance and law, and literature and film, psychiatry has operated as a frame for articulating the tensions surrounding decolonization and development. Its languages have figured in many of the critical questions of the postcolonial era, including debates over the place of the welfare state in resource-poor countries, immigration and citizenship, and the nature of the ongoing relationship between France and its former colonies, and they have resonated in three principal registers. In the Maghreb, a new iteration of the discourse of development that began in the age of colonial *mise en valeur* has emerged in psychiatrists' engagement with the difficulties of practice in a developing-world setting. In France, discussions about deracination and migration have forced a resurfacing of a vocabulary of pathological maladaptation and the tensions between Islam, republicanism, and global modernity. On both sides of the Mediterranean, a lexicon of psychological normality and pathology has tinged engagements with the traumatic dimensions of decolonization and negotiations of the postcolonial moment.

What is novel in the postcolonial era is that both French and North African voices have contributed to these debates. An audible exchange has replaced the Algiers School's efforts to speak for the Muslim, as two recent films by North African directors make clear. Abdellatif Kechiche's dramatic film *La faute à Voltaire* (2000) tells the story of a Tunisian immigrant in Paris.[1] Jallel Brahimi is the oldest son of a large

191

family whose father has recently died. As the only viable breadwinner, he strives to support his family by working in the French capital. The strategy works, at least at first. Through false pretenses, Jallel attains refugee status and a three-month visa as well as a bed in a shelter, and he soon falls in with both a local community of established Arab immigrants and his marginal but good-hearted cohabitants at the shelter. He also falls in love with Nassera, a temperamental Franco-Tunisian single mother and café waitress. Yet the difficulties of life on the margins of legality soon become clear. With no work authorization, his strategies for economic survival are meager, and he must constantly dodge the police. Jallel proposes to Nassera, a French citizen, as a means of attaining legal status, and she agrees to marry him for the fee of 30,000 francs. On the wedding day, however, Nassera abandons Jallel. He collapses into an unshakable depression, bedridden and able neither to eat nor to communicate. His friends at the shelter provide him with false papers and admit him to the Hôpital Esquirol, a psychiatric facility in the Paris *banlieue*, where he remains under treatment for several weeks.

The film toys with many of the central precepts that marked ideas about race, mentality, and immigration through the twentieth century. Jallel's story recalls the cautionary tales of psychiatrists who saw in immigration a force of great potential instability and a profound mental hygiene risk. A secular Muslim, Jallel drinks to excess in an early scene and spends hundreds of francs in a drunken blackout. Economically marginalized and desperate to stay in France, he resorts to petty crime to support himself, collapses under the stresses of life in urban postmodernity, and finds himself confined in a mental hospital. A cursory reading of the film casts Jallel in the light of the Algiers School, whose practitioners often warned of the moral degradation, incipient criminality, and precarious mental state of the immigrant. Yet Kechiche effectively writes back to these discourses by inserting Jallel in a complex web of forces and fleshing out his character beyond the two-dimensional stereotypes of colonial psychiatrists. Jallel's drinking is incidental—he is caught in a moment of frivolity and forgets himself only once in the film. His petty crime is a victimless means of economic survival—he sells produce in the Métro and roses to couples in restaurants and cafés. His confinement makes clear that he is the only sane character in the hospital, and he comes to serve as a moral guide for other inmates. He becomes entangled in a difficult relationship with Lucie, a pregnant prostitute whom he meets at the hospital, but he winds up being a protective figure for her rather than merely a sex partner, saving her from her own impulsive tendencies. At the end of the film, Jallel is arrested and deported, but Kechiche has made clear that he is an innocent victim of economic circumstance and is among the few honest and stable characters populating the urban landscape of working-class Paris.

Malek Bensmaïl's 2004 documentary *Aliénations* tackles a different topic. Dedicated to Bensmaïl's father, a psychiatrist who died in 2002, the film follows a series of diverse patients through their experiences in a psychiatric hospital in Constantine. In many ways, this could be any psychiatric hospital. Most patients suffer from various psychotic disorders, including bipolar disorder, schizophrenia, and major depressive psychosis, for which they take haloperidol, Phenergan, and a range of other drugs. Scenes depict the rituals of medication and resistance, meetings in which physicians negotiate drug regimens with patients, and patients who promise to take their medication if only they are released to their families. Patients talk of their desire to leave the hospital and start their lives again. The film also shows patients who are afraid to leave the hospital—who only feel safe in the presence of their psychiatrists—as well as visits by tormented families that reveal the tenderness and sadness surrounding mental illness in the modern world.

Yet the patients' conversations reveal that this is still clearly a psychiatric ward in a developing Muslim country. There is constant discussion of unemployment and underemployment. The politics of terrorism and the state are a preoccupation of many of the patients. One is an Islamist who claims that he had been persecuted because of his religion. Another, who constantly sings the refrain from the American song "We Are the World," believes that he can bring peace to Algeria simply by meeting with radical Islamists, Americans, and Algerian politicians and convincing them of the virtues of nonviolence. There is extensive talk about religion: quoting from the Qur'an, discussion of *j'nun*, and constant reference to God's will ("Insh'Allah"). There are both official and unofficial efforts to incorporate local healing traditions into a medical regimen: patients frequently attempt to cure each other, and in one scene a Muslim cleric meets with a patient, holding his hand on the patient's forehead and reading therapeutic verses from the Qur'an. In contrast with the hospital in Kechiche's film, segregation by sex is strictly enforced, and preservation of gender roles is a principal concern of the patients. Women discuss domestic life and the politics of the welfare state, while men discuss global politics and terrorism. In a moment of apparent anxiety about the emasculating effects of madness and confinement, one patient tells the barber shaving him to "leave me a bit of moustache—I'm still a man!"

Bensmaïl's film accomplishes at least two goals. On a local and overt level, it examines the difficulties of providing effective psychiatric care in a developing world setting. It reveals that despite the dedication of the hospital's staff, the economic obstacles facing Algerian psychiatry are overwhelming. Yet the film also explores more pervasive problems facing Algeria and the Maghreb in the postcolonial era. By exploiting the trope of the wisdom of the fool, the film draws on patients' utterances and the content of their delusions to reveal truths of decolonization and development in North Africa. Frequent references to terrorism, state violence, and a yearning for peace among the patients draws the viewer's realization to the central paradox of psychopathology in Algeria: that madness is both the origin and the outcome of a political situation shaken by the traumatic violence of a decade of civil war, itself a renegotiation of the savage brutality of the war for independence.

Taken together, the films point to this chapter's central theme: the utility of psychiatry as a site of condensation for the dilemmas of decolonization. Jallel's migration and Bensmaïl's attention to the meager resources of public psychiatry in Algeria highlight the devastating economic realities of the postcolonial moment in North Africa that followed the flight of French capital. Both films also elaborate the themes of resistance that predominated in the work of wartime intellectuals such as Fanon and Kateb Yacine. By revealing the complexity of their characters and the multiple factors that shape mental breakdown, the films indicate the importance of listening to the patient as a means of scaling the barriers to cross-cultural treatment. They speak to the problems of dislocation and deracination that have been central to the postcolonial experience for both France and the Maghreb. Above all, they highlight the critical traumas of political violence that have marked the Mediterranean world in the aftermath of colonization, including powerful tensions between France and its former colonies and the legacy of colonial and civil wars in Algeria, and the ways in which psychiatry offers not only a therapeutic tool but also an object of inquiry for understanding them.

Development and Its Discontents: Decolonizing Psychiatry in the Maghreb

The decolonization struggles of the 1950s witnessed the Algiers School's struggle for its very existence. The Algerian war temporarily heightened interest in the school's work, but France's loss forced the dissolution of the group. Although he continued publishing widely, Antoine Porot retired from teaching and moved back to France in 1946. In the next fifteen years he was followed by many of his students. Jean Sutter, who had taken Porot's place at the Algiers Faculté, took up practice in Marseille, and Porot's son, Maurice, relocated to a faculty position at Clermont-Ferrand, while other colonial psychiatrists landed in Paris, Strasbourg, and other French cities.

The most prominent trace that colonial psychiatrists left behind in the 1950s and 1960s was the Maghreb's psychiatric infrastructure. France's transfer of the hospitals and clinics of its North African colonies to local administrators took place under the threat of anticolonial violence—as per the famous dictum, for example, that in the summer of 1962 the French were forced to leave Algeria either carrying suitcases or packed in coffins— but also at a curious juncture in the history of modern psychiatry. The period that witnessed widespread decolonization also experienced an early wave of enthusiasm for the deinstitutionalization of psychiatry. The introduction of chlorpromazine (Thorazine in the United States, Largactil in Europe) in France in 1952 and in the United States in 1954 had provided an effective alternative to confinement for schizophrenia, long recognized as the most unmanageable and chronic of psychiatric disorders. As a result, confinement increasingly appeared an outdated concept by the late 1950s, a sensibility that gave rise to the deinstitutionalization movement and the development of community psychiatry as an alternative to asilary confinement. Combined with the emergence of a countercultural underground that witnessed in mental illness the creative possibilities stifled by bourgeois conformity and capitalist mandates, a newly invigorated antipsychiatry movement agitated for an end to the asylum. Prominent publications such as Erving Goffman's essays on total institutions and Foucault's analysis of modern psychiatry as a dark side of the Enlightenment project fueled the fire.[2]

Strategies for decolonizing psychiatry in the Maghreb took many forms. The promotion of Muslim staff psychiatrists to administrative positions was an initial step, as was the renaming of many institutions: the Hôpital Psychiatrique de Blida became the Hôpital Frantz Fanon, for example, and the Hôpital pour les Maladies Mentales de la Manouba became the Hôpital Razi, named for the great medieval medical theorist. Other reforms were more substantive and difficult. In all specializations, the training of physicians in the new postcolonies was an essential step toward medical independence. In Algeria, such training had begun during the decolonization struggle. As Fanon famously noted in *A Dying Colonialism*, the French military had weaponized medicine in the course of the Algerian War, prohibiting access to medical supplies and greatly limiting access to care for Algerians. Faced with a desperate need for medical staff to serve its growing army, the FLN trained its own. Beginning in 1959 the FLN launched a covert program for the basic training of medics and nursing staff, known as the Écoles Militaires d'Infirmiers, and sent promising future physicians to already-independent Morocco, Tunisia, and Egypt for crash courses in medicine, surgery, and public health management. The goals of these

programs were modest: they sought merely to stem the tide of losses in the
FLN's army to disease and wounds. Yet they formed the basis for medical
education in the postcolonial era in three ways. They greatly expanded
Algeria's medical ranks by opening education to those to whom such training was largely prohibited under the colonial state. They also welcomed
significant numbers of women into these ranks. Finally, by emphasizing
primary care, they provided Algeria with a medical corps trained for the
immediate needs of an underdeveloped state. These reforms, initiated in a
circumstance of dire military necessity, were reflected in the demographics
and priorities of the Algiers Medical Faculty in the post-independence era,
which dramatically increased its enrollment of both Algerian Muslims and
women.[3]

Such reforms, as well as similar programs in Tunisia and Morocco, enabled the former colonies to meet many of their immediate medical needs.
Yet resources were far more limited for psychiatric care, despite the fact
that the Maghreb faced problems similar to those that confronted psychiatrists in Europe and the United States. By the 1950s overcrowding had
devastated North African institutions' ability to provide effective patient
care. It forced French authorities to turn away all but the "most dangerous" patients even before decolonization initiated a shortage of staff and
economic resources for the hospitals.[4] With independence the problem
worsened. A year before formal independence in Tunisia, for example,
Manouba's new director, Sleïm Ammar, complained that the hospital
housed 770 patients in its 555 beds. In 1956 the situation was worse still,
with more than 1,000 patients vying for space and medical attention. The
hospital's former French director lamented that "*encumbrance* is indeed the
plague of psychiatric hospitals and Manouba is far from an exception on
this front": patients in threadbare gowns now lived and ate in bathrooms
or outdoor cages.[5]

Despite the fading appeal of large institutions as therapeutic tools in the
industrialized world, however, they represented the only real resource for
managing mental illness for the Maghreb's emerging nations. Amid political turmoil and precarious economic circumstances, experiments with
community psychiatric clinics represented a low priority for postcolonial
administrators. In the clinics' place psychiatrists in Algeria, Tunisia, and
Morocco advocated an extensive medicalization of psychiatric care, an apparent step in the opposite direction of the therapeutic vogue that pervaded
the global north in the period. Authorities undertook this project by embracing the optimism that accompanied newly won independence, struggling to unshackle psychiatric institutions from the stigma that surrounded
them, and recognizing the limitations that constrained their efforts.

Psychiatrists across the Maghreb issued similar complaints and advocated similar programs. In Tunisia, the first of France's former colonies to attempt postcolonial medical reform, optimism quickly gave way to serious concern about a newly independent African nation's capacity to cope with the inevitable difficulties of the transition to self-sufficiency. Noting in 1956 that mental illness had reached severe proportions in Europe and the United States, Sleïm Ammar inveighed that "the problems of mental health" were no "less significant in non-industrialized countries." In underdeveloped regions, factors such as malnutrition, unemployment, epidemic illnesses, and "insecurity about the future" compounded the etiological factors found in the industrialized world: Ammar predicted that Tunisia "would soon count one dangerous 'lunatic' for every 1000 citizens."[6] Ammar also blamed colonialism for contributing to this mounting crisis.[7] Despite the fact that Tunisia was "relatively privileged in comparison with a number of Afro-Asiatic nations, our country remains nevertheless strained by the burdensome heritage of the past and by the weight of classic medico-social scourges that characterized the colonial period." To cope with this problem, Ammar proposed a major investment in psychiatry. His plan was reminiscent of the projects of the 1920s and 1930s: it entailed a move away from "traditional asilary structures" toward the implementation of psychiatric wards in general hospitals, the extension of outpatient services, legal reform, and a central coordination of state mental health resources.[8]

Thus, at the same time many Western therapists encouraged the decentralization and downscaling of psychiatric medicine, Ammar proposed a greater medicalization in the name of modernization. Ammar's program characterizes psychiatrists' responses to underdevelopment across North Africa in the postcolonial era. Such projects demonstrated eerie parallels with the modernization theory that swept postwar intellectual circles in the 1950s and 1960s. Based in the successes of the Marshall Plan and on the research of economic historians such as W. W. Rostow, modernization theory proposed that the development of industrial sectors held the power to bring the poor agrarian countries of the global south into economic modernity. The idea undergirded extensive development projects sponsored by both the United States and the Soviets well into the 1970s. Yet two major flaws undermined these projects. They typically focused on major programs such as dam construction, airports, and urban planning, while dedicating little attention to less glamorous yet critical infrastructure such as education and primary health care. They were thus often difficult to maintain and relied on extensive and often illusory foreign expertise to ensure a modicum of sustainability. More often, as in the case of psychiatry and many other public health and medical sectors, projects based in modernization theory resulted in shoddy copies of already outdated Western institutions and programs. A fetishization of the "stages of economic growth" effectively mandated the postcolonial world's passage through an industrial modernity that Europe and the United States had already experienced, even as future growth pointed toward the development of a new economy based on electronics and information technologies. In a similar way the "stages of psychiatric growth" appeared to mandate bringing an obsolete system to fruition rather than moving toward deinstitutionalization at the same pace as the north.

As late as the 1970s, such projects had still not materialized. In Rabat in 1975, the psychiatry professor Taieb Chkili echoed Ammar's criticism of colonial psychiatry's failures. The Berrechid hospital, he argued, was a "monster" based on a "retrograde conception of psychiatry." Of the hospital's 2,200 beds, "2,000 [were] immobilized by chronic patients." Many of these patients had been confined in Berrechid since the colonial era. Chkili even suggested "destroying" the hospital and beginning from scratch. Chkili labeled existing psychiatric legislation "seriously insufficient" for Morocco's needs, and he proposed the implementation of "centers for the detection of mental illness," "mental hygiene, juvenile, and geriatric dispensaries," and "centers for intermediary social readaptation between the hospital and social reintegration."[9]

The Algerian psychiatrist Mahfoud Boucebci raised similar concerns about psychiatric practice in dismal facilities. Yet in contrast with Ammar, who argued that the pressures of life in a modernizing society led to rising caseloads, Boucebci pinned this problem on Algerians' increasing confidence in native practitioners of Western biomedicine. In a 1975 article Boucebci claimed that the postcolonial era had witnessed a "hyperinvestment in the doctor and his message . . . with a tendency to ask the psychiatrist to be the healer of all 'ills.'"[10] Fanon had outlined a similar phenomenon in his essay on medicine and colonialism of 1959. The weaponization of medicine inspired an increased confidence in its efficacy among Algerians, whereby formerly "noncompliant" patients carefully adhered to the strictest of regimens. This was a classic example of the "dying" influence of colonialism for Fanon, according to which the sites of greatest resistance became uncontroversial when appropriated by Algerians as central components of a revolutionary arsenal.[11]

In contrast with those in Tunisia and Morocco, Algerian mental health networks had developed substantially in the immediate postcolonial era. The Blida hospital, now a university medical center, still represented the cornerstone of Algerian mental assistance, but new hospitals and clinics had opened in Oran and Algiers. Yet despite Algerians' rising confidence in psychiatric medicine, Boucebci argued, Algeria's existing structures were wholly "inadequate" to meet the country's needs. The problem of training effective practitioners with minimal resources—a universal one in underdeveloped countries—was paramount.[12] Yet Boucebci also considered education in Europe to be a problematic solution for Algerian psychiatry students. The European obsession with psychological testing should be "rejected," he insisted, because these tests were inappropriate and inadequate for Algerian populations, a point Fanon had made twenty years earlier.[13]

The call for the medicalization of psychiatric institutions in postcolonial North Africa was therefore not necessarily a call for the reinstatement of the colonial order of things. Nor was it an appeal to the medical knowledge of the industrial world. Instead, psychiatrists such as Ammar, Chkili, and Boucebci came to propose a negotiation between traditional and modern forms of patient care in the postcolonial Maghreb. Throughout the Maghreb critics of the psychiatric status quo raised the possibility of integrating traditional healing into modern therapy. As one Moroccan journalist described them, psychiatric hospitals were "vicious circles": they were insufficient structures for social reintegration that left recovered patients as "alienated" as they had been before hospitalization.[14] To these critics, a revival of traditional healing practices suggested a plausible means of treating patients within their own cultural parameters.

This concern reflected a general predicament of the Maghreb's postcolonial societies. As colonies that had experienced the full force of France's "civilizing mission," they had existed on the threshold of modernity for much of the twentieth century. If anything, the postcolonial period exacerbated the stresses that plagued a colonial lycéen such as the Moroccan student Mohamed S., who felt as if he were constantly pulled "in two directions." Much of the revolutionary call to action had entailed a rediscovery of the Muslim past. Although the independence movements of Algeria and Tunisia were far from Islamist, they nevertheless drew attention to Muslim culture as a valid alternative to a Gallic modernity. The readoption of Arabic as an official language and an increased investment in Muslim civil law gave a further impetus to these tendencies. Yet a burgeoning Islamism emerged in powerful tension with the secularism of the nationalist movements. This was especially the case in Tunisia, when the new president, Habib Bourguiba, closed the Zitouna mosque's theological university, promoted women's rights, and was filmed drinking to the health of his people in the middle of the day during Ramadan, acts that amounted to the direct provocation of Tunisia's Muslim clerics.[15]

Differences among revolutionaries were at least apparently set aside during many of the independence struggles. In Algeria, despite constant infighting that brought the FLN to the brink of internal collapse, the group maintained the illusion of a united front and burst into open internecine war only in the wake of liberation. As Benjamin Stora has noted, the FLN's victory "paradoxically" revealed its impotence and the limits of the widespread support it had claimed.[16] Independence thus brought an intense struggle for power that exploded in the course of the 1960s with the birth of a new Islamist movement that established a firm presence on the political scene within a decade. The paranoia of the nascent regime, its efforts to rewrite Algerian history as a tool of political legitimation, and a widespread intolerance of dissent created a chilling atmosphere in postcolonial Algeria in which the violence of peace succeeded the violence of anticolonial war.

The works of the Algerian author Rachid Boudjedra point to the intersection between this struggle for the heart of Algeria and efforts to remake psychiatry. Like Bensmaïl's film *Aliénations*, Boudjedra's novel *L'insolation* (Sunstroke) uses the device of the madman as a subversive character who points to the insanity of the world around him.[17] The book's narrator, Mehdi, is a philosophy professor at an Algerian lycée who writes from his bed in an Algerian psychiatric hospital, the fictitious Hôpital L'Ermitage in a city that appears to be Algiers. There are two explanations for Mehdi's confinement. Mehdi believes that he has been hospitalized as a result of sunstroke, which assailed him after he deflowered a student, Samia, on a nearby beach. His nurse and physician, however, refuse to believe the story and insist that a suicide attempt brought him to the hospital. Regardless of the origins of his hospitalization, Mehdi's tale reflects a deeply disordered society in the throes of postcolonial anguish.

The narrative draws heavily on intertextual references that reflect both the author's and the central character's positions as torn between Western modernity and an Algerian national tradition.[18] Boudjedra, born in a village near Constantine in 1941, came of age during the Algerian war. In the 1960s he married a Frenchwoman and took a position as a philosophy teacher at a lycée in Blida. He later relocated to Paris, where he wrote his first two novels, *La répudiation* and *L'insolation*. The first novel is an Algerian man's confession of his family history to his French lover, a history deeply scarred by his father's repudiation of his mother and the family's subsequent disintegration, which ends in the protagonist's confinement in an asylum. *L'insolation* continues many of these themes—some characters are almost identical to those in the first—and elaborates the Oedipal tensions outlined in *Répudiation*. Yet *Insolation* is also clearer in its references than the early novel, which include Camus and Kateb Yacine as well as

Freud. Mehdi is an Algerian Meurseault, bound to his fate by a crime committed on a beach under the Algerian sun. Unlike Meurseault's murder of an Arab, however, Mehdi's crime is his willing complicity in Samia's effort to dishonor her family by losing her virginity outside of marriage.

It is his participation in this act that points both to the pathologies of Algerian society and to Kateb's influence. Seeing the blood flow from between Samia's legs takes Mehdi to the imagined scene of the rape of his mother by Siomar, his "uncle," a wealthy landowner. Like Nedjma, he is conceived in an act of violence; like Kateb's mother, Yasmina, it is Mehdi's mother, Selma, who bears the physical and emotional pain of this violence of which she cannot speak. Siomar silences her and convinces Djohâ, a poor ex-revolutionary, to marry her as a means of diverting attention from the scandal of the rape. Djohâ raises Mehdi as his own child, yet Mehdi discovers the truth of his conception on his own wedding night. Devastated by hatred and betrayal, Mehdi courses in his narrative between the scene on the beach and the rape of his mother while punctuating the story's hallucinatory strains with lucid intervals in the hospital. Yet here the pathological scenario becomes further complicated. The seduction of Samia took place in the presence of an old black man—himself a reference to the black murderer of Si Mohktar in *Nedjma*—who looked upon the couple with scorn.[19] Finding Samia in a state of postcoital celebration, he sacrifices a small goat as a means of saving her: dripping the goat's blood over her, he says, "Go wash yourself. You have lost nothing. Blood has replaced blood."[20] Yet despite this rectification, Mehdi remains haunted by what he has done, which he links to the rape of his mother, despite Samia's willing engagement in the act. Moreover, Samia disappears after the seduction: it remains unclear whether she drowns in the sea while bathing or Mehdi murders her out of contempt for his own actions. The threat of recrimination by a group of Islamists investigating Samia's fate, the Membres Secrets du Clan, also assails Mehdi during his confinement. This threat is the chief source of his delirium of persecution, which leads him eventually to suicide.

With his references to the blinding Algerian sun and death on the beach, to rape and seduction, and to the violence of the father, Boudjedra self-consciously links the novel to Camus and Kateb. In so doing he betrays ambivalence toward both past and future. He is riven between France and Algeria, the West and Islam. Scornful of the French colonial legacy—he derides Siomar as a profiteer of the colonial period and laments the "seven-year war"—Mehdi finds no security in the Algerian present, with its brutal infighting. Camus and Kateb are thus even more appropriate, for each of these authors was tormented by the Algerian predicament: Camus, torn between republican humanism and his colonial heritage; Kateb, eager for liberation but distraught by the violence of Algeria's rebirth. For Boudje- dra, as for Kateb, the figure of the insane patient is the only sensible filter for the madness of a society caught between an oppressive tradition and a seductive but alien modernity.

Psychiatry offers a metaphor for state power and a space for expressing the paranoia that shaped the collective mentality of a postcolonial soci- ety. Boudjedra's novel contains no references to medical treatment in the hospital—only a sense of the hospital as a space of a deep and ineradicable pathology and a tool for giving voice to postcolonial discontents. The text thus reflects not only the tensions of early nationhood but also the predica- ment of psychiatry in a developing context. Psychiatrists themselves were caught between a colonial past that tainted their institutions and an uncer- tain future. Mental health services in the postcolonies were on the verge of collapse, dilapidated "monsters" of the colonial era besieged by a new generation of patients who broke down in a moment when anxiety, fear, and violence had replaced the promise of independence.

This was the context for a "medicalization" of psychiatry that sought the introduction of effective patient care into institutions that had decayed from their "luxurious" peaks in the 1930s. Medicalization could mean the use of effective medications, bringing a modern biochemical approach to psychiatry, or it could mean the introduction of what one physician called "alternative methods," including the trance and group therapies practiced by organizations such as the Hamadsha.[21] In Algeria, Boucebci suggested that psychiatrists must give careful consideration to these therapies even as they attempted to institute biomedical techniques in their fledgling institu- tions.[22] Likewise, in the 1970s Sleïm Ammar began experimenting with healing ceremonies such as the *hadra*. Although he never practiced them himself, he attended such ceremonies while wearing a white lab coat—a conscious effort both to make institutional psychiatry less threatening to Tunisian Muslims, and to demonstrate biomedical psychiatry's increas- ing tolerance of pluralist approaches to mental illness in postcolonial Tunisia.[23]

The reconsideration of these local knowledges of illness represented a significant departure from the past. With few exceptions, colonial psychi- atric reforms had targeted such practices for eradication. In many cases, North Africans themselves attempted to banish the activities of the healing brotherhoods. For liberal nationalists such as Bourguiba, who cast them- selves in a Western model, popular Islam was an embarrassment that re- flected a society in decline rather than an emerging national culture. For radical Islamists such as Sheik Abdelhamid Ben Badis, the architect of an

Islamist nationalist movement in Algeria during the interwar period, the brotherhoods represented an intolerable corruption of Islam. Even Sleïm Ammar and many of his colleagues saw these practices as barbaric and antimedical: Ammar, for example, demonstrated a marked contempt for local healing practices in the immediate aftermath of independence. In 1955, for example, he considered them a risk factor for mental illness in their own right, arguing that "even if the persistence of maraboutism, with its various practices of sorcery, magic, and collective trances, does not create psychopathology, it at least contributes to its spread." Only in the 1960s and 1970s did he acknowledge the potential efficacy of certain traditional therapies.[24]

The postcolonial resurgence of interest in local knowledge about sickness and healing is important both for an expanded view of what constitutes "medicalization" and for its marked departure from a similar interest during the colonial period. The Algerian anthropologist Nadia Mohia believes that the adoption of Western biomedical techniques in developing countries can be a profound detriment to patients. Writing of the installation of a modern psychiatric hospital near Tizi-Ouzou in Kabylie, she argues that psychiatry is a critical site for exploring the development state because it reveals the "perturbations that are rocking it and . . . the multiple contradictions it is forced to confront." Such institutions occupy a "paradoxical status": modern psychiatry's presence is a sign of "development," but its practices crystallize mental illness. Whereas traditional therapies tended to reinsert the patient into the community by using the social group to validate the patient's experience of illness and to negotiate a social position, biomedical psychiatry's function was more often to remove the patient from the community. In postcolonial Kabylie, nearly 80 percent of patients who came to the psychiatric hospital did so through the referral of traditional seer-healers; yet their families brought them there not for a "cure," but strictly for medication to reduce violent agitation. Admission to the hospital, however, entailed a change of social status. One went from being a member of the community to being a "mental patient." The hospital, "far from curing or simply struggling against mental illness," is instead "an institution that produces it and officially consecrates it," with the effect that the illness becomes "a defect that must be hidden from others." The community comes to see these attitudes as signs of modernity and readily adopts them. Mohia cites the case of a woman at the hospital whose sons refuse her demands to seek healing through pilgrimage and consultation of a *marabout*: as fully Westernized Algerians, "they prefer their mother to be a 'mental patient' rather than a possessed woman so as not to tarnish their social prestige."[25]

Mohia's and others' focus on local belief systems differs profoundly from colonial psychiatrists' interests in the same phenomena.[26] For psychiatrists such as Suzanne Taïeb, such ideas were themselves both cause and symptom of mental disorder, as well as mental artifacts that offered insight into the modal personality of the North African Muslim. More recent efforts have focused instead on the opportunities local belief systems present for ameliorating the realities of care in a developing world setting. Because many of these practices draw heavily on the social and familial milieux as therapeutic tools, they constitute a localized form of community psychiatry and present opportunities for social reintegration that are often impossible to implement in formal hospital settings.

Among the more successful of these programs was Essedik Jeddi's "door" project at the Razi hospital in Tunis in 1981. By this period, the hospital was in a condition of utter decay. In 1981 alone, three patients died of neglect, one by drowning in a bathtub; another's body was only found six months after the patient's death. Suicides were frequent.[27] In an effort toward reform, Jeddi and a team of medical students took aim at the hospital's "Pinel" ward—ironically, a lockdown facility for schizophrenic patients. Jeddi and his students encouraged their patients to remove the door that led to the ward's ECT chamber, which for them had been a menacing symbol of their confinement and powerlessness. After removing the door, patients "painted their feelings" on it, expressing their outrage at the threshold of their isolation: as one patient claimed, they "transformed it and made it lovely . . . and beautiful to look at." More than a symbolic gesture, this action and the subsequent introduction of art, occupational, and dance therapy attempted an integration of the patient's body and mind as an effort toward resocialization. Combined with the development of a regular market at which patients sold agricultural goods to the local community, the experiment represented a cutting-edge therapy for schizophrenia that has since received critical acclaim from European psychiatrists.[28] The subject of a documentary, *Al Baab* (The Door), the project inspired further art- and music-therapy projects that aimed at reconnecting patients with social practices and promoting patients' happiness as a fundamental human quality.

The therapeutic strategy behind this and similar efforts relies on simplicity, a factor as responsible for their success as any culturally specific dimension such attempts contain. A return to local ideas about health and healing entails the incorporation of sustainable forms of care with strong community support by virtue of their familiarity. Yet they also rely on the interpretation of culture as a central component of healing. Interpretation in these cases is a form of mediation: the search for a middle ground in which doctor and patient meet on equal footing, at least epistemologically. Practitioners such as Jeddi have developed therapeutic means that constitute their patients as enfranchised subjects, rather than objects of inquiry. In encouraging patients to paint their feelings about confinement on a broken door, Jeddi is listening to his patients' expression of their symbolic world of illness in their own terms. It is no accident that many of the Maghreb's most reformist practitioners in the postcolonial period have been trained in psychoanalysis as well as psychiatry: Jeddi is a Lacanian by orientation, while Mohia's larger project is the development of a "psychoanalytic anthropology."

For all its problems, psychoanalysis places the patient's subjectivity at the center of the clinical encounter. It grants the patient a crucial role in the cure because it mandates listening to the patient. Doctor and patient are engaged in the act of interpreting the patient's illness as a means of negotiating the patient back to health. As the psychiatrist and anthropologist Arthur Kleinman has argued, such practices facilitate effective healing because they grant validity to the patient's illness complex—the totality of the patient's experience of a disvalued social state—as well as to the symptoms of disease or disorder. By incorporating ethnographic and psychoanalytic methods into a therapeutic program, these projects have thus attempted to varying degrees of success to restitute patients to themselves, rather than to an abstract ideal of social normality.

Recentering Science: Ethnopsychiatry in the Global City

Immigration and a concomitant social, cultural, and political globalization have figured among the most critical legacies of decolonization in France. Although Paris has been a cosmopolitan city at least since the early modern era, France is now more than at any point in its history a global society. As Paul Silverstein has recently argued, decolonization has produced a "transpolitical space" from the former colonizing and colonized nations of France and Algeria.[29] This transformation, which began during the colonial era and first gradually, then rapidly increased in its extent, has dramatically reshaped French politics and culture since the late twentieth century. Immigration and its effects have called into question the concepts of nation, citizenship, and Frenchness itself, fostering a crisis of identity for both immigrant populations and the host society. Many of the central debates that mark French politics, economics, and culture stem from or involve issues of immigration, multiculturalism, and religion, forcing a reconsideration of France's place in Europe and the world. Problems of unemployment, debates over European unification and a European constitution, battles over laicism, fears of a rise in urban insecurity, and transatlantic diplomatic relations each find a touchstone in the major demographic and cultural shifts that France has experienced and attempted to negotiate in the aftermath of decolonization.

These debates have also become new flashpoints for psychiatry and its political interventions. As in the colonial era, psychiatry in particular, and the behavioral sciences more broadly, have seized the opportunity to exercise their authority through extensive commentary on the critical social problems of the present. In controversies over Muslim girls wearing headscarves in French public schools, the radical polarization of French politics, and the sentiment of rising insecurity linked to immigration in periurban France, psychiatrists and psychoanalysts have offered elaborate interpretations designed to sway public debate. In so doing ethnopsychiatrists have prodigiously developed the legacy of their colonial forebears, yet they have also taken their profession in a new direction. Where colonial psychiatrists intervened regularly in public debates about colonial policy, ethnopsychiatrists in a globalizing France have remade themselves in the model of engaged Parisian intellectuals. The contemporary era has thus involved a recentering of ethnopsychiatric science: a return of a discipline from a colonial periphery to a Parisian center, as well as a recasting of the debate over the administrative ideologies of assimilation and association for a postcolonial context.

Among the most immediate effects of the Algerian war's disastrous ending was what came to be called the "exodus." The horrific turns of events that marked the period from 1959 to 1962 forced an already painful split between France and Algeria into a traumatic severing of space, family, and culture. The rise of the settler terrorist-mercenary OAS, the Organisation de l'Armée Sécrète, and the generals' putsch of the early 1960s, in which four commanders split from the French army to lead new regiments fighting for the maintenance of a French Algeria, led Algeria into a new state of civil war, with Europeans fighting Europeans. The Evian Accords of spring 1962 brought an ostensible end to the war, yet the violence continued well into the summer, for the OAS failed to disband completely and the FLN continued deadly reprisals on both Europeans who remained in Algeria and the *harkis*, the Algerians who had fought on the side of the French. Both of these populations constituted the bulk of the waves of "repatriation" that besieged France in the summer of 1962, as hundreds of thousands crossed the Mediterranean into France—most of them for the first time.

The exodus from Algeria destroyed the coherence of the Algiers School and much of its work. The school's practitioners were among the hundreds of thousands of Europeans who found difficult their transition to life in the metropole. Most quietly continued their work as psychiatrists in new settings and experienced the downside of assimilation into a vast metropolitan profession: the loss of status as representatives of a school of thought. Although they continued to publish extensively, the end of empire had undercut their life's work as interpreters of the colonial predicament, and their work now focused much more on the problems of general psychiatry and the training of students. Their research on the tensions between "primitive mentality" and Western modernity, whose validity now dated to a bygone era, had its greatest impact among psychiatrists investigating marginal populations within the hexagon: for example, psychiatrists who studied the persistence of witchcraft beliefs among peasant populations were among those who cited colonial psychiatrists' works most extensively.[30]

Yet in many ways, the work of the repatriated psychiatrists bore significant potential relevance to France's changing demographics. The mass northward migration of many former colonized subjects accompanied the exodus of the *pieds-noirs*. North African immigrants had populated the French urban landscape for decades. Many contract workers and soldiers who came to France during the First World War stayed on in the interwar period, while others joined them seeking better employment than could be found in exploitative colonial settings. During the Algerian war immigration intensified as many uncommitted North Africans sought to avoid the violence that surrounded them in Algeria. But the upsurge in North African immigration in the postcolonial era was unprecedented. *Harkis* seeking refuge from the bitter reprisals of the FLN in the aftermath of the war were among the first populations to move northward. They were soon followed by economic refugees fleeing a postcolonial wasteland of underdevelopment that the French had left behind in Algeria, Tunisia, and Morocco. By the 1970s, a relaxation of immigration policy encouraged still further waves of male North Africans to relocate in France seeking a living wage and the means to support their families at home in the Maghreb.

French responses to immigration have varied in the course of the twentieth century as the makeup of the immigrant population has changed. In the interwar period, for example, groups such as the Action Française feared for French traditions in the face of an onslaught of Polish and other Eastern European migrants, while a growing North African population in the metropole also drew the attention of politicians, police, and other authorities.[31] Yet the sheer scale of postcolonial immigration facilitated a resuscitation of the language and principal themes of the work of the Algiers School in a wider political culture. As a substitute for the colonial

other, relegated to the past as a painful memory, the neocolonial population of immigrant workers and their families in periurban Paris, Marseille,
and Lyon have become a new foil for the ordering of French identity, a
phenomenon that has contributed to a resurgence of many of the worst
excesses of colonial language and the scientific arsenal mobilized in its
defense.[32]

The figure of "the Arab" holds a special place in the imagination of immigration. As the historian Yvan Gastaut has argued, among the "indifference and even contempt" with which the French have received other immigrant populations, "nothing equals the extent of passionate hostility" that
they have directed at North Africans. Public opinion polls conducted in the
1980s demonstrated that the term "Arab" conjured in the public imagination the figure of the working-class North African immigrant rather than
any of a range of other stereotypes, including the archetypal Palestinian,
the oil sheik, or the mullah. This figure of the Arab also contained a profound ambivalence. On the one hand was the idea of the harmless but lazy,
ignorant, possibly thieving Arab worker, what Gastaut calls the image of
the "good Arab"; on the other was the figure of the born criminal and terrorist. Where the "good Arab" displayed a near inadaptability to modern
life and French culture, the "dangerous Arab" actively threatened public
safety. A "wanted" poster displayed throughout France in the early 1980s
encapsulated this sentiment. Depicting a sneering, hook-nosed, musta-
chioed caricature of an Arab wearing a fez, the poster declared

> WANTED: MOHAMED BEN ZOBI, born in Algeria, residing in France. THIS
> MAN IS DANGEROUS! Susceptible of: MURDER! RAPE! THEFT! BURGLARY! To
> find him do not go far: all around you there are 700,000 JUST LIKE HIM![33]

Although there was no direct reference to the work of colonial psychiatrists in this and other popular images of North Africans in France, artifacts
like this poster, crime novels, and media representations of the sexualized
and dangerous Arab drew on a lexicon established and scientifically backed
by the work of the Algiers School. The distance from Don Côme Arrii's indictment of the North African Muslim as a rapist and murderer who could
not escape the innate criminal impulsivity of his being to the popular image
of the thieving fanatical Arab of the *banlieue* was minuscule.

Yet by the 1970s, psychiatrists themselves had departed dramatically
from these theses. Much of this falling-away related to the simultaneous
migration and implantation in France of French-educated Maghrebian
practitioners who contested the popular image of the deracinated Muslim
as shadowy figure of urban danger in French society. By pointing to the

difficulties of the male immigrant's material circumstances, the pressures of his social position as family breadwinner, the isolation of immigrant life (even in an immigrant community), and the omnipresence of a dehumanizing racism, psychiatrists speaking for the immigrant produced a language divorced from mainstream public opinion that attempted to restitute the humanity of the migrant subject. In contrast to its uses under colonialism, in the postcolonial era, psychiatry, as practiced and theorized by assimilated Muslim doctors, served as a tool not of marginalization, but of reincorporation.[34]

The predicament of the immigrant worker has been one of psychosocial fragmentation. In the formulation of the Tunisian psychiatrist Essedik Jeddi, the immigrant was torn between two sets of expectations and cultural framings. For his family in North Africa, the worker in France represented economic hope and future salvation. Once in France he met with the powerful and fragmenting ambivalence of the host society. The worker, reduced from human subject to corporal entity, found simultaneous acceptance and rejection: he was accepted as a laboring body but rejected as a dangerous Arab body. As a cog in the machinery of postwar capitalism, the laboring migrant's body was essential to economic growth; but as a potential rapist and murderer, his body generated fear among the French population. These constant tensions shaped what Jeddi called a generally "psychogenic social milieu" of the migrant worker. Any sickness, accident, or traumatic injury exacerbated the steady psychological pressures on the migrant and set environmental predisposition on a disastrous course toward breakdown. The assault on the body that resulted from any of these events reduced the laborer to the status of invalid body and illegitimate subject: his body lost its legitimacy as a laboring unit, while the trauma also alienated the migrant worker from his high status in the family.[35]

This ambivalence of the body—a site of vulnerability and a site of danger, a marker of difference and an empty tool of capitalism—has also marked the work of the Moroccan author Tahar Ben Jelloun. Born in Fez in 1944, Ben Jelloun studied philosophy in Tangiers and Rabat and taught in Morocco before emigrating to France on a fellowship in 1971. His novels and essays have assessed the situation of North African immigrants and racism in France with a brutal honesty.[36] Yet much of his assessment of the situation of migrant workers comes less from personal experience than from his work at the Université de Paris VII, where he earned a degree in social psychiatry in 1975. His thesis explored the psychological tensions of the immigrant worker from the perspectives of sexuality, isolation, and the political economy of desire, and in so doing radically interrogated French attitudes toward immigration and the dangers of the immigrant's body.

For Ben Jelloun immigration represented a continuation of the political economy of colonial exploitation. It was the product of an illicit union between the dominant classes of France and the Maghreb. Under colonialism, "contempt for the other and the ethnocide of intolerable difference" left North Africans "dispossessed of their identity" and their resources: "Their body was the only thing left to them. Naked. It was given to the disposition of production." In colonialism's aftermath the capitalist classes made a new industry of immigration, placing the worker "in a political situation that opposes him both to the possessing class of his own country and to the Western dominant class that purchases the force of his labor." This link of "complicity" sustained French capitalism while simultaneously "depriving the country of origin of a strong and combative working class," and thereby "curtailing the class struggle" in the developing world.[37]

Neocolonial capitalist exploitation, by compelling the Maghreb's vital workforce into emigration, thus stood as the ultimate cause of economic misery and underdevelopment in North Africa, which in turn fed the social and psychological misery of the immigrant forced into the system. Workers who sold their labor through immigration also abandoned their "cultural, familial, affective, and sexual homes." The function of a host society was thus the dehumanization of the subject through the deracination of desire. The immigrant worker became an empty body, one stripped, in the language of capital, to its bare form as a tool of labor. Ripped from its family, the body's placement in a hostile society proscribed normal desire. In the host society "one doesn't want to know if these bodies desire." Instead the imagination "uses them and fills them with evil" by endowing them with "a sexual violence that can only be satisfied through perversity, rape, and crime." Transplantation "separated [men] from their lives so as better to extract the force of their labor," but also to the end of "annihilating their memories and fettering their capacity to become desiring subjects."[38]

Case histories demonstrated the economic and social pressures that drove the psychological breakdown of immigrant workers. E. S., for example, an Algerian immigrant, told a typical story:

> I was married in Algeria in 1962. When you get married, you have to feed your family, so I came to France. I worked as a manual laborer. I saw my wife for two weeks every three years. It was only in 1970 that I stayed three months in my country. After this, my wife got pregnant.

Forced into migration as an economic refugee of underdevelopment, E. S. was also forced into social isolation, where he experienced the pressures

of "forced abstinence and an increasing repression of [his] sexual drives."
By resorting to a prostitute, he caught a "woman disease," which resulted
in his sterility and impotence. As a result E. S. could not return to face his
wife and child. Emasculated, he experienced the lot of the immigrant's
sexual misery: his "existential autonomy fissured, disturbed, his ego vacil-
lating, his personality crumbling," he was a victim of his body's "betrayal"
of his subjectivity.[39]

E. S. represented for Ben Jelloun the classic example of the fragmented
immigrant psyche, destroyed by the psychological pressures of isolation,
racism, and the silencing of desire. Although the 1970s witnessed an increasing attention to the economic plight and social misery of refugee
populations in the *bidonvilles* (shantytowns) and public housing projects of
periurban Paris, Lyon, and Marseille, the "less visible but equally evident
misery" of "solitude in the street, in the bedroom, in sleep" was unspeakable in French society. This silence condemned the immigrant to experience emotionally "a silent trial": met with the contempt of the host society,
condemned as an incipient rapist and murderer, he resorts to the company
of a prostitute who also despises him, and he despises her in turn. She can
"give him nothing but her own misery, her own distress." The immigrant
thus "closes his fly over this absence and leaves the sinister room to go back
to the street, the street of anguish." Sexual disorder, Ben Jelloun acknowledged, was common enough in the Maghreb; but it was "the host environment, rich in pathogenic factors," that typically "unleashed the crisis" in
the immigrant worker. "Even if an individual embarks for France with a
'solid core of ontological security,'" Ben Jelloun argued, "conditions join
forces to attack this solidity and to bring him little by little toward this real
feeling that many consultants have expressed, that of death: the death of
the soul before that of the body."[40]

The *habitus* of the host society ultimately produces the immigrant's sick
body, and in turn, his sick mind. As the sociologist Abdelmalek Sayad has
argued, following Jeddi and Ben Jelloun, the immigrant becomes by virtue
of his displacement an alienated body. He literally is his body, as constituted in his strength as a laborer and through the biological difference that
his body signifies. The fact of emigration begins a process of "individuation" that compounds the body's contradictions and complexities, making
it a repository of meanings and a source of psychological pressures. Conceived as a part of the social and familial group in the country of origin,
the body becomes individuated through social functions of capitalism and
the specific forms of alienation that apply to the immigrant. The compartmentalization of "individualized time" through industrial work-discipline,
the feeling of constant surveillance as a living symbol of difference in a

contemptuous host society, and the new conception of the body as a laboring tool and as a system of biological needs rather than as a social unit force an alienation from the body that is always both a source of survival and a site of potential vulnerability.[41]

The immigrant body is for Sayad an epistemological aberration. It loses and gains meanings in the process of emigration. Its coherence destroyed by the act of displacement, it is individuated through social practice in France. Life in a typical immigrant *foyer*, or shelter, inscribes the body with new meaning. Eating and sleeping are no longer collective acts, but the means of meeting biological necessities. In place of dining as a family, the immigrant eats alone, with his food that is closed in his locker, with his knife, fork, plate, and napkin. He sleeps alone in a cot, rather than in a bed with his wife. Yet the immigrant only discovers this individuation when "he is dispossessed of his body," whose new meanings are inscribed from without. His body is invested with the fear of a society that watches and polices his every move; his body is itself the source of betrayal as it signals his danger to a watchful society through its signs of difference. It is the instrument of labor, and thus the tool of economic viability, but it is also the "site and expression of illness." The onset of any meaningful illness or injury calls the body's productive capacity—for the immigrant, its only source of meaning and belonging in a host society that constitutes the body through economic relations—and thus the immigrant's very "existence" into question. The immigrant is therefore always menaced by his body and its vulnerability. The paranoia that surrounds every illness, however minor, and that invades the immigrant's encounter with state medicine that threatens to deport him as an invalid, thus signals to the French doctor a process of somatization: "When the 'body' speaks and speaks too much, it is surely because the 'head' . . . is 'sick.'" The medicine that "refuses" to "read and diagnose in his body (and only in his body) the signs of his illness" denies his citizenship by denying his "right to sickness," and does so "to the end of making him a 'madman.'"[42]

For these social analysts it was not a "primitive" mentality or a conflict between French modernity and Islamic tradition that constituted a "Muslim new wave" of immigrant madness. It was rather an epistemological, structural, and socioeconomic construction of the immigrant as a contradictory body that stressed him to the breaking point. The immigrant body was caught between opposing forces of self and other: it was socially constructed as an empty vessel for conveying the fears of a society steeped in fantasies of colonial violence and constituted through the immigrant's phenomenological experience as a space of vulnerability and desire. The immigrant's body was a site of contestation made manifest in its visible difference and the attention it called to demographic change in French society, and as a stinging wound that served as a constant reminder of the loss of empire. In place of the Algiers School's psychiatry of the body, which somatized mental and behavioral difference in a pathological brain, a new psychiatry of the body as practiced in the metropole reconceived the immigrant's psychological dislocation as the product of a new corporal fact torn by ambivalence and intolerance, which were themselves products of displacement in late capitalism and its transition to postcoloniality.

The dominant trend launched by North African analysts of the psychopathological structures of immigration was one of incorporation in two senses. By highlighting the importance of differentiation and alienation as social pressures, psychiatrists pointed to the body as a critical space of tension in the formation of immigrant identity. But they also incorporated the Muslim immigrant in another way. By pointing to a new series of facts that shaped identity, they stripped away the particularism that had shrouded psychiatric study of the Muslim since the colonial era and absorbed the North African immigrant into a humanity construed as universal. The factors at play in determining the immigrant's psychopathology were neither biological nor cultural; they belonged neither to the brain nor to religion. Instead, the social fact was operative. Economic marginalization, exile and isolation, the experience of a body both raced and sexed as different: these phenomena were not particular to the Maghrebian worker, but pertained in many cases and shaped both identity and behavior. As such, these interpretations operated as part of a new project of assimilation that sought to invest the Maghrebian immigrant with full humanity. If psychological disturbance was a product of exile or sexual repression, of poverty or the experience of prejudice, then it was a mental sequela of emotional trauma rather than the particular product of a pathological brain structure or culture.

Yet this contention quickly became part of a searing debate in therapeutic circles as a new attempt to interpret the relationship between culture and psychiatry through the lens of difference emerged. In 1966 the psychologist Marie-Cécile Ortigues and her husband, the anthropologist Edmond Ortigues, published their sensational volume *Oedipe africain*. The book reviewed four years of Marie-Cécile's psychoanalytic practice at the Fann psychiatric clinic in Dakar, along with attempts to explain differences in Senegalese patients' presentations and experiences of illness from those of European patients through reference to culture. The text pointed to "sensible differences" in the "rate of development, type of psychosomatic balance, social adaptation, and reaction modes" of Senegalese and Europeans.[43] Each of these, combined with educational, familial, and historical differences, contributed to a clinical picture with the potential to depart radically from the middle-class European model that many psycho-analysts had taken as representative since Freud. Yet although the project bore superficial resemblances to works by colonial psychiatrists such as Porot in Algeria or Carothers in Kenya in its emphasis on difference, the Ortigueses departed radically from their colonial forebears in both their objectives and the assumptions they brought to their work.

In contrast with their predecessors, the Ortigueses greatly limited the scope of their project and the applicability of their findings. They insisted, for example, that their research had no capacity to "explain the psychology of the average African nor to link certain particularities of mores to a hypothetical 'base personality.'"[44] Instead they proposed simply the exploration of a single critical psychoanalytic concept—the Oedipus complex—in an urbanizing Senegalese milieu in an attempt to gauge both the possible universality of the concept and the potential for its adaptation in moving away from the model European family. Through the analysis of nearly two hundred patients, they concluded that a form of the Oedipus complex existed in Senegal, but one that bore only a faint resemblance to that described by Freud as essential to infantile psychological and sexual development. Because the father in much of Senegalese society approximated the position of ancestor rather than a rival for the mother's love, competition was transferred to brothers, including both biological siblings and those who played similar roles in the child's family.[45] The authors also noted a critical difference between the "classic" and the "African" Oedipus concerning guilt. Guilt over the complex's violent and sexual drives and their objects was central to the splitting of the ego that marked resolution of the complex in the West. Yet guilt operated differently in Senegalese culture, provoking instead "an anxiety over the abandonment of the individual by the group." A range of factors informed this difference; critical among them was the importance of social attitudes toward gender in the shaping of ideas about the mother and the father. "If the Oedipal question is resolved otherwise than how it is in Europe, that is because from the outset it has not been posed in the same terms."[46]

The Ortigueses also insisted that "racial" or biological differences played no role in transforming the Oedipus complex in Senegalese society. Rather, an elastic yet deeply influential "culture"—defined principally through social relations, education, and typical family patterns in the community the Ortigueses studied—was the operative factor. This perspective toward their patients reflected a widening trend that merged ethnology and psychiatry in new ways. Whereas a number of therapists and social scientists had begun intense efforts to inscribe increasingly diverse populations

into universalizing systems—by highlighting factors such as political economy that shaped the psychological reactions of given populations—others
launched an impassioned defense of the understanding of multicultural
differences as critical for the interpretation and treatment of mental illness in non-Europeans. By drawing heavily on ethnographic methods and
data, this new ethnopsychiatry advocated treating patients within their
cultural idioms—whether Western or Wolof—and retooling therapeutic
objectives accordingly. Unlike ethnopsychiatric studies of the interwar
period (including those of the Algiers School), which borrowed from the
ideas of armchair and veranda ethnographers such as Lucien Lévy-Bruhl,
the new works incorporated the findings of intensive fieldworkers, including Claude Lévi-Strauss and practitioners of the American "culture of
personality school" such as Ruth Benedict and Margaret Mead, which
pointed less to essentializing difference and more to the role of cultural
practice in the organization of behavior and mentality.

Among the key figures to shape a postcolonial ethnopsychiatry was
Georges Devereux. Devereux was no stranger to crossing cultural boundaries. Born in Hungary, trained in France as an anthropologist by Marcel
Mauss in the 1930s and as a psychoanalyst by Marc Schlumberger in the
1940s, he then moved to the United States, where he studied at Berkeley
and underwent analysis at the Menninger Clinic in Topeka, Kansas.[47] Despite having published in anthropological and psychiatric journals before
his arrival in America, it was in Topeka that Devereux came to promi-
nence. The standard treatment offered at Menninger in the 1940s and
1950s combined psychotherapeutic strategies with medical examination.
Devereux broke with this program by leaning heavily on both his anthropological and psychoanalytic backgrounds. In his landmark study *Reality
and Dream: Psychotherapy of a Plains Indian*, Devereux followed the path
blazed by his fellow Hungarian analyst Géza Roheim in his work with
Australian aboriginal peoples. Like Roheim, Devereux focused on dream
interpretation, his patient's sexuality, and the operation of transference in
the analytic setting. On one level he therefore embraced the treatment of a
non-Western patient with Western therapeutics. But he also accounted for
the patient's understanding of his own predicament through reference to
his tribal history as well as his personal history.[48]

Devereux recognized that treating patients across cultures complicated
the distinction between ideas of the normal and the pathological. Ethnopsychiatry, by Devereux's definition, entailed the "coordination of the
concept of 'culture'"—the dominant concept in 1960s ethnology—"with
the paired concepts 'normal' and 'abnormal.'"[49] Yet it also necessitated the
practitioner's acknowledgment of his or her own stake in the therapeu-

tic relationship, a function of countertransference. Whereas the behavioral sciences had traditionally emphasized the neutrality of the observer,
Devereux argued that such distance and objectivity were impossible to
attain. Instead, the data generated by psychiatric, psychoanalytic, and
ethnographic study invariably confronted the researcher with a range of
anxieties. Rather than confounding such study, Devereux insisted, the
observer's anxieties (and defenses against them) were a critical element of
behavioral science research that deeply informed the observer's interpretations. Drawing heavily on Lévi-Strauss's *Tristes tropiques* and Georges
Balandier's *Afrique ambiguë*, Devereux noted that close attention to the
countertransferential relationship in therapeutic environments provided
deep insight into these interpretations and held the potential to render the
clinical encounter more sympathetic and therefore more effective at facilitating a cure, especially in practice across cultural divides.[50]

Devereux's consideration of countertransference marks the most significant departure of his work from that of the Algiers School. It was precisely
this sort of attention to the observer's cultural and social position and the
ways in which the colonial situation complicated the doctor-patient relationship that was absent from the work of Porot and his students, and that
could have mediated a degree of the tension that prevailed in the colonial
clinic. Yet it is also important to note that for Devereux, such mediation
did not entail the abandonment of a Western paradigm: one should never,
he argued, "identify oneself with the shaman." Instead, one should strive
toward a complementarist ethnopsychiatry. A proper analysis should not
aim to produce some abstraction of an average middle-class American or
European; instead, it should "reveal to the patient a means of reattaching
himself to the normal structure of his ethnic personality." The goal of
ethnopsychiatry, for Devereux, is to explain a system of thought in the language of the practitioner's own culture—that is, to be an ethnographer—
while using the patient's potential self, rather than a Western, universalist
ideal of "health," as a model for a cure. Such a model takes aim at both
ethnocentrism—the idea that the patient can only be cured from within a
cultural tradition—as well as abstract universalism—the idea that all subjects are potentially interchangeable, regardless of culture.[51]

In 1964 Devereux returned to Paris, where he began instructing students in anthropology and psychoanalysis. Among these students was
the leading proponent of ethnopsychiatry in contemporary France, Tobie
Nathan, until recently the director of the Centre Georges Devereux at the
Université de Paris VIII in Saint-Denis, which he opened in 1993. The
center employs a team of psychiatrists, psychologists, anthropologists, and
healers to treat the mentally ill in Paris's diverse immigrant population.

The facility, imagined as an ethnopsychiatric utopia, is designed for training and research in ethnopsychiatry as well as clinical practice. In a typical session, the patient and his or her family come to the center through referral by a social worker, a psychologist, or a general practitioner. The referring authority presents the case to a group of anthropologists and linguists as well as clinicians. At least one of these is ideally a native of the patient's region, who is certified in France but who speaks the patient's language as a mother tongue and is conversant with the therapeutic traditions of the region, whether rural Morocco or a West African city. The sessions last an average of two to three hours and are often conducted through the interpretation of the regional specialist.

The goal is to make the patient less an object and more the subject of medical intervention. As Nathan has recently argued, ethnopsychiatry's mission is to concern itself "with the singular nature of the patient's suffering." The "psychotherapeutic space" opened between patient, interpreter, and healer accounts for the world in which the patient operates, the "things" and "objects" that organize a local tradition's system of thought and therapy.[52] As one account describes the phenomenon, the group discussions "create a transitional space where the clinician's interventions mediate the collective symbolic worlds of the immigrant's country of origin and of France."[53]

This model, which Nathan pioneered at the Hôpital Avicenne in the *banlieue* city of Bobigny, attracted immediate interest in therapeutic and intellectual circles upon the publication of Nathan's book *La folie des autres* (The Madness of Others) in 1986.[54] Immigration from the former colonies had become a fixture of French social, cultural, and political life, with new generations of children born to immigrant families raising a host of debates over citizenship. France's global cities of Paris, Lyon, and Marseille also now sheltered rising numbers of migrant workers who had spent most of their adult lives in France. In addition, the rumors and reports of widespread delinquency permeating the immigrant neighborhoods of the *banlieues* raised important questions about the role of behavioral and social science in the management of France's apparent transition to a multicultural society. Nathan's work had strong explanatory and therapeutic potential for a society experiencing rapid demographic change. As one critic in *Libération* framed the question, "How can one stay the same when everything is changing?" Moreover, "how does one find a cure for a traumatic neurosis when one is Maghrebian or African and when nothing prepares you [*sic*] for a psychoanalytic cure?"[55]

Yet by virtue of its efforts to situate patients in their cultural milieux, Nathan's work also reinforced the notion of cultural difference as the ori-

gin of pathology. This was especially the case by the 1990s, when rising
fears of "insecurity" linked to immigration and experiences with terrorism
prompted a widespread social and political interrogation of France's immigration "problem."[56] Terrorist attacks in European cities in the late 1980s
and again in 1995, the explosions of sectarian violence in Algeria after the
cancelled 1992 elections, and the split in European public opinion over the
first Gulf War in 1991 raised questions about a culture war in the making
between the "West" and "Islam" in which difference and displacement
figured prominently.[57] The careful scrutiny of ethnopsychiatric claims and
assumptions that followed in the wake of these debates prompted a reassessment of the field both in the French press and in academic research,
in the course of which many have accused Nathan of breaking with the
key tenets of Devereux's therapeutic philosophy and even of favoring
the "ghettoization" of minority populations. The engagement between
Nathan and his colleagues' insistence on the importance of ethnicity as a
critical determinant of difference and the work of those who have defended
universalist positions has given language about assimilability and acculturation a new valence in a globalizing era.

Critics have accused Nathan of applying to immigrant patients in his
Saint-Denis clinic a binding pan-culturalism with potentially grave political and therapeutic consequences. As one of Nathan's former interns has
argued, in many cases an illness, however complex and whomever it strikes,
has universal implications. Writing in *Les temps modernes*, Zerdalia Dahoun cited the case of an immigrant woman who experienced a "dysfunc-
tion in her relationship with her new baby" as a classic example in which
Nathan's group privileged the issue of migration and minimized what she
considered the patient's fundamental problem: "There are postpartum
psychoses everywhere in the world, in Mali and in France, whether the
context involves migration or not. Yet they foreground the migrant character of the mother and her cultural references, even though this was above
all a case of psychotic pathology."[58] Others insisted that even where immigration was central to a case at hand, it was often the stresses of exile rather
than the "ethnic" or cultural dimensions of the patient's disorders that
merited the most clinical attention. For the psychoanalyst Fethi Benslama,
the therapist's role in such cases is thus not "to send them back on a flying
carpet in the direction of their culture," but instead to pay close attention
to the "internal histories of their displacement, to find its memory, to recognize its significations of rupture."[59] To ignore the individual dimensions
of exile is akin to ignoring the realities of life in a marginalized community
as critical stressors: to forget that many consultants at the Centre Georges
Devereux "live in overpopulated and wretched conditions, are confronted

with the pressures of unstable employment and the impermanence of their visa status, and face situations of racism and discrimination" by focusing on these patients' culture of origin, the anthropologist Didier Fassin has asserted, is to "negate" the patient's "existence" in favor of his or her culture.[60]

Other critics have noted that to focus on the condition rather than the personal experience of exile is to miss some of the most important dimensions of illness in a migrant population. Many patients have left their cultures of origin because of traumatic experiences; to return them there as a matter of course, even metaphorically, could potentially exacerbate rather than ameliorate their disorders.[61] The more productive route, Dahoun argues, is to "discern the place that exile holds in the history of the subject and the value it retains in his recounting as a traumatic event" in its own right. To consider "the psychopathology of the migrant as different from general psychopathology" also contributes to a "doubling" of the patient's exile: it entraps the patient in languages of alterity both in society and in "psychiatric knowledge."[62]

In a psychoanalytic scenario, an overemphasis on the patient's cultural origins risks enhancing the patient's resistance to therapy. As Dahoun indicates, "the cultural can become a screen" that conceals the patient's base neurosis: the patient's "interminable digressions on his customs satisfy the analyst's curiosity and transform the sessions into an anthropology course."[63] More seriously, an overemphasis on culture as a factor in pathogenicity or pathoplasticity often views the cultural as "monolithic."[64] In one journalist's words, "Reduced to his sociocultural being, man is stripped of his reason, that is, what renders him capable of moving across cultural codes."[65] Nathan's emphasis on a "radical differentialism" converts the ethnic origin into "an irreducible and immutable dimension of the person."[66] Nathan himself has argued for a strict compartmentalization of populations as a means of avoiding the pathogenic dangers of abrupt cultural homogenization. "In societies with high rates of immigration, we must favor the development of ghettos—yes, I say loud and clear—we must favor the development of ghettos so as not to force a family to abandon its cultural system."[67] Statements such as these have led many to accuse Nathan of defending cultural integrity at all costs. In his defense, Nathan has argued that his detractors have been motivated by a knee-jerk leftism that rejects anything that denies the universalist principles of French republicanism or by a defense of intolerant psychoanalytic models of subjectivity that reject pluralism.[68]

The question of culture and psychiatry in the context of the global city has thus provoked an unlikely debate among the academic and therapeutic

Left in France that is reminiscent of similar arguments during the colonial era. Between the late nineteenth century and the outbreak of the Second World War, an intellectual struggle between right-leaning "physicalists" such as Porot, who drew on the legacy of Broca's anthropology, and left-leaning "culturalists" such as the ethnographers and philosophers who founded the Musée de l'Homme in the late 1930s (including Paul Rivet and Marcel Mauss), marked the colonial debate. Whereas those who proposed that physical causes meant an irremediable difference between European and colonial populations and their potential value as citizens, those on the cultural side advocated assimilationist measures to absorb the colonized into a "greater France" of a hundred million subjects. At present, only the radical Right maintains this emphasis on physical distinction, and a new line between cultural preservationists and universalists has recast the debate in new terms. On the one side are those who have readopted an "assimilationist" argument that advocates the inclusion of a diversifying population into the eternal project of republican citizenship. By applying the ostensibly "universal" concepts of Freudian psychoanalysis and Marxian political economy to non-Western populations, they have claimed a broad equality that eradicates difference in the name of human nature. On the other side, practitioners such as Nathan have taken the "associationist" line by claiming to adapt medicine to suit a multicultural society that values differences.

The former group has not rejected ethnopsychiatry in principle. Instead, they have claimed to be redirecting ethnopsychiatry to its modern roots in Devereux's work. To an extent, they have taken a line similar to that of American medical anthropologists such as Arthur Kleinman and the group behind the journal *Culture, Medicine and Psychiatry*.[69] Ethnography in this view offers a useful tool for investigating the patient's worldview and providing for an "empathic listening" but stops short of "using the technique of the healer."[70] As the psychoanalyst Daniel Sibony has argued, "There is a difference between reinscribing people into their origins as a means of including them and helping them to recognize their origins so that they can depart from them or come back to them; in short, so that they can engage with them."[71] They have thus claimed to value cultural difference in the manner of the Ortigueses in *Oedipe africain*: to understand the essential role that ethnicity and culture have in shaping illness while eschewing an "exoticizing and above all ineffective culturalization," a position that has in turn fed the production of psychoanalytic studies of migrant populations and their societies of origin—a search for the *Oedipe maghrébin*—that draw heavily on the Ortigueses' model.[72]

Both of these perspectives have highly problematic elements. The promise of universalism is of course a mask for the advocacy of Western systems. One can only be "universal" by subsuming the particular to the notion that any individual represents an abstraction of the nation, as in the official policy of *intégration* framed by the 1993 Pasqua Laws, which refused to recognize individual ethnic differences as specific political constituencies.[73] By contrast, the particularist rejection of any "psychiatry outside of culture" smacks of the possibility of both "relativizing all of psychiatry" and "psychiatrizing all of culture."[74] Bruno Latour rightly notes in his defense of Nathan that ethnopsychiatric practice provides a radical contestation of Western biomedical ideas about universality and objectivity—that Nathan's focus on the healing power of local belief systems sheds a powerful light on the local dimensions of "science" itself.[75] Yet Nathan's own language is eerily reminiscent of the words of colonial psychiatrists such as Charles Bardenat and André Donnadieu, whose work rejected the possibility of cultural adaptation of the Muslim. Nathan's claim that "Medicine and the School" are the "chief machines for the scraping away of cultural systems"—and that they pose great risks to the mental stability of immigrant populations—reiterates the notion of "civilization psychosis" that led many colonial psychiatrists to advocate for a severe limitation on colonial education, as does the hypothetical case that Nathan invokes: "To place a three-year-old Soninké born in France but cradled as a Soninké, breastfed, and raised in a Soninké manner abruptly into school and wait for him to adapt to it is to know nothing of psychical function." Such an action is "shameful! At this age, it is totally impossible to manage effectively the process of mediation between two cultures and two languages."[76] Although intended as a defense of "Culture with a big C," as Nathan puts it, this effort to preserve the integrity of the ego by preserving its cultural roots has the taxidermic rhetorical effect of locking the immigrant into a fixed position in a fluid society.

Epilogue: "Let Me Tell You My Story"

Immigration and the making of a global society; tragic underdevelopment and the creation of generations of economic refugees: these have been the respective legacies of decolonization in France and North Africa. Each of these phenomena has probed repeated interrogations of the major themes of the colonial era. How, for example, to continue the republican project in a postcolonial and multicultural society, where efforts by populations to embrace their differences appear to undermine the project itself? How has the overt racism of the colonial period transmuted into the implicit (and at times explicit) racism that greets North African immigrants in an inhospitable society nevertheless dependent on their labor?[77] On the North African side, the bitterness with which the many manifestations of France's "civilizing mission" were received has tainted development projects for the Westernization of medicine, while economic depression has exacerbated stress throughout the population. Meanwhile, struggles between largely secular administrations and rising Islamist movements in Tunisia, Morocco, and especially Algeria have resuscitated the internecine struggles of the resistance movements of the early twentieth century, raising questions about the pathways of development in a postcolonial era. These legacies of colonialism have deeply marked psychiatry in both France and the Maghreb. Whether in the struggle to handle the intellectual and social difficulties presented by immigration, or in the question of how to manage scarce health resources, psychiatry has been a flashpoint for postcolonial disputes. Yet it is perhaps in the shared legacy of France and the Maghreb—their ongoing relationship as a "transpolitical" space and their common memories of the colonial experience—that psychiatry has been most relevant.

The shadow of violence that has darkened memories of trauma and loss in France and Algeria was the central theme of the first meeting of the Société Franco-Algérien de Psychiatrie (Franco-Algerian Psychiatric Society), which I attended in October 2003. Held in Paris at the Hôpital Européen Georges Pompidou, the meeting was part of "Djazaïr," the celebratory "year of Algeria" sponsored by the French Ministry of Culture, and the congress welcomed some two hundred participants for discussions of "Sufferings and Memories" linked to the Algerian War. Papers by French and Algerian psychiatrists, sociologists, historians, and writers addressed a range of topics, including the epidemiology of post-traumatic stress disorder among former combatants and civilians on both sides of the war, colonial nostalgia, the effects of the violence for postcolonial generations, the repetition of the war's violence in acts of terror, and the continuing importance of the war in both French and Algerian cultural memory. The presentations made clear that psychiatry remains a critical touchstone for examining the emotional charges that surround the postcolonial relationship between France and the Maghreb, while they also showed that the decolonization of psychiatry, like the decolonization of memory, has remained incomplete.

Discussions ranged widely, from typical case histories of PTSD in soldiers to epidemiological data that supported startling conclusions. In his introductory presentation, the meeting's president pointed to the case of "Roger," a former French soldier, for whom sleep was a chronic trial by ordeal: "Every night for forty years, I have nightmares where I see mutilated bodies." Yet in contrast with Vietnam, the apartheid crisis in South Africa, and the genocides of the Khmer Rouge, Rwanda, and Kosovo, psychiatrists had paid little attention to Algeria. Such was the result of a "collective repression" that silenced discussions "of this 'dirty war' in which summary executions, round-ups, torture, and rape comprised the combat arsenal," in one psychiatrist's words.[78] For the Algerian side, Mohammed Bedjaoui, a former president of the International Court of Justice, recounted the mechanisms of repression that exacerbated the stress of memories of violence. Just as "napalm burned eight thousand villages" during the war, it also "burned the wounded memories" of Algerians: "Torture, rape, cruel, degrading and inhumane treatments were repressed as if by deliberate but desperate will, a will to forget so as to reconstitute a painfully injured physical or moral integrity."[79] The meeting was designed as a means of overcoming this repression and to begin a process of "calm analysis of the determinants of psychotraumatic consequences of these events."[80]

One of the keynote speakers at the meeting was the historian Benjamin Stora, who has studied official and unofficial repressions of the memory of the Algerian war in depth.[81] Stora argued that there are three principal locations of memory of the war in the French population, each with a different stake: soldiers, who remember the war as a traumatic phenomenon that forever destroyed their youth; former settlers, who imagined the war as a violent disruption of their sun-filled lives in Algeria; and France's immigrant populations. Yet Stora, a native of Constantine born in 1954, also pointed to the ways in which these guardians of memory had transferred their experience and its affective charge to new generations born during and after the war. Other presentations and discussions powerfully echoed this theme. As *Le Monde* reported in 2000, nearly one in four French veterans of the war manifested a form of PTSD; yet this figure said nothing of the war's other victims: civilian populations and the families of combatants. Maïssa Bey, an Algerian author, invoked this dimension of the problem in her paper "The Scars of History," in which she recounted the torture and execution of her father in an attempt to "reconstitute" the "primal scene" of this memory "in the detective's sense of the term."[82]

The notion of traumatic violence shaping the cultural memory of a second generation is not surprising. It is almost to be expected, especially when the violence in question is constitutive of a national identity forged in conflict; the Holocaust and the Six-Day War contribute similarly to the identity of modern Israel and the shape of its geographic boundaries. Yet it is curious that the cases presented at the French-Algerian psychiatric meeting were near replications of Frantz Fanon's famous case histories that figured prominently in *The Wretched of the Earth* forty years earlier.

Fanon's passionate study of the war's wounded detailed the stories of victims, perpetrators, and bystanders. The torturer who beat his wife and
children at home and his Algerian victim were both casualties of the conflict, as were the young Frenchwoman who overheard her father beating
Algerians in her basement, the Algerian man who heard while imprisoned
of his wife's gang rape by French soldiers, and the young Algerian boys
who beat their European playmate to death "because he was French." The
psyches of these victims of war, Fanon argued, had been forged in violence. In Fanon's account, many responded to therapy. But the silence that
has surrounded the war's memory has perpetuated the social repression
of these and other traumas, leaving these wounds to fester. As *Le Monde*
reported in its account of the conference, "most" of these trauma victims
"are reluctant to seek help."[83]

What was remarkable about the meeting was that it served as a forum
for the public revisitation of the personal traumas of speakers, discussants,
and audience members. Official silences about the war had begun to crack
in the years preceding the conference. The Algerian presidential elections
of 1999 called attention to the war's legacy in the French press, and a law
passed that year officially recognized that "the war without a name," the
"events" of 1954–62, had actually taken place. Likewise, the publication in
2001 of General Paul Aussaresses's memoir of torturing Algerian suspects
sent shock waves through the press and prompted claims for reparations
and indictments.[84] Yet the conference's papers and subsequent discussions
offered a medium for personal confession and grievance. Throughout the
meeting, roughly a quarter of the questions and comments offered after
the presentations opened with the remark, "Let me tell you my story."
These comments came from both French and Algerians. They came from
the children of French soldiers who told of their fathers' nightmares and
personal violence. They came from the children of Algerian revolutionaries who told of their fathers' disappearances. They reflected the perspectives of *pieds-noirs* who had lost their homes through exile, and of Algerians
who had lost their families through round-ups and *ratonnades*. On both
sides, they told the story of a war's capacity to tarnish multiple generations
with its impermissible memory.

The conference was thus both a scholarly meeting and a historical artifact. The medical findings presented at the meeting revealed for nearly the
first time the extent and the persistence of the psychic wounds of the Algerian war. Yet the meeting's themes also highlighted the ways in which psychiatry remains a critical frame for exploring France's and North Africa's
shared legacies of colonial violence and postcolonial transition. The airing
of a new French generation's shame over the war's conduct, expressed as

a traumatic memory, points to France's displacement from stewardship of empire to global society, from a role of aggression and expansion to one of perceived besiegement by both an expanding Muslim population and the reach of American multinational capitalism.[85] The sentiment of outrage, fear, and loss that marks generations of Algerians, immigrants, and their children born in the war's aftermath reveals the long shadow of violence that continues to darken the relationship of the Franco-Algerian trans-political space. Psychiatry also offers a new language for the *pieds-noirs'* simultaneous expression of nostalgia and victimization by their forced exile in the aftermath of the Evian Accords in 1962. As the epidemiologist Sylvaine Artéro noted in her presentation at the meeting, the *pieds-noirs* of the region near Montpellier show far higher rates of depression, anxiety, and dementia than their native French counterparts of similar ages and economic levels.[86] The genetic insularity of the cohort offers one possible explanation (especially for high rates of Alzheimer's disease). But other possible risk factors include the traumatic experience of a population forced into exile and resettlement in an alien society that frequently rejected them as racists, terrorists, and torturers.[87]

The mental decay of this cohort of repatriated *pieds-noirs* is a critical site of memory, a scar of the traumatic past that marks France and its former colonies in the Maghreb. The Blida hospital, too, is an important site of colonial memory that both reflects and betrays its complicated past. By the 1990s, with Algeria's immersion in a new decade of civil war, Blida had become better known as a seat of the Groupe Islamique Armée, the radical Islamist faction that arose in response to the FLN's cancellation of the 1992 elections, than as a space of mental illness and healing. The city's Centre Hospitalier Universitaire Frantz Fanon is in a state of near ruin, having decayed from its origins as a prominent symbol of colonial *mise en valeur* and a utopian symbol of postcolonial development. The reformist touches that marked the hospital to its critics as overly luxurious in the 1930s, as well as those introduced by Fanon in the 1950s, are barely visible as fossilized traces, worn away by overuse and a dearth of funding. Its soccer fields are now barren dirt lots with a scattering of weeds, the goals missing their nets and corroded. Paint flakes from the walls and the rusting bars covering the windows in lockdown wards. The hospital is overcrowded with chronic patients, some of whom have been confined there since Fanon's day. A 2002 documentary filmed at the hospital shows a number of aging women patients suffering from dementia in a dusty courtyard, their heads shaven in an attempt at delousing, pressing their faces against the camera lens as they stare intently at their reflections: the hospital has no mirrors, and the women have not seen themselves for decades.[88] The hospital has become what its founders and caretakers, including Antoine Porot, Frantz Fanon, and Mahfoud Boucebci, had most hoped to avoid: a warehouse of madness that recalls the asylums of the late nineteenth century rather than a vestige of colonial investment and a sign of a progressive outlook on psychopathology.

Psychiatry and its objects of inquiry offer privileged windows into the postcolonial experience. It is a field with rhetorical uses as both setting and subject for authors such as Rachid Boudjedra and the filmmakers Abdellatif Kechiche and Malek Bensmaïl. As in Fanon's writings during the war, the psychiatric setting offers a powerful means of telling the story of a world in disarray. The patient as character represents a marginal subject. Yet the act of marginalization itself is critical for examination of the normal and pathological dimensions of the social and political orders of things. In the case of Kechiche's character Jallel, the experience in the hospital reveals the madness of a society that polices and rejects many of its most dedicated citizens. In the Algerian stories of Bensmaïl and Boudjedra, the schizophrenic patient provides a vessel for exploring the fragmentation of societies in development that are riven by their colonial pasts. The patient's voice, incompletely silenced during the colonial era, returns in these narratives to its full volume, with its capacity to speak the truth about the madness of violence and trauma, of memory and loss, phenomena that remain the critical stumbling blocks in the postcolonial relationship of France and the Maghreb.

Conclusion
Pills and Paving Stones, Centers and Margins

We've found a trick that works.
House physician, Sainte-Anne Hospital, Paris, 1952

A startling discovery rocked the psychiatric world in early 1952. It involved the treatment of Philippe Burg, an archaeology student at the École du Louvre who had been confined at the Centre Hospitalier Sainte-Anne, Paris's largest mental hospital, for several years. In the late 1940s Philippe, who lived with his mother in the Rue de Vaugirard, stopped attending classes and began to disappear for days at a time. At one point officials at the Musée Guimet discovered him sitting naked in the lotus position in front of a statue of the Buddha. After a short stay at Sainte-Anne, hospital officials released him to his mother's custody. Shortly thereafter, suffering from the cold one night, he set fire to the books in his room. He returned to Sainte-Anne, where his condition worsened. Insulin treatments had little effect, and because of increasing amounts of glucose needed to bring him out of his daily comas, his weight ballooned to nearly three hundred pounds. Psychiatrists despaired of his case as he entered a catatonic state. On a hunch, his treating physician placed Philippe on a new drug with which psychiatrists at the hospital were experimenting. After adjusting the dose to compensate for his massive size, the drug began to take effect. He began to speak again, became animated, and when his mother visited he recognized her for the first time in years. For his mother, it was as if "he had been brought back to life." As a trial, he left the hospital with his mother for lunch at the Closerie des Lilas and a stroll in the Jardin du Luxembourg; soon thereafter he began to go on home visits for days at a time.[1]

According to his treating physician, the psychiatrist and pharmacologist Jean Thuillier, Philippe's recovery was the result of a new "trick that worked." The drug was a compound called 4560 RP—better known as chlorpromazine. The compound was an antihistamine that proved to be the first effective treatment for schizophrenia. Jean Delay, professor and chair of the department of psychiatry at the hospital, tested the drug repeatedly on the hospital's most desperate cases, the apparently incurable and violent schizophrenic men on his colleague Pierre Deniker's locked ward. As Delay and Deniker's initial publications noted, the drug calmed manic patients.[2] It sometimes eliminated auditory hallucinations and delusions and almost always reduced their frequency. In contrast with the barbiturates that psychiatrists had traditionally used for these cases, it tranquilized patients without putting them to sleep. It brought catatonic patients back to the world around them. For Thuillier, a colleague of Delay and Deniker's, "the results obtained with chlorpromazine could be measured in the psychiatric hospitals in decibels"; even those who lived in the neighborhood surrounding Sainte-Anne noticed a drop in the cries and screams that emerged from behind its walls after 1952.[3]

Chlorpromazine virtually transformed psychiatry in industrialized countries overnight. Although hospitals had already begun downsizing, chlorpromazine and other antipsychotic drugs prompted greater advocacy among physicians and psychiatrists for outpatient treatment of even the most recalcitrant cases. As the chemical management of psychopathology increasingly replaced both confinement and psychotherapy over the next several decades, community psychiatry, for all its failures, replaced asylum psychiatry as the dominant mode of treatment, shifting the field's major spheres of influence away from universities and state hospitals and toward pharmaceutical giants in the private sector. According to the historian and psychiatrist David Healy, the explosive growth of the antidepressant industry finds its origins in the pharmacological revolution that chlorpromazine and its successors initiated.[4]

The story of chemical innovation in psychiatry relates to the historical trajectory of the Algiers School in several ways. Colonial psychiatrists marked their position on the cutting edge of their field by seizing the initiative on many of the most important innovations of the early twentieth century. They were the first to implement entire networks of psychiatric care structured around the principle of mental hygiene and prophylaxis. They made Algiers the undisputed center for the study of the relationship between mental illness and race, what Henri Aubin called a pragmatic "ethno-psycho-pathology." While Paris struggled under the occupation and its aftermath, psychiatrists in the Maghreb prodigiously developed the somatic treatment of mental disorders, pushing its limits, testing its safety and efficacy. By publishing countless articles and prominent textbooks for physicians and psychiatrists in France and the colonies, colonial psychiatrists established their relevance to the discipline and made names for themselves and their institutions as leaders in the field.

Yet the most lasting innovation of the century literally passed them by. It was only by a historical accident that the chlorpromazine story was centered in Paris and not in Tunis or Algiers. The first tests of chlorpromazine's immediate antecedent took place in Tunisia. Henri Laborit, a surgeon stationed at the Sidi-Abdallah naval hospital in Bizerte, had begun conducting experiments to control surgical shock. He theorized that placing the body in a form of artificial hibernation by lowering its temperature might help to stabilize physiological systems and started using antihistamines, a new class of drug that emerged in the early 1940s, to reduce the risks of hypothermia and its stresses on the body.[5] With his colleague Pierre Huguenard, he developed a "lytic cocktail" designed both to sedate and to stabilize the patient during surgery. He also noticed what he called a "euphoric quietude," even "indifference," in patients who had exhibited high levels of stress before administration of the cocktail. As he noted in an interview in the early 1970s, at this point he asked a "psychiatrist to watch me operate on some of my tense, anxious, Mediterranean-type patients." The psychiatrist, whom Laborit never named, "agreed" that "the patients were remarkably calm and relaxed." However, Laborit noted, "I guess he didn't think any more about his observations as they might apply to psychiatric patients."[6]

The Tunisian psychiatrist missed a substantial opportunity. Restationed in Paris, Laborit brought the cocktail to the Val-de-Grâce hospital, where he and several colleagues synthesized the new antihistamine 4560 RP (for Rhône-Poulenc, which licensed the drug as Largactil, named for its broad spectrum ["large action"], or effect on many systems).[7] Psychiatrists working under Jean Delay at Sainte-Anne began experimenting with the drug immediately. With a wave of publications in the early 1950s, Delay and Deniker became psychiatry's new luminaries. Rhône-Poulenc sent Deniker and Laborit to the United States and Canada on missions to spread the word about new possibilities in the field. An international congress on chlorpromazine that Delay hosted in Paris in 1955 combined with these missions to draw global attention to Sainte-Anne as the undisputed center of a new biochemical paradigm for the management of madness.

The development of chlorpromazine is but one of the historical circumstances that shaped the rise and decline of the Algiers School as a scientific center on the imperial periphery. The expansion of European settlement in the Maghreb in the late nineteenth and early twentieth centuries created a demand among administrators both for understanding the psychological consequences of migration to new environments and for knowing the mindset of the colonial other. This second demand intensified in the course of the First World War as imperial conscripts changed the face of the French military. Psychiatrists' advocacy for colonial investment in the interwar period merged seamlessly with a reiteration of the "civilizing mission" that sought to remold the colonies through the assimilation of infrastructure. The decolonization struggles of the 1950s, however, marked a new period for the Algiers School as it fought for its very existence. The Algerian war temporarily heightened interest in the school's work, and military and police authorities looked to Porot, Sutter, and their colleagues for insight into the "Arab mind" and the psychological dimensions of the insurgency. France's loss, however, forced the repatriation of the group and its dissolution into the existing psychiatric infrastructure of the metropole.[8]

But the story of chlorpromazine indicates that the physical disbanding of the school was only one circumstance that ended the group's influence. At the height of the decolonization struggles in the Maghreb—with Moroccan independence and the outbreak of the Algerian war in 1954 and the formal granting of Tunisian independence in 1956—psychiatry itself began to move in different directions from those that marked the school's major contributions. As with much of medicine, where antibiotics, antihistamines, and analgesics had transformed the management of illness, a new biochemical psychiatry replaced the racially and ethnically centered configurations of normality and pathology that marked the biocultural psychiatry of the colonies. Entities such as dopamine and norepinephrine replaced "acute mania" and "external action phases" as the critical factors in determining health and illness. A pathbreaking development that might have carried colonial psychiatrists to new heights in the postcolonial era thus literally slipped through their fingers with Laborit's move from Bizerte to Val-de-Grâce. During the 1950s colonial psychiatrists performed only a small handful of studies on the new drug, and even these were either speculative studies or reviews, with only one empirical study performed at Blida.[9] Although Algiers would never have replaced Paris, Delay and Deniker's apotheosis at the moment of imperial disintegration ensured that the colonial periphery could no longer rival the center.

The chemical revolution in psychiatry brought a further ironic dimension to the story of the Algiers School by the late 1960s. As with many other therapeutic innovations, the optimism that surrounded its moment of inception was short-lived. The neuroleptics' psychological and neurological side effects quickly detracted from their promise.[10] Critics seized on chlorpromazine in particular as a chemical straitjacket that assaulted the personality; the more conspiratorially minded saw antipsychotics as a mechanism for breeding conformity in a capitalist society. Along with techniques such as electroshock and lobotomy, chlorpromazine became a rallying cry for the antipsychiatry movement. Motivated by the denunciations of psychiatric practice in the works of Fanon and Foucault, student revolutionaries in Paris adopted an antipsychiatric platform in 1968. The movement was indiscriminate, aiming its paving stones at both the racial psychiatrists of the Algiers School and the chemical revolutionaries such as Delay as representatives of an oppressive society and profession.[11] Despite the fact that Fanon embraced many orthodox psychiatric practices, including the administration of strong medications and ECT, antipsychiatrists throughout the industrialized world brought attention to his work, and in turn to the Algiers School. As David Macey, citing Eldridge Cleaver, has argued, by the end of the 1960s "every brother on a rooftop" in America could quote Fanon; by extension, they also knew about Porot and psychiatry as instruments of colonial power.[12] The psychiatrists who had sought a global spotlight as the drivers of innovation finally received the world's attention as the architects of a racist order.

The words of Frantz Fanon, Kateb Yacine, and countless patients whose voices creep through the stifling filters of their case histories provide a form of critical witnessing. They lay out in clear terms the violence of the colonial medical encounter and offer a powerful testimony born of experience, a glimpse of the desperate struggle of the marginal against the forces of science and the state. But in their foregrounding of violence they obscure the utopianism that guided colonial psychiatrists, as well as the colonial project itself, through the early twentieth century. Rather than a counterweight to colonial excesses, this outlook was their counterpart. Optimism marched in step with domination, as did innovation with dehumanization. The institutional structures that Antoine Porot and his students implemented throughout French North Africa developed a backwater into an avant-garde center for psychiatric science. The warm reception of their work by the leading lights of the profession—references to their pioneering efforts in mental hygiene, praise of their ethnopsychiatric research, the widespread publication and glowing reviews of their texts—indicates that by 1954 the group had come close to achieving its

goal. Yet they accomplished this work at often profound cost to their patients. The emancipatory promises of psychiatric social engineering in the
colonial state, of daring new therapies with the potential to liberate minds
from devious bodies, were belied by a pervasive belief in the irremediable
nature of the North African mind.

Perhaps ahistorically, we tend to follow Fanon and Kateb in regarding
colonial psychiatrists as marginal figures, politically motivated agents of the
colonial state, and an insult to science. This book has pointed to the truths
of these claims. But it is crucial to remember that this was not the source
of colonial psychiatrists' fall from grace. Their work met the accepted gold
standards of psychiatric science for much of the twentieth century. It fell
out of favor not because attitudes had shifted, but because their profession
itself had changed. Such ideas and practices—for instance, when a racist
organization nudged French psychiatry in disturbing new directions—are
embarrassing episodes in the history of the disciplines, yet they also offer
a useful space for examining science and its contexts, and the historical
circumstances of practices in centers and at the margins.

Notes

Introduction

1. Du Camp, *Nil*, 39.

2. Lamartine, *Voyage en Orient*, 305–6.

3. Flaubert, *Première éducation sentimentale*, 242.

4. See Said, *Orientalism*; also Lowe, *Critical Terrains*, esp. 75–101.

5. Fanon, *Dying Colonialism*, 121.

6. Fanon, *Wretched*, 296.

7. Osborne, *Nature*; Conklin, *Mission to Civilize*; also Wilder, *French Imperial Nation-State*.

8. See, e.g., Stoler, "Rethinking Colonial Categories," and *Race*.

9. See esp. Basalla, "Spread of Western Science"; Goonatilake, "Modern Science."

10. Latour, *Pasteurization*, esp. 140–45. On the changing historiography of colonial science, see Palladino and Worboys, "Science and Imperialism"; Pyenson, "Cultural Imperialism." Key examples include Adas, *Machines*; Harrison, *Climates and Constitutions*; MacLeod, "On Visiting"; Pelis, "Prophet"; Prakash, *Another Reason*; and several essays in MacLeod, *Nature and Empire*.

11. See esp. Rabinow, *French Modern*; Wright, *Politics of Design*.

12. John Colin Carothers of Mathari Mental Hospital in Nairobi, Kenya, attracted some significant attention with a range of publications, but his case was anomalous; see McCulloch, *Colonial Psychiatry*; Sadowsky, *Imperial Bedlam*; and Vaughan, *Curing Their Ills*. For India, see Ernst, *Mad Tales from the Raj*, and Mills, *Madness, Cannabis, and Colonialism*.

13. Concerning the last example, see Goldstein, *Console and Classify*, 297; she notes that provincial deputies objected that the law governing the confinement of the insane was "cut to the measure of the capital" and only applied "with great difficulty to the provinces," where facilities remained sparse.

14. Boigey, "Étude psychologique," 9.

15. Conklin, *Mission to Civilize*; Sherman, "Arts and Sciences."

16. Terracini, *Si bleu le ciel*, 112–13.

17. Apter, "Out of Character," 502–3.

18. Benslama, "Identity as a Cause," 44.

19. Bhabha, *Location of Culture*; McClintock, *Imperial Leather.*

20. See esp. chapters 5 and 6.

21. As an exception, there was a group of European expatriate analysts in Casablanca who served only Europeans; see Bennani, *Psychanalyse au pays des saints.* On Fanon's own position with regard to psychoanalysis, see esp. Gates, "Critical Fanonism"; Macey, *Frantz Fanon.*

22. The literature on physical anthropology, biology, and race is too vast to cite here; for a few salient examples, see Schiebinger, *The Mind Has No Sex?* and *Nature's Body*; also Gould, *Mismeasure of Man.*

23. "Papiers d'agents pièces annexées à la correspondance d'Alapetite avec Peretti de la Rocca et pièces diverses," Institut Supérieur d'Histoire du Mouvement National, Manouba (henceforth ISHMN): Quai d'Orsay 8, d. 2, fol. 223.

24. See Kateb, *Européens, "Indigènes" et Juifs*; Lorcin, *Imperial Identities* and "Imperialism, Colonial Identity, and Race"; Pelis, "Prophet for Profit." For a more sympathetic view of these developments, see Micouleau-Sicault, *Les médecins français.*

25. Lorcin, "Imperialism, Colonial Identity, and Race," esp. 655; see also Turin, *Affrontements culturels.*

26. Gallagher, *Medicine and Power*, 82.

27. See Katz, "The 1907 Mauchamp Affair"; also Paul, "Medicine and Imperialism."

28. See esp. Kocher, *De la criminalité.*

29. Trenga, *Âme arabo-berbère*, 9.

30. Lemanski, *Hygiène du colon*, 571; and Escande de Messières, *Psychologie des coloniaux*, 8.

31. Ernst, *Mad Tales from the Raj.* For a more detailed analysis of these and other works, see Keller, "Madness and Colonization."

32. Vaughan, *Curing Their Ills*; Sadowsky, *Imperial Bedlam*; see also McCulloch, *Colonial Psychiatry.*

33. Bégué, "Un siècle de psychiatrie française"; Berthelier, *Homme maghrébin.*

34. Bennani, *Psychanalyse au pays des saints*, 239.

Chapter 1

1. Lwoff and Sérieux, "Sur quelques moyens," 171.

2. Pierson, "Assistance psychiatrique."

3. Postel, *Génèse de la psychiatrie*, 57; see also Weiner, *Comprendre et soigner.*

4. Postel, *Genèse de la psychiatrie*, 95; see also Daumezon, "Lecture historique"; Foucault, *Histoire de la folie*, 593–96; Swain, *Sujet de la folie.*

5. Jean Comaroff, "'Diseased Heart of Africa'"; Gilman, *Picturing Health.*

6. Vergès, "Chains of Madness."

7. Maupassant, *Vie errante*, 201–4.

8. Ibid., 204–8.

9. Lorcin, "Rome and France," 296–97. The idea of a link to the Roman past also played a role in the establishment of misguided policies; as Swearingen, *Moroccan Mirages*, 28–34, has noted, the idea that Morocco was the "granary of Rome" influenced disastrous policies based on inflated notions of agricultural capacity.

10. See Lorcin, "Rome and France," 315–27, and *Imperial Identities*, 196–213.

11. Goldstein, *Console and Classify*.

12. Esquirol, cited in Morel and Quétel, "Thérapeutiques de l'aliénation," 317. See also Goldstein, *Console and Classify*, 287–92.

13. This account is drawn from Desruelles and Bersot, "Assistance aux aliénés en Algérie," 97; Edmond Doutté, *Magie et religion dans l'Afrique du Nord* (Algiers: Jourdan, 1909; reprint, Paris: Maisonneuve, 1984); Crapanzano, *Hamadsha*; and other texts cited below.

14. See, e.g., Peter Gran, "Medical Pluralism"; also Greenwood, "Cold or Spirits?," as well as essays in Longuenesse, *Santé, médecine et société*.

15. Dols, *Majnun*, 124; see also Cloarec, *Bimaristans*.

16. Larguèche, *Ombres de la ville*.

17. See, e.g., Conklin, *Mission to Civilize*.

18. Variot, "Une visite," 537.

19. Voisin, "Souvenirs," 90.

20. Bouquet, "Aliénés en Tunisie," 11, 17, 24.

21. Ibid., 67.

22. Ibid., 51; emphasis in original.

23. CADN—Tunisie, 1er versement 1538.

24. Bouquet, "Aliénés en Tunisie," 28, 50–51, 53–55.

25. Ibid., 56–62.

26. Ibid., 71, 110, 116–17.

27. *Congrès*, Dijon (1908) 2:243–45.

28. *Congrès*, Tunis (1912), 1:7.

29. Ibid., 2:21–25.

30. Ibid., 1:56, 73.

31. Ibid., 1:58, 65–66, 74; italics in the original.

32. *Code pénal tunisien*, chapter 4, sec. 2, art. 38.

33. *Journal officiel tunisien* 38, no. 37 (8 May 1920): 745.

34. *Journal officiel tunisien* 42, no. 43 (28 May 1924): 719.

35. Régence de Tunis, Protectorat Français, *Procès-verbaux, IVe session (Décembre 1925)* (1926), sec. française: 20 December 1925, 150; hereafter cited as GCT.

36. GCT, sess. IV (December 1925), sec. indigène, 98.

37. Ibid., sec. française, 20 December 1925, 144.

38. Ibid., sec. française, 22 December 1925, 324, 337, 345; 23 December 1925, soir, 370.

39. Even, "Protection de la santé publique "; MAE, Tunisie 1917–40, No. 301, P-73-1, doss. no. 1, 5–6.

40. Ibid., doss. no. 7, 48–49.

41. Perrussel, cited in Mignot, "Journées médicales Tunisiennes," 163.

42. ANT, Tunis, série E, 607 9/1, no. 14: letter from Résident-Général to Contrôleurs-Civils, 15 April 1921.

43. Ibid., no. 72: letter from Contrôleur-Civil de Kairouan to Résident-Général, 12 August 1921.

44. Ibid.

45. Stoler, *Race*, 39.

46. Prakash, *Another Reason*, 130–32; also Cohn, "Census."

47. Letter from Ministère de l'Hygiène, de l'Assistance, et de la Prévoyance sociale (MHAPS) to Ministère des Affaires Etrangères, 8 March 1924; MAE: Tunisie 1917–40, No. 304, P-73-1; GCT IV (December 1925), sec. française, 23 December 1925 (soir), 370.

48. Letter from Lucien Saint to Aristide Briand, 26 November 1921; MAE: Tunisie 302, P-73-2 (Hôpitaux 1917–29).

49. Rapport général de la Commission des Travaux Publics et de l'Administration générale, GCT V (December 1926), 21 December 1926.

50. Luccioni to M. le Conseiller, 8 October 1951; CADN Maroc-Protectorat, Direction de l'Intérieur 615.

51. "Les maristanes au Maroc avant le Protectorat"; CADN Maroc-Protectorat, Direction de l'Intérieur 615; emphasis in the original.

52. Georges Sicault, article manuscript on "Santé Publique": CADN, Maroc-Protectorat, Secrétariat Général du Protectorat 141, 1.

53. L'oeuvre de la santé publique au Maroc (Paris: Copernic, 1951), 5–6; emphasis in original.

54. Sicault, "Santé publique," 3.

55. See Rabinow, French Modern, 284–87.

56. Raynaud, Étude sur l'hygiène, 46.

57. Ibid., 54–55.

58. Lwoff and Sérieux, "Sur quelques moyens de contrainte," 169–71.

59. Lwoff and Sérieux, "Aliénés au Maroc," 471, 473, 475.

60. Congrès at Tunis (1912), 1:75.

61. Letter from Lwoff and Sérieux to Ministère des Affaires Etrangères, 29 December 1918; MAE: Maroc 1283, M-63-3 (Hygiène publique, Services sanitaires, Aliénés 1918–26).

62. Ibid., correspondence from 19 November 1921 to 4 October 1926.

63. Memorandum number 1013 from Ministère des Affaires Etrangères to Lyautey, 15 June 1922; and letter from Urbain Blanc to Ministère des Affaires Etrangères, 4 February 1926, and response of 13 February 1926; MAE: Maroc 1283, M-63-3.

64. Anonymous report from Grand Orient de France to Ministère des Affaires Etrangères; ibid.

65. Letter no. 1971 from Lyautey to Ministère des Affaires Etrangères, 19 August 1925; ibid.

66. Congrès at Rabat (1933), 1:56, 58, 73.

67. Périale, "Formations neuro-psychiatriques," Paris médical, 84–85.

68. See Osborne, Nature.

69. See Lorcin, "Imperialism"; Turin, Affrontements culturels, esp. 142–50, 313–18.

70. Voisin, "Aliénés en Algérie," 491.

71. Ibid., 492.

72. Barbier, "Fous et le mal de mer," 228–29.

73. See Foucault, Histoire de la folie, 15–66.

74. Gérente, "Discussion," 45.

75. Gérente and Colin, "Réforme," 1, art. 50.

76. Meilhon, "Aliénation mentale," 357–58; see also Bégué, "Un siècle de psychiatrie française," and Berthelier, Homme maghrébin.

77. Levet, "Assistance des aliénés algériens dans un asile métropolitain," *AMP* 67 (1909): 45–67 and 239–49, at 56, 50, 52, 58–59, and 243–44, respectively.

78. Livet, "Aliénés algériens," 26.

79. See Bégué, "Un siècle de psychiatrie française," 98, and Berthelier, *Homme maghrébin*, 31–33.

80. See Kocher, *De la criminalité*, and Meilhon, "Aliénation mentale," pt. 1, 178.

81. Livet, "Aliénés algériens," 34–35, 43.

82. Rouby, "Un aliéné arabe."

83. See Rouby, "Aliénés arabes" and "Aliénés en liberté."

84. Fanon, *Wretched*, 296–304.

85. Sauzay, "Assistance aux psychopathes," 38.

86. Arrii, "De l'impulsivité criminelle," 51.

87. Vadon, "Assistance médicale, " 28.

88. Desruelles and Bersot, "Assistance aux aliénés en Algérie."

89. Maréschal, "Réflexions," 73.

90. On challenges to the French tradition, see Dean, *Self.* See also Roudinesco, *Bataille de cent ans.*

Chapter 2

1. Macey, *Frantz Fanon*, 212.

2. Cheula, *Hier est proche d'aujourd'hui*, 22.

3. See Macey, *Frantz Fanon*, 212; also Cherki, *Frantz Fanon*, 89.

4. With very few exceptions: see, for example, the 1918 case involving the transportation of a pig farmer from Indochina to France outlined in Centre des Archives d'Outre-Mer, Aix-en-Provence (hereafter CAOM)—Indochine NF 1748.

5. Huot, "Aliénation mentale," esp. 18.

6. On Bien-Hoa, see R. Lefèvre, "Assistance psychiatrique en Indochine."

7. Steeg to Lutaud, cited in Gouvernement Général de l'Algérie, *Comptes rendus des Assemblées financières algériennes, Session extraordinaire de 1923* (Algiers: Société anonyme d'imprimérie rapide, 1923), 66 (30 November). Hereafter AFA.

8. See, e.g., Mabille, *Notice sur l'asile des aliénés.*

9. Mabille-Saliège report, cited in Sauzay, "Assistance aux psychopathes," 15.

10. AFA 1923, Session Extraordinaire: 30 November, Colons, 70.

11. Sauzay, "Assistance aux psychopathes," 18–19.

12. For examples of Steeg's ideological stance on colonial development, see Cohen, "Colonial Policy"; Gershovich, "Ait Ya'qub Incident."

13. Collot, *Institutions de l'Algérie*, 218–19.

14. Baldacci, *C'était ainsi*, 103.

15. AFA 1923, Session Extraordinaire: 30 November, Colons, 74.

16. See Goldstein, *Console and Classify*, 276–321.

17. Toulouse, "Hôpitaux et services," 165.

18. Toulouse, "Ligue de Prophylaxie et d'Hygiène Mentales," n.d., n.p., AN, F22 529.

19. Toulouse and Dupouy, "De la transformation," 83.

20. Toulouse, "Ligue de Prophylaxie et d'Hygiène Mentales."

21. See, e.g., Nolan, *Visions of Modernity.* On the relationship between mental hygiene and Taylorism, see Schneider, "Scientific Study of Labor."

22. Toulouse and Dupouy, "Services ouverts," 5–6, AN F22 529.

23. Toulouse, *Problème de la prophylaxie mentale*, 21.

24. Toulouse, "Ligue de Prophylaxie et d'Hygiène Mentales."

25. See Béguin, "Machine à guérir."

26. See Toulouse, "Conduite de la vie," 3: "Without a doubt, the prevention of these diseases is primarily physical, because they are contagious. Yet the individual, through life discipline of a mental order, can do much to avoid such ills."

27. See, e.g., Kohler, *Lords of the Fly* and *Landscapes and Labscapes*; Kuklick and Kohler, *Science in the Field*; Latour, "Give Me a Laboratory"; Secord, "Crisis of Nature."

28. AN F22 529.

29. Foucault, *Society Must Be Defended*, 242–54.

30. Toulouse, "Problème de la prophylaxie mentale," 7, 13.

31. AN F22 529: Toulouse, "Ligue de Prophylaxie et d'Hygiène mentales," unpublished brochure (27 February 1921).

32. "Centre de psychiatrie et de prophylaxie mentale," 9, AN F22 529.

33. Toulouse and Dupouy, "Organisation générale," AN F22 529.

34. On the psychiatric community's response to the League's proposals, see Wojciechowski, *Hygiène mentale et hygiène sociale*, esp. vol. 2, *La Ligue d'Hygiène et de Prophylaxie Mentales et l'action du docteur Edouard Toulouse (1865–1947) au cours de l'entre-deux-guerres*.

35. Latour, *Pasteurization of France*, 144–45.

36. Sauzay, "Assistance aux psychopathes," 32.

37. J. Lépine, "Organisation de l'assistance aux aliénés en Algérie: Rapport de la Commission de 1924," cited in its entirety in Sauzay, "Assistance aux psychopathes," 33–36, at 34.

38. Sauzay, "Assistance aux psychopathes," 35–36.

39. Fanon, *Wretched*.

40. See esp. Berthelier, *Homme maghrébin*.

41. A. Porot, "Question des injections mercurielles."

42. Maréschal and Lamarche, "Assistance médicale," 394.

43. Michaux, "Professeur Antoine Porot," 71–72.

44. A. Porot, *Manuel alphabétique de psychiatrie*, 642–43. Despite the fact that this volume still bears Porot's name as editor, much of its content has been completely revised; yet he is still remembered as a pioneer in launching open services.

45. A. Porot, "Résultats," 112.

46. Antheaume, "Chronique," and erratum note, "Évolution de l'assistance psychiatrique," ibid., 148 n. 1.

47. Monnais-Rousselot has noted parallel disparities in clinical services in French colonial Indochina; see *Médecine et colonisation*.

48. Bouquet, "Aliénés en Tunisie," 109–13.

49. Régis, "Assistance des aliénés," 181.

50. Antheaume, "Communiqués," 101.

51. *Congrès* at Tunis (1912), 1:73.

52. Ibid., 1:195–97, at 197.

53. A. Porot, "Résultats," 112.

54. AFA 1923, Session Ordinaire: 19 June, Plénière, 367; AFA 1923, Session Extraordinaire: 30 November, Colons, 66.

55. AFA 1923, Session Extraordinaire: 1 December, Indigènes, 72. On relative representation in the assemblies, see Collot, *Institutions de l'Algérie*, 218–19.

56. AFA 1924, Session Ordinaire: 3 June, Non Colons, 427.

57. AFA 1923, Session Extraordinaire: 30 November, Colons, 77.

58. Ibid., 73.

59. AFA 1924, Session Ordinaire: 12 June, Colons, 776; AFA 1924, Session Ordinaire: 3 June, Non Colons, 431.

60. AFA 1925, Session Ordinaire: 23 June, Plénière, 814; AFA 1926, Session Ordinaire: 4 June, Non Colons, 1140.

61. AFA 1929, Session Ordinaire: 15 June, Plénière, 575.

62. AFA 1923, Session Extraordinaire: 30 November, Colons, 77.

63. See, e.g., Cohen, "Colonial Policy," 371–76.

64. Quoted in Stora, *Histoire de l'Algérie coloniale*, 71.

65. Prochaska, *Making Algeria French*, 155.

66. Ageron, *Histoire de l'Algérie contemporaine*, 60; see also Bourdieu and Sayad, *Déracinement*.

67. Lorcin, *Imperial Identities*, 167–213; see also Ageron, *Histoire de l'Algérie contemporaine*, 38–54; Prochaska, *Making Algeria French*, 206–29.

68. As practiced in other French colonies such as West Africa, associationism referred to governance through native elites. The notion of coexistence perhaps better encapsulates the relationship between colonizer and colonized in Algeria, because the inclusion of Algerian Muslims in any but the most local levels of governance remained practically implausible given the extent of French settlement in the colony. On this distinction, see Shepard, "Decolonizing France." On the two policies more generally, see Betts, *Assimilation*.

69. Bonneuil, *Des savants*, 16, 40.

70. Conklin, "Redefining 'Frenchness,'" 71.

71. Scott, "Colonial Governmentality." For manifestations of this problematic in French colonial contexts, see esp. the work of Horne, "In Pursuit of Greater France"; Rabinow, *French Modern*; Wright, "Tradition" and *Politics of Design*.

72. As in many colonial contexts: see Prakash, *Another Reason*, as well as Stoler, *Race*, for examples drawn from British India and the Dutch East Indies. Citation from Prakash, 130–32.

73. See Féry, *Oeuvre médicale*, 33–34.

74. "Création en France d'une Commission d'hygiène mentale coloniale." See also "Arrêté Ministériel" and "Commission d'hygiène mentale."

75. AFA 1923, Session Extraordinaire: 29 November, Non Colons, 11.

76. AFA 1928, Session Ordinaire: 19 June, Plénière, 575.

77. AFA 1929, Session Ordinaire: 15 June, Plénière, 567–68.

78. See, e.g., Viollette's characterization of the situation in Gouvernement Général de l'Algérie, Direction de l'Intérieur, *Assistance et l'hygiène publique*.

79. Maurin, *Khenchela*, 64.

80. Antoine Porot and Raphaël Lalanne, "Note sur l'Assistance des aliénés en Algérie et l'asile en construction à Blida," in AFA 1928, Session Ordinaire: Programme de la session et procès-verbaux de l'assemblée plénière, 74–78, at 75.

81. AFA 1928, Session Ordinaire: 19 June, Plénière, 573.

82. AFA 1928, Session Ordinaire: 13 June, Non Colons, 815.

83. Morton, *Hybrid Modernities*, 6, 176–215.

84. See, e.g., Çelik, *Urban Forms*; King, *Colonial Urban Development* and *Urbanism*; Mitchell, *Colonising Egypt*.

85. See chapter 1.

86. Citation from Çelik, *Urban Forms*, 114–15; see also 38–39, 130–31.

87. Gervais, "Oeuvre sociale," 493.

88. AFA 1923, Session Extraordinaire: 30 November, Colons, 76.

89. Cited in Sauzay, "Assistance aux psychopathes," 39–41.

90. On the beginnings of modern hospital design, see Pinel, *Clinical Training*.

91. A. Porot, "Assistance psychiatrique."

92. Porot-Garnier report, in AFA 1929, Session Ordinaire: Programme de la session et procès-verbaux de l'assemblée plénière, 20–35; on 24.

93. On the imagined violence of the Muslim psychopath, see chapters 1 and 4.

94. A. Porot, "Assistance psychiatrique," 88. By 1933, new studies of this phenomenon had been published by Porot and his student Don Côme Arrii; see Arrii, "De l'impulsivité criminelle," as well as A. Porot and Arrii, "Impulsivité criminelle chez l'indigène algérien," both of which I discuss at length in chapter 4.

95. Porot-Garnier report, 22.

96. Ibid., 33–35.

97. A. Porot, "Assistance psychiatrique," 90.

98. Porot-Garnier report, 25.

99. On Carde's administration of French West Africa, see Conklin, *Mission to Civilize*, esp. 212–45. For the reorganization of Algerian public health, see CAOM, Alg GGA 9X184: esp. Gouvernement Général de l'Algérie, Direction de la Santé Publique, *Developpement*.

100. Lasnet, "Communication," 1308.

101. A. Porot, "Oeuvre psychiatrique," 362.

102. "Instruction sur le fonctionnement des Services de Psychiatrie de 1re ligne dans les hôpitaux d'Alger, Constantine et Oran," 10 August 1934, in Gouvernement Général de l'Algérie, Direction de la Santé Publique, "Organisation."

103. "Arrêté instituant un contrôle technique permanent."

104. AFA 1929, Session Ordinaire: 23 May, Colons, 220, 222.

105. AFA 1929, Session Ordinaire: 15 June, Plénière, 579.

106. AFA 1928, Session Ordinaire: 19 June, Plénière, 576.

107. AFA 1929, Session Ordinaire: 15 June, Plénière, 574.

108. Ernst, *Mad Tales*.

109. A. Porot, "Assistance psychiatrique," 86.

110. Latour, *Pasteurization of France*, 142–45.

111. AFA 1934, Session Ordinaire: 30 May, Non Colons, 419.

112. On other attempts to revisit the past, see Maier, *Recasting Bourgeois Europe*; Roberts, *Civilization without Sexes*.

113. AFA 1932, Session Extraordinaire: 26 October, Plénière, 671–72.

114. A. Porot, "Assistance psychiatrique," 92.

Chapter 3

1. Périale, *Maroc à 60 kms à l'heure*, 234, and "Formations neuro-psychiatriques," 86; "Le traitement des aliénés en Algérie," *L'echo d'Alger*, 3 July 1933, 3. See also Vadon, "Assistance médicale des psychopathes," 13, 51.

2. "L'hôpital psychiatrique de Blida a été inauguré hier par M. le Gouverneur Général Le Beau," *La dépêche algérienne*, 9 April 1938, 2; Yvonne Lartigaud, "Avec les fous à Blida-Joinville," *Algér républicain*, 14 October 1947, 1.

3. "L'hôpital psychiatrique de Blida a été inauguré hier par M. le Gouverneur Général Le Beau," *La dépêche algérienne*, 9 April 1938, 2.

4. "Une grande belle oeuvre française," *La dépêche tunisienne*, 19 February 1931, 2.

5. When citing published case histories, I have used the names and abbreviations supplied by the author. In archival cases, I have concealed patients' identities to protect their and their descendents' privacy.

6. Soumeire, "Meurtre," 43–46.

7. Gouvernement Général de l'Algérie, Direction de la Santé Publique, "Services d'assistance sociale"; AAP: B 5072[3].

8. A. Porot, "Services hospitaliers," 802, 794; emphasis in original.

9. Wright, *Politics of Design*, 3. See also Rabinow, *French Modern*, 277–319.

10. Périale, "Formations neuro-psychiatriques," 86.

11. Vadon, "Assistance médicale," 13, 51.

12. GCT XI (February–March 1932), Sec. française, 149.

13. "Avec le Congrès des neurologistes, M. Georges Le Beau inaugure l'hôpital psychiatrique de Blida-Joinville," *L'echo d'Alger*, 9 April 1938, 4.

14. AFA 1938 (Ordinaire, Plénière), 431, 435.

15. "Rapport sur l'assistance publique," 27 June 1934, Gouvernement Général de l'Algérie, Conseil Supérieur du Gouvernement, session ordinaire de juin 1934, 168; "Fonctionnement de l'Assistance psychiatrique en Algérie," AFA 1936 (Ordinaire, Plénière), 833–37; "Fonctionnement de l'Assistance psychiatrique en Algérie," AFA 1937 (Ordinaire, Plénière), 410–12.

16. GCT XIV (October–November 1935), 67.

17. Pierson, Response to Aubin, *Congrès*, Algiers (1938): 187–89.

18. A. Porot, "Oeuvre psychiatrique," 363.

19. Pierson, Response to Aubin, *Congrès*, Algiers (1938): 187–89.

20. Ibid.; also A. Porot, "Oeuvre psychiatrique," 366.

21. Ministère de la Santé Publique: Internement des aliénés. Correspondence Générale: Circulaire aux Caïds, 20 November 1936; ANT E 607, 9/2, no. 1.

22. Demande d'internement, Commissaire Divisionnaire, Chef de la 4ème Région de Police to Caïd at Sousse, 9 June 1937; ANT E 607, 9/2, no. 27.

23. Bardenat, "Criminalité et délinquance," pt. 1, 324.

24. M. Porot and Gentile, "Alcoolisme et troubles mentaux," 130.

25. A. Porot, "Oeuvre psychiatrique," 366.

26. Donnadieu, "Alcoolisme mental," 163–64.

27. The idea among Destouriens that the French might facilitate heroin distribution in the social milieux most favorable to resistance against colonial authority is extremely significant, regardless of the truth of the accusations. This sentiment parallels accusations that the CIA facilitated the crack explosion in American cities in the late 1980s: see Turner, *I Heard It through the Grapevine*, 137–64, 180–201.

28. Maréschal, "Héroïnomanie en Tunisie," 255–57.

29. GCT XIV (1935), Sec. française, 369.

30. Pressman, *Last Resort*, 154.

31. See Rhodes, "Subject of Power," 56.

32. *Code pénal tunisien*, chapter 4, sec. 1, art. 38.

33. Guiraud, *Code de procédure pénale*, chapter 4, sec. 1, art. 38.

34. See, e.g., Acker, *Creating the American Junkie*.

35. Bardenat, "Criminalité et délinquance," 475.

36. Ibid., 326.

37. Ibid., 321.

38. See, e.g, Sutter, *Épilepsie mentale*, as well as A. Porot and Sutter, "'Primitivisme.'"

39. Sutter, "Une famille des psychopathes."

40. Ibid., 40.

41. Demassieux, "Service social psychiatrique"; hereafter cited parenthetically in the text as "SSP."

42. More recently, see Fuller, *Don't Let's Go*. For historical studies, see Ernst, *Mad Tales*; Jacob, "Psychiatrie française"; Anderson, "Trespass Speaks"; Fabian, *Out of Our Minds*.

43. Margain, "Aliénation mentale."

44. Lorcin, *Imperial Identities*, esp. 196–213.

45. Escande de Messières, *Psychologie des coloniaux*, 17–18. See also Lemanski, *Hygiène du Colon*, and Joyeux, *Hygiène de l'Européen*.

46. Gouvernement Général de l'Algérie, Direction de la Santé Publique, "Oeuvre française," 1, 31; Aix-en-Provence, Centre d'Archives d'Outre-Mer, Algérie, GGA, 9X184, DSP.

47. As opposed to fewer than a third of the Algerian patients; see, among other sources, A. Porot, "Oeuvre psychiatrique."

48. Lunbeck, *Psychiatric Persuasion*; Kunzel, *Fallen Women*.

49. See Foucault, *History of Sexuality*, and "Governmentality." See also Donzelot, *Policing of Families*; Schaefer, *Children in Moral Danger*.

50. For a listing of the dozens of programs operative in Algiers alone, see Union des Institutions Privées de Protection de la Santé Publique et d'Assistance Sociale du Dpt. d'Alger, "L'Effort Social Algerois: Alger et ses oeuvres bienfaisantes" [1942]; CAOM, Algérie, GGA, 9X194.

51. Donnadieu, "Situation actuelle."

52. E.g., M. Porot and Duboucher, "Guerison."

53. A. Porot, "Oeuvre psychiatrique," 364.

54. Several histories of psychiatry dwell on this problem. Most informative is Braslow, *Mental Ills and Bodily Cures*. See also Valenstein, *Great and Desperate Cures*; Shorter, *History of Psychiatry*.

55. M. Porot, "Cardiazol" and "Cardiazol-Test."

56. M. Porot, "Insulinotherapie," 311.

57. Kalinowsky and Hoch, *Shock Treatments*, 37–51, 91–94; see also Pressman, *Last Resort*, 158.

58. Cerletti and Bini, "Elettroshock," 266.

59. See Yealland, *Hysterical Disorders*; see also Brunner, "Psychiatry, Psychoanalysis, and Politics."

60. Cerletti, "Old and New Information," 90–91.

61. Lapipe and Rondepierre, "Essai d'un appareil français" and "Électro-choc (2e note)"; Plichet, "Électro-choc."

62. Baruk et al., "Etude expérimentale," 81.

63. Poitrot, "Considérations," 220.

64. Maréschal, Ben Soltane, and Corcos, "Résultats," 341–43. In a brief *aperçu historique* on electroshock, Ebtinger referred to this meeting of the Congrès as an *étape marquante* in the history of electroshock; *Aspects psychopathologiques*, 25.

65. Maréschal et al., "Résultats," 345.

66. Cited in Bouzgarrou, " À propos d'une expérience," 24; emphasis in original.

67. Igert and Viaud, "Bilan," 218; A. Porot et al., "Réflexions," 329–31, 336; emphasis in original

68. Houssin, "Un cas de confusion," 228.

69. M. Porot, "Electrochoc"; M. Porot and Bisquerra, "Note préliminaire."

70. M. Porot and Cohen-Tenoudji, "Tuberculose." Also M. Porot, "Electrochocs et cardiopathies."

71. Igert and Viaud, "Bilan d'une année d'électro-chocs," 219.

72. Maréschal, Ben Soltane, and Corcos, "Résultats," 341–43.

73. M. Porot and Descuns, "État actuel," 532. Braslow has determined, for example, that physicians performed 245 lobotomies at Stockton State Hospital in California in the same period (1947–54), but this hospital held nearly 5,000 patients. Blida, by contrast, housed only 2,200 patients in 1955.

74. Ibid., 139–40.

75. Carrère, "Nécessité," 280–81. Also Jean Mons to Contrôleurs Civils et Chefs de Bureau des Affaires Indigènes, 22 June 1949; ISHMN (Nantes), 1960B, 2, no. 578; Section d'État, Circulaire no. 19 C PM/SE, 13 August 1949; Caïd at Mateur to Premier Ministre, 16 December 1949; and Ministère de la Santé Publique to Premier Ministre no. 1897, 21 March 1950; ANT 607, 9/3, nos. 17, 21–22, 26.

76. Cited in Bouzgarrou, "À propos d'une expérience," 24.

77. Ammar, "Assistance aux aliénés en Tunisie," 26; Ministère de la Santé Publique, "Note d'Audience," 26 December 1949. ISHMN (Nantes), 1960B, 2, fol. 643; Maréschal, "Réflexions," 70–71.

78. Dequeker et al., "Aspects actuels," 11–12, 14.

79. Couderc, "Assistance psychiatrique dans le Département d'Oran (Algérie)," 19.

80. M. Porot and Descuns, "État actuel," 532.

81. Ibid., 535.

82. Ibid., 537.

83. CAOM: Gouvernement Général de l'Algérie (GGA), Département d'Alger 1K751, doss. 2, sous dérogation. Because these files are classified until 2017, I have changed names to protect the privacy of patients and their families. For the same reason, the authors of letters to government officials cannot be specified.

84. These cases are drawn from CAOM: GGA, Alger, 1K751, doss. 2 and loose files. For Tunisian examples, see ANT, SGGT, Série E 607, 9/2, no. 12, and E 607, 9/3.

85. Fanon, *Dying Colonialism*, 121; hereafter cited parenthetically in the text as *DC*.

86. On Western biomedical approaches to disease, see esp. Kleinman, "What Is Specific," 1:15–23; also Eisenberg, "Disease and Illness," 11; Rosenberg, "Framing Disease."

87. Foucault, *Histoire de la folie*, 614–23.

88. Sadowsky, *Imperial Bedlam*, 49; see also Rhodes, "Subject of Power."

89. Taïeb, "Idées d'influence," obs. 32.

90. Doutté, *Magie et religion*, 36, 38.

91. Crapanzano, *Hamadsha*, 5; also Taoufik Adohane, "Un remède," and "Nourrisson médusé."

92. Crapanzano, *Hamadsha*, 178–82.

93. See Geertz, "Common Sense," 78.

94. Crapanzano, *Hamadsha*, 149–68.

95. See especially Pandolfo, *Impasse*. Rabinow includes an account of an Aïssawa *hadra* in his *Reflections*, 50–58. Maraboutism is common in some West African Islamic communities as well; see Soubeiga, "Syncrétisme," 54–64; Fall, "Marabouts," 82–87.

96. Douglas, *Fountains*, 53.

97. Ibid., 185.

98. Rabinow, *Reflections*, 50.

99. For the political assault on maraboutic tradition in post-independence Tunisia, see Schilder, *Popular Islam*, 73. See also Crapanzano, *Hamadsha*, 7.

100. Valensi, *Tunisian Peasants*; see also Schilder, *Popular Islam*, 13–35.

101. Taïeb, "Idées d'influence"; cases hereafter cited parenthetically in the text as Taïeb.

102. Bégué and Berthelier both cite Taïeb's thesis as a turning point in the evolution of ethnopsychiatric theory about Algerians. This is doubtful: although she certainly moved far beyond her colleagues in her efforts to understand Algerian and Tunisian subjects on their own terms, the Algiers School's imprint remains clear in the general conclusions she proffers. Her ethnographic approach signals a departure, but at the same time, her findings that "primitivism" and "intellectual poverty" mark an essentialized North African psychology are of a piece with A. Porot and Sutter, especially because she cites Lévy-Bruhl and Blondel throughout the thesis. See Bégué, "Un siècle de psychiatrie française," 217–19; Berthelier, *Homme maghrébin*, 125.

103. As in the case of a tubercular man who never received treatment and died in the hospital after eight years of suffering from the disease: Bardenat, "Criminalité et délinquance," 329.

104. Sadowsky, *Imperial Bedlam*, 75.

105. CAOM 1K751.

106. Taïeb, "Idées d'influence," 26.

107. Braslow introduces the analogy of a language barrier in the relationship between doctors and patients in American state mental hospitals in *Mental Ills and Bodily Cures*, 47.

108. *Congrès*, Rabat (1933), 66.

109. See Osborne, *Nature*; Warwick Anderson, "Immunities"; Comaroff, "Diseased Heart."

110. See esp. Stoler, *Race*; Clancy-Smith and Gouda, *Domesticating Empire*.

111. *Congrès*, Rabat (1933), 66.

Chapter 4

1. Donnadieu, "Psychose de civilisation," 30–37.

2. Ibid., 35.

3. Cohen, *French Encounter*.

4. Bégué, "Un siècle de psychiatrie française"; Berthelier, *Homme maghrébin*; see also Bulhan, "Revolutionary Psychiatry of Fanon."

5. Fanon, *Wretched*, 296.

6. Jacob, "Psychiatrie française."

7. Moreau (de Tours), "Recherches sur les aliénés."

8. Although the theory lived on in different contexts; see Anderson, "Trespass Speaks."

9. Kocher, *De la criminalité chez les Arabes*, 103–6.

10. Ibid., 133, 169–77, 181. Although Bégué and Berthelier discuss Kocher's constitutionalist thesis, they ignore these observations about sexuality.

11. Of 184 convictions between 1879 and 1881, the Cour d'Assises in Algiers found 162 Arabs and only 22 Europeans guilty of violent crimes; ibid., 103–6.

12. Meilhon, "Aliénation mentale chez les Arabes," pt. 1: 17–18.

13. Ibid., pt. 2: 180–83.

14. Ageron, *Histoire de l'Algérie contemporaine*, 60.

15. Marie, "Conférence," 16 March 1907, 1.

16. Ibid., 19 March 1907, 6.

17. Ibid., 22 March 1907, 4, 9–10; 19 March 1907, 25.

18. Ibid., 26 March 1907, 4. See also Le Bon, *Psychology of Peoples*.

19. Marie, "Conférence," 29 March 1907, 4–7.

20. Ibid., 28.

21. Marie, "Rapport sur la question des asiles coloniaux," 3–4.

22. Trenga, *Âme arabo-berbère*; also Trenga, *Sur les psychoses*, 7–15.

23. Trenga, *Âme arabo-berbère*, 211.

24. Ibid., 214.

25. See Lorcin, *Imperial Identities*.

26. See Prochaska, *Making Algeria French*; also Lewis, "Company of Strangers."

27. Even Meilhon, who distinguished Arabs from Kabyles, still tended to overlook these differences: despite his emphasis on "a great distinction [that] must be established among our *indigènes*," he generally assimilated the groups to one another in "Aliénation mentale chez les Arabes," 23–24.

28. Ibid., 14–16; emphasis in original.

29. Ibid., 37, 46, 69n.

30. A. Porot and Hesnard, *Psychiatrie de guerre*, 59–60.

31. Ibid., 63. See also A. Porot, "Notes."

32. A. Porot, "Notes," 377.

33. Le Bon, *Psychologie des foules*; see also Nye, *Origins of Crowd Psychology*.

34. A. Porot, "Notes," 378–83.

35. See Landau, *Juifs de France*, esp. 161–85 and 211–51.

36. Bégué, "Un siècle de psychiatrie française," 211; Berthelier, *Homme maghrébin*, 85.

37. Adas, *Machines as the Measure of Men*, 345–401.

38. See, e.g., Clifford, *Predicament of Culture*; also Kucklick, *Savage Within*; Torgovnick, *Gone Primitive*, esp. 105–18.

39. Although he had intended to entitle the 1910 volume *Primitive Mentality*, he noted that "at that time the expressions 'mentality,' and even 'primitive,' were not current terms as they are to-day"; Lévy-Bruhl, *Primitive Mentality*, 11.

40. Ibid., 431.

41. Ibid., 29–30, 431–42. Lévy-Bruhl even took issue with the term "primitive" itself: he argued that term was "inappropriate" but "nearly indispensable" for describing "members of the most simple societies with which we are familiar"; *Fonctions mentales*, 2 n.

42. Jude and Augagneur, "Utilité de l'étude."

43. Ibid., 266.

44. Martin, "Mentalité primitive indigène," 93, 104.

45. Peyre, "Maladies mentales aux colonies," 185–98, 212.

46. See Foster, "Primitive Scenes."

47. See Clifford, *Predicament of Culture*, 61; Conklin, *Mission to Civilize*, 197.

48. Rubenovitch, "Notion d'évolution," 89.

49. Freud, *Totem and Taboo*.

50. Roheim, "Psychoanalysis of Primitive Cultural Types"; see also Rose, *On Not Being Able to Sleep*, 125–48.

51. See esp. Roudinesco, *Bataille de cent ans*, I.

52. Lauriol, *Quelques remarques*, 55–56.

53. Dumas, "Mentalité paranoïde," 759.

54. Lévy-Valensi, "Mentalité primitive et psychopathologie," 685.

55. Bursztyn, *Schizophrénie*, 74.

56. Ibid., 75; this real is not the Lacanian real: here Bursztyn opposes external reality and the metaphysical.

57. Dean, *Self*, 43–45, 51–53.

58. See especially Lacan's medical thesis, *De la psychose paranoïaque*. Lacan asserted that paranoia represented a manifestation of complex structures within the personality rather than the "all or nothing of mental decay" that preoccupied orthodox psychiatry, but he still attributed violent outbursts to the condition; see Lacan, "Problème du style" and "Motifs du crime." See also Dean, *Self*, 42–48; Roudinesco, *Jacques Lacan*, 31–51; Roudinesco and Plon, "Paranoïa."

59. Martin, "Mentalité primitive indigène," 101.

60. See, e.g., Wallon, "Oeuvre de Lévy-Bruhl."

61. *Congrès*, Rabat (1933): 64–65.

62. *Congrès*, Brussels (1935): 38.

63. Marie, "Rapport sur la question des asiles coloniaux," 4.

64. Aubin, "Esquisse," 174.

65. See Prochaska, *Making Algeria French*, 155.

66. Arrii, "De l'impulsivité criminelle," 19.

67. Ibid., 33–35.

68. Bégué is careful to note this as well; see "Un siècle de psychiatrie française," 152–54, 175–78.

69. Arrii, "De l'impulsivité criminelle," 40–41.

70. Macey, "Algerian with the Knife," 165.

71. A. Porot and Arrii, "Impulsivité criminelle chez l'indigène algérien," 588–611.

72. See Barthes, *Critical Essays*, 186–87. For histories of the *fait divers*, see Walker, *Outrage and Insight*; Kalifa, "Tâcherons de l'information."

73. See Walkowitz, *City of Dreadful Delight*.

74. Stora, *Histoire de l'Algérie coloniale*, 54–58; see also Bourdieu and Sayad, *Déracinement*.

75. Arrii, "De l'impulsivité criminelle," 13.

76. Sutter, *Épilepsie mentale*, 132. See also Bégué's discussion of Sutter's thesis in "Un siècle de psychiatrie française."

77. A. Porot and Sutter, "'Primitivisme,'" 226.

78. Ibid., 234; see also Bardenat, "Criminalité et délinquance dans l'aliénation mentale chez les indigènes algériens," pts. 1 and 2.

79. A. Porot and Sutter, "Primitivisme," 234.

80. See Fanon, *Wretched*, 301; Bégué, "Un siècle de psychiatrie française," 201–13; Berthelier, *Homme maghrébin*, 83–85; Macey, "Algerian with the Knife," 165; McCulloch, *Colonial Psychiatry*, 107.

81. See Cohen, "Colonial Policy," 379–82.

82. See Bhabha, "Mimicry and Man."

83. Bardenat, "Criminalité et délinquance," pt. 1, 319–20, 332–33.

84. J. C. Carothers of Nairobi was an exception, although he too only began formal psychiatric training years after he became director of Mathari Mental Hospital; see McCulloch, *Colonial Psychiatry*, 137–46.

85. Courbon, review of A. Porot and Sutter, "Primitivisme."

86. Charpentier, review of A. [*sic*] Porot, "Alcoolisme en Algérie"; Sutter, review of Taïeb, "Idées d'influence."

87. Charpentier, review of Aubin, "Test évolutif."

88. Charpentier, review of Aubin, "Epilepsie psychique."

89. Review of Aubin, "Mensonge."

90. Charpentier, review of Sutter, "Indigènes nord-africains au combat."

91. Charpentier, review of M. Porot et al., "Situation familiale."

92. A. Porot et al., *Manuel*, 217; hereafter cited parenthetically in text.

93. Plichet, review of A. Porot et al., *Manuel*.

94. Charpentier, review of A. Porot et al., *Manuel*, 649–50.

95. Porot and Bardenat, *Psychiatrie médico-légale* and *Anormaux et malades mentaux*.

96. Porot and Bardenat, *Anormaux et malades mentaux*, 63.

97. See Michel, "Algériens à l'hôtel à Paris." The "psychopathology" to which the author refers is the hostility metropolitan hoteliers and employers constantly directed at North Africans. See also Delore, Lambert, and Marin, "Enquête."

98. Alliez and Descombes, "Réflexions," 153.

99. Daumezon, Champion, and Champion-Basset, "Étude démographique et statistique," 106.

100. Daumezon, Champion, and Champion-Basset, *Assistance psychiatrique aux malades mentaux*, 8, 15, 94.

101. Hirsch, "Criminalité des nord-africains en France," 129; emphasis in the original; hereafter cited parenthetically in the text as "CNA."

102. "Papiers d'agents pièces annexées à la correspondance d'Alapetite avec Peretti de la Rocca et pièces diverses," ISHMN (Quai d'Orsay), 8, dossier 2, fol. 223.

103. Borel, "Nord-Africains malades mentaux."

104. Fanon, *Dying Colonialism*, 124 n., 135, 139 n.; *Wretched*, 284, 288.

105. Porot and Bardenat, *Anormaux et malades mentaux*, 155–56. Porot and Bardenat admitted, however, that they "only envisage[d] xenophobia here as a

strictly individual behavior or reaction . . . and not as a collective movement or uprising against occupants."

106. Porot and Bardenat, *Psychiatrie medico-légale*, 305.

107. Maurin, *Khenchela*, 189–90.

108. See Fanon, *Dying Colonialism*, 69–97.

109. SHAT 10 H 346: A. Fossey-François, "Historique de l'action psychologique en Indochine de 1945 au 20 juillet 1954," 1.

110. On the American use of psychological warfare in the Second World War, see Dower's classic *War without Mercy*.

111. SHAT 10 H 346: Rapport de mission du Capitaine Jacques C. Giraud, de l'Infantérie Coloniale, 14 August 1953.

112. Fossey-François, "Historique," 18.

113. SHAT 10 H 346: État-Major Interarmées de Forces Terrestres [EMIFT]: Section d'Action Psychologique Stage de Guerre psychologique. Exposé du Capitaine Caniot de la Section Technique de l'Armée sur "Quelques enseignements de la guerre psychologique en Indochine," n. d. (1953).

114. See Kayanakis's somewhat problematic *Algérie 1960* for a general narrative of the program's history.

115. SHAT 10 H 346: EMIFT: "Quelques Enseignements de la Guerre Psychologique en Indochine."

116. Centre des Archives d'Outre-Mer, Aix-en-Provence (CAOM), SAS/DOC/5: "Memento de l'Officier d'Action Psychologique en Algérie," Appendix 5: "La psychologie de coeur," 2; SHAT, 1 H 2409 1: "Extrait d'un compte-rendu de stage en AFN établi par des officiers stagiaires de la 70e promotion de l'École Supérieure de Guerre."

117. SHAT, 1 H 2409 1: "Extrait d'un compte-rendu de stage en AFN établi par des officiers stagiaires de la 70e promotion de l'École Supérieure de Guerre."

118. SHAT, 1 H 2411: Secrétariat d'État aux Forces Armées "Terre," État-Major de l'Armée, 3e Bureau, "Notice d'Information sur la defense intérieure du territoire et la guerre psychologique," Section II: "Notions de guerre psychologique adaptées à l'Algérie," 3 November 1956 (hereafter "Notions de guerre psychologique").

119. SHAT, 1 H 2409 1: "Fondements scientifiques de la guerre psychologique."

120. "Notions de guerre psychologique," 46.

121. SHAT 1 H 2411: "Comment obtenir des renseignements d'un prisonnier de guerre." On interrogation during the Algerian War, see Talbott, *War without a Name*; Maran, *Torture*; and Branche, *Torture et l'armée*.

122. SHAT 1 H 2460 1: Letter from Colonel Juigner, Chef du Secrétariat Permanent du Comité d'Action Scientifique de Défense nationale, to M. le Chef du Cinquième Bureau, Alger (à l'attention du Lt. Col. Garde): "Étude sur la mentalité des musulmans," 1959.

123. Alleg, *Guerre d'Algérie*, 2:383. On the SAS, see Mathias, *Sections administratives spécialisées en Algérie*; also Lacoste-Dujardin, *Opération Oiseau Bleu*.

124. "Memento de l'Officier d'Action Psychologique en Algérie," 5; emphasis in original.

125. Ibid.

126. Ibid., Annexe V, 1.

127. SHAT 1 H 2411: "Comprendre et agir," 4.

128. SHAT 1 H 2411: "Contribution de l'Armée à l'oeuvre de pacification: Annexes."

129. "L'oeuvre de la France en Afrique du Nord fera l'objet d'une leçon spéciale dans toutes les classes," *Le Monde*, 2–3 February 1958.

130. Manue, "Guerre psychologique."

131. SHAT 1 H 2411: "Enseignements à tirer sur campagne d'Algérie," memorandum 5238 from General R. Quenard to 10ème Région Militaire, Commandement des Troupes et Services des Territoires du Sud Algérien."

132. "Étude sur la mentalité des musulmans."

133. CAOM, SAS/DOC/5: "Plan type de panneau pour hall d'information."

134. "Une notice officielle fixe les règles de l'action psychologique' dans les camps d'hébergement," *Le Monde* (23 January 1958), 4.

135. Ibid.

136. SHAT 1 H 2411: "Les étudiants en psychologie s'interrogent sur l'utilisation de leur science."

137. Amrouche, "Aspects psychologiques," 287–88; Ferhat Abbas, "Au-delà de l'action psychologique," in *Guerre et révolution d'Algérie: La nuit coloniale* (Paris: Julliard, 1962), 21–41. For a French critic's reaction to *action psychologique*, see Duquesne, *Algérie ou la guerre des mythes*.

Chapter 5

1. Foucault, *Birth of the Clinic*. A small sampling of works informed by Foucauldian understandings of biopower includes those by Agamben, *Homo Sacer*; Stoler, *Race*; Donzelot, *Policing of Families*; and Rabinow, *French Modern*.

2. Bulhan, *Fanon and Oppression*, esp. 207–25; Geismar, *Fanon*; Gendzier, *Frantz Fanon*, 76; McCulloch, *Black Soul*, esp. 101–7; Youssef and Fadl, "Political Psychiatry." Although Ehlen, *Frantz Fanon*, 107–23, admits that Fanon most likely never "unchained" patients at Blida, he largely subscribes to the image of Fanon as a superhuman "liberator of minds."

3. McCulloch, *Black Soul*, 83, 101, 104; Youssef and Fadl, "Political Psychiatry," 529.

4. See Hansen, "Fanon, Revolutionary Intellectual"; Geismar, *Fanon*, 163.

5. Youssef and Fadl, "Political Psychiatry," 530.

6. Julien, *Black Skin*.

7. Fanon, *Pour la révolution africaine*.

8. Fanon, *Wretched*, 296.

9. Ibid., 309.

10. Khanna, *Dark Continents*, 150.

11. Scheper-Hughes, *Death without Weeping*, passim; see also the reiteration of her ideas in the introduction by Das and Kleinman and in the essays by Ramphele in *Violence and Subjectivity*.

12. Fanon, *Wretched*, 305–6.

13. Boigey, "Étude psychologique," 6; italics in the original.

14. Chérif, "Étude psychologique sur l'Islam," 353–54, 358, 361, 363.

15. On colonial education, see Scham, *Lyautey in Morocco*, 144–61; Bidwell, *Morocco under Colonial Rule*, 237–57; Colonna, *Instituteurs algériens*; Turin, *Affrontements culturels*.

16. Bernard, *Conflit franco-marocain*, 2:135.

17. Fanon, *Wretched*, 58–60.

18. Chraïbi, *Passé simple*, 208.

19. Memmi, *Statue de sel*, 119–28.

20. Bardenat, "Criminalité et délinquance," pt. 1, 332–33.

21. Memmi, *Colonizer and Colonized*, 124; henceforth cited in text as *CC*.

22. Farmer, "On Suffering."

23. Farmer, *Infections and Inequalities*, esp. 76–82.

24. Amrouche, "Aspects psychologiques du problème algérien," in *Un Algérien s'adresse aux Français*, 288–92.

25. Fanon, *Wretched*, 288.

26. "Notes pour une esquisse de l'état d'âme du colonisé," in *Un Algérien s'adresse*, 49–51; orig. in *Etudes méditerranéennes*, 1958; "La France comme mythe et comme réalité," in ibid., 55; orig. in *Le Monde*, 11 January 1958. Duquesne, *Algérie ou la guerre des mythes*, 90–101, 116–17, argued that this psychological assault produced stronger results in Algeria's European community than in the indigenous population: the repeated assertion that Muslims were "lazy, liars, thieves, etc." may have produced an "inferiority complex" in Algerians, but more effectively it "justified the privileges of the settler."

27. A. Porot and Hesnard, *Expertise mentale militaire*, 14.

28. Sutter, *Épilepsie mentale*, 132.

29. Fanon, "Rencontre," 2.

30. Ammar, "Folie à travers les âges," 1–4. My pagination pertains to an off-print of the article conserved at the Institut de Belles Lettres Arabes, Tunis.

31. On Nazi medicine, see Proctor, *Racial Hygiene*, and Burleigh, *Ethics and Extermination*, esp. 113–25; for an exploration of the complicated legacy of Nazi medicine, see Harrington's incisive "Unmasking Suffering's Masks." For the origins of French antipsychiatry in this era, see Meyer, "Antipsychiatrie."

32. Police Spéciale des chemins de fer et des ports, Tunis, to SGGT, no. 741, 27 June 1919; Commissaire Spécial to M. le Directeur de la Securité, 18 March 1919; Ministère de l'Intérieur—Police Spéciale des Chemins de Fer et de la Frontière to Commissariat Général et al., no. 2054, 17 May 1919; and Ministre de l'Intérieur to MAE, no. 3169, 12 August 1919 in ANT E: 550, d. 30/15, sd. 1780.

33. "Rythme paradoxal," 18. See also Saida Douki, "Rapport concernant la demande de rehabilitation de feu le docteur Salem Esch-Chadely," Esch-Chadely Papers, unpaginated.

34. Esch-Chadely, "Rythme paradoxal," 18. In an article published in *L'etendard tunisien* (25 January 1929), Esch-Chadely criticized Arrii's thesis on Algerian criminality as "scientific heresy and a grotesque lie"; cited in Douki, "Rapport."

35. Arrêté of 20 June 1934. See the subsequent debate over the position in the proceedings of the Grand Conseil de la Tunisie XV (October–December 1936), Conseil Supérieur, 358, 362.

36. Dr. Dupoux, "Note sur Monsieur le docteur Salem ben Ahmed Ech Chadly," 13 May 1939. ANT E 609, d. 7.

37. Mahmoud el Matéri, "A l'asile de Manouba," *Tunis-soir*, 9 November 1936, 2.

38. *Nahdha*, 7 December 1936; cited in Administration Tunisienne: Compte-rendu de la presse arabe. ANT E 553, d. 3/2, fol. 151.

39. GCT XV (October–December 1936), Conseil Supérieur, 358, 362. See also Esch-Chadely to M. Lagrosillière, 28 April 1939. ANT E 609, d. 7.

40. Interview with Newine Eschadely (Tunis, 14 May 2000); Douki, "Rapport"; Ben Youssef, "Docteur"; M. Ennabli, cited in Bouzgarrou, "À propos d'une expérience," 4.

41. Kateb, *Poète*, 14.

42. Kateb, *Polygone étoilé*, 182.

43. E.g., Aresu, introduction, xiv.

44. Yacine, "Poésie et vérité," 39.

45. Estimates range between 1,000 and 45,000 victims in the reprisals; see Horne, *Savage War*, 27.

46. Ibid.; Kateb, "Poésie et verité," 39.

47. Arnaud, *Recherches*, 2:493–94; also Mathilde la Bardonnie, "Un tramway nommé Yacine," *Libération*, 21 October 1999.

48. Kateb, "La femme sauvage/1," in *Oeuvre en fragments*, 164.

49. Kateb, "La rose de Blida," 9.

50. *Nedjma*, 225–26; henceforth cited in text as *N*.

51. An aspect at which Arnaud has hinted: see *Recherches*, 2:415–16.

52. *Cadavre encerclé*, in *Cercle des représailles*, 62–63.

53. Abdel-Jaouad, "'Too Much in the Sun.'"

54. Freud, "Mourning and Melancholia," 246, 244.

55. Abdel-Jaouad, "'Too Much in the Sun,'" 24.

56. Taïeb, "Idées d'influence," 78.

57. Freud, "Mourning and Melancholia," 243.

58. Kleinman and Kleinman, "Appeal of Experience," 10.

59. Farmer, *Infections and Inequalities*, 5; also "On Suffering and Structural Violence," 273–76.

60. Agamben, *Homo Sacer*, passim.

61. Biehl, "Vita," 131.

62. Fanon, *Dying Colonialism*, 120–45.

63. Ibid., 128.

64. Kateb, *Cadavre encerclé*, 62–64.

65. Dequeker et al., "Aspects actuels," 11–18.

66. See esp. Macey's account of these experiments in *Frantz Fanon*, 227–39.

67. "Lettre au Ministre-Résident" (1956), in *Pour la révolution africaine* (Paris: Maspéro, 1964).

68. Bouzgarrou, " À propos d'une expérience," 12, 19–20, 26.

69. Fanon and Geromini, "Hospitalisation."

70. See Macey, *Frantz Fanon*, 241–301.

71. Fanon, *Wretched*, 304.

72. SGGT to Dr. Dupoux, Direction de l'Assistance et de la Santé Publique, 3 May 1939; Dupoux, "Note"; in ANT E 609, d. 7; see also Douki, "Rapport." On the nationalist movement in the 1930s, see Kraiem, *Mouvement national*; also Garas, *Bourguiba*, 43–120. On the beginnings of this movement in the 1920s see Schaar, "Creation."

73. "Un Algérien s'adresse aux Français," in *Un Algérien s'adresse*, 31.

74. Chérif, *Histoire*. The chapter on Ibn Omran was reprinted as Chérif, "Médecine arabe en Tunisie."

75. Gallagher, *Medicine and Power*, 83–101.

76. Résidence-Générale, Direction des Contrôles, "Notice: Docteur Ahmed Chérif," n. d. ISHMN (Nantes), 1960B d. 1, fol. 313–14.

77. Ammar, "Folie à travers les âges," 1–4.

78. This is the first violent scene *chronologically*, although it appears twenty pages after the second in the text.

79. Fanon, *Wretched*, 305–6.

80. See Chatinières, *Dans le Grand Atlas marocain*, vii–viii.

81. Ibid., i–viii; Kateb, "Ce pays est un grand hôpital," in *Oeuvre en fragments*, 391–93.

82. Arnold, *Colonizing the Body*, 9.

83. Thanks to an anonymous reviewer for sharing this insight.

84. I draw here on the notion of the evidentiary "fragment" employed by Pandey, "In Defense of the Fragment," esp. 28–30.

Chapter 6

1. The film was released as both *Poetical Refugee* and *Blame It on Voltaire* in American festivals.

2. Goffman, "Characteristics" and *Asylums*; Foucault, *Histoire de la folie*; and Laing, *Divided Self* are foundational texts of the antipsychiatry movement. But see also Swain, *Sujet de la folie*; Castel, *Ordre psychiatrique*.

3. For an outline of the EMIs and the specific problems of wartime medicine in Algeria, see Amir, *Contribution*; see also Khiati, *Histoire de la médecine*.

4. Ministère de la Santé Publique to Premier Ministre no. 1897, 21 March 1950; ANT 607, 9/3, no. 26.

5. Ammar, "Assistance aux aliénés en Tunisie," 26; Maréschal, "Réflexions," 70–71.

6. Sleïm Ammar, "Rapport de la Commission de l'Hygiène Mentale et l'Assistance Publique," presented at the Premières Journées Médico-Sociales Tunisiennes, Tunis, 2–3 June 1956; Ammar Papers.

7. Although he later lauded Porot for some of his accomplishments; see Ammar, "Antoine et Maurice Porot."

8. Ammar, "Assistance psychiatrique moderne: Principales données et perspectives. Introduction générale à un programme d'action à long terme en Tunisie," Extrait de *La Tunisie médicale* (1962): 1–7; Ammar Papers. See also "Les desordres psychiques dans la société tunisienne: Leur évolution et fréquence en fonction des transformations socio-économiques et culturelles depuis l'indépendance," Extrait de *La Tunisie médicale* (1964), unpaginated; Ammar Papers.

9. Chkili, "Assistance psychiatrique," 345–47; see also Larheribi, "Maladie mentale."

10. Boucebci and Yaker, "Aspects généraux," 357.

11. Fanon, *Dying Colonialism*, 120–45.

12. See Bakiri, "À propos de l'organisation."

13. See Fanon and Geromini, "TAT en milieu maghrébin."

14. Daoud, "Chez les fous," 24.

15. Benslama, *Psychanalyse*.

16. Stora, *Histoire de la guerre*, 82.

17. See Boutet de Monvel, *Boudjedra l'insolé*; Harrow, "Metaphors for Revolution."

18. Alemdjrodo, *Rachid Boudjedra*, explores some of these connections, as does Boutet de Monvel, *Boudjedra l'insolé*.

19. Alemdjrodo, *Rachid Boudjedra*, 63–64.

20. Boudjedra, *Insolation*, 27.

21. Ziou Ziou, "Psychiatrie moderne?," 52.

22. Boucebci, *Maladie mentale*.

23. Interview with Cherifa Ammar (Tunis, 16 May 2000). See also Ben Rejeb, "À propos de la transe psychothérapeutique."

24. Ammar, "Assistance aux aliénés en Tunisie," 8. For Ammar's change in attitude, see "Désordres psychiques" and "Troubles mentaux en Tunisie."

25. Mohia, "Pratiques traditionnelles," 57–58.

26. For other examples of interest in Maghrebian healing practices, see Adohane, "Nourrisson médusé" and "Remède pour les pensées"; also Lheimeur, "À la croisée d'une rencontre."

27. See Loussaief, "Assistance psychiatrique en Tunisie."

28. Jeddi, *Al Baab*. See also Devisch and Vervaeck, "Doors and Thresholds"; Bouzgarrou, "À propos d'une expérience "; and Jeddi et al., "Corps et asile." The reforms were also followed in the Tunisian press: see Baraket, "Pour une psychiatrie ouverte"; Khélil, "Drames"; and a series of short articles in *Le phare*, November–December 1981.

29. Silverstein, *Algeria in France*, 2.

30. See, e.g., Léger, Péron, and Vallat, "Aspects actuels de la sorcellerie"; Jacquel and Morel, "Sorcellerie et troubles mentaux."

31. Rosenberg, "Republican Surveillance," and Lewis, "Company of Strangers," have expertly studied immigration in this period. See also Noiriel, *Creuset français*, and Taguieff, "Face à l'immigration," among others.

32. Silverstein, *Algeria in France*, 6.

33. Gastaut, *Immigration et l'opinion*, 111–14.

34. For a different interpretation of the historical relationship between psychiatry and immigration in France, see Meriem, "Sociologie et psychiatrie."

35. Jeddi, "Aspect sociogène."

36. See esp. Ben Jelloun, *Hospitalité française*.

37. Ben Jelloun, *Plus haute des solitudes*, 11, 51.

38. Ibid., 12–15.

39. Ibid., 18.

40. Ibid., 15, 175–8.

41. Sayad, *Double absence*, 255–303; the essay, titled "La maladie, la souffrance et le corps," was originally presented in 1980 at the meeting of the Société de Psychologie Médicale de Langue Française in Marseille.

42. Ibid., 292, 260, 302–3.

43. Ortigues and Ortigues, *Oedipe africain*, 13–14.

44. Ibid., 10.

45. Ibid., 126. See also Riesman, "Person and Life Cycle," esp. 75–80.

46. Ortigues and Ortigues, *Oedipe africain*, 303–4.

47. On Devereux's biography, see Roudinesco's preface to Devereux, *Psychothérapie d'un Indien des Plaines*, 8–28.

48. Devereux, *Reality and Dream*.

49. Devereux, *Basic Problems*, 3–4.

50. Devereux, *From Anxiety to Method*.

51. Roudinesco, in Devereux, *Psychothérapie d'un Indien des Plaines*, 24–26.

52. Nathan, "Psychothérapie et politique," 152, 154, 159.

53. Kirmayer and Minas, "Future of Cultural Psychiatry," 442.

54. Nathan, *Folie des autres* and *Influence qui guérit*.

55. Pascale Werner, "Tobie Nathan: Psychanalyser l'exil?" *Libération*, 26 November 1986, 46.

56. For recent interventions on these topics, see Fenech, *Tolérance zéro*; Rudolph and Soullez, *Insécurité*; and opposing views from Wacquant, "Sur quelques contes sécuritaires," and Tissot and Tévanian, *Stop quelle violence*.

57. See the special issue of *Esprit*, *Les cahiers de l'Orient: Paysages après la bataille, contre la guerre des cultures*, June 1991, esp. Mongin, "Guerre des cultures"; Benslama, "À propos de l'*Oumma*"; Stora, "Maghreb face à l'Europe."

58. Dahoun, "Us et abus," 225.

59. Benslama, "L'illusion ethnopsychiatrique," *Le Monde*, 4 December 1996, 14.

60. Fassin, "Ethnopsychiatrie," 169.

61. Sibony, "Tous malades."

62. Dahoun, "Us et abus," 249.

63. Ibid., 245.

64. Ibid., 232.

65. Alain Policar, "La dérive de l'ethnopsychiatrie," *Libération*, 20 June 1997, 13.

66. Fassin, "Ethnopsychiatrie," 152; see also Fassin, "Politiques de l'ethnopsychiatrie."

67. Nathan, *Influence qui guérit*, 190.

68. Nathan, "Psychothérapie et politique," 137.

69. Kleinman, "Anthropology and Psychiatry," and *Patients and Healers*; see also Good, "Culture and DSM-IV."

70. Dahoun, "Us et abus," 251.

71. Daniel Sibony, "Tous malades de l'exil," *Libération*, 30 January 1997, 5.

72. Bennegadi, "Anthropologie médicale clinique," 445; also Elfakir, *Oedipe et personnalité*; in literature, see Bonn, "Roman maghrébin."

73. This has been a critical problem for feminist scholars. For a cogent analysis of how a similar logic has undergirded the debate over sexual difference and *parité* in France, along with comments about its parallels in France's immigration policies, see Scott, "French Universalism," esp. 38–40.

74. Tobie Nathan, "Pas de psychiatrie hors les cultures," *Libération*, 30 July 1997, 4; Laplantine, *Ethnopsychiatrie*, 6.

75. See Latour, *Petite réflexion*.

76. Nathan, *Influence qui guérit*, 191.

77. Stora, *Transfert d'une mémoire*.

78. Rouillon, introduction; Taleb, interview.

79. Bedjaoui, "Allocution."

80. Rouillon, introduction.

81. Stora, *Gangrène et l'oubli*.

82. Florence Beauge, "350,000 anciens d'Algérie souffriraient de troubles psychiques liés à la guerre," *Le Monde*, 28 December 2000, 8; Maïssa Bey, "Les ci-

catrices de l'histoire," paper presented at the Premier Congrès de la Société Franco-Algérien de Psychiatrie, 4 October 2003; also Bey, *Entendez-vous dans les montagnes*.

83. Philippe Bernard, "L''agonie psychique' des anciens d'Algérie," *Le Monde*, 7 October 2003, 12.

84. Aussaresses, *Services spéciaux*; an excerpt of the book appeared in *Le Monde* in November 2000.

85. On this transition, see Ross, *Fast Cars, Clean Bodies*; and, more recently, de Grazia, *Irresistible Empire*.

86. Artéro et al., "Prévalence des troubles psychiatriques." Subsequently published as Ritchie et al., "Prevalence of DSM-IV Psychiatric Disorder."

87. See Shepard, "Decolonizing France"; Stora, *Transfert d'une mémoire*; Buono, *Pieds-noirs de père en fils*; Kramer, "Pieds-noirs."

88. Abdenour Zahzah, *Frantz Fanon: Mémoire d'asile* (Algeria, 2002).

Conclusion

1. Cited in Thuillier, *Ten Years*, 111.

2. See, e.g., Delay, Deniker, and Harl, "Utilisation."

3. Thuillier, *Ten Years*, 113.

4. Healy, *Creation of Psychopharmacology*.

5. Laborit, "Sur l'utilisation de certains agents pharmacodynamiques"; and Laborit, "Thérapeutique neuro-végétative."

6. Swazey, *Chlorpromazine in Psychiatry*, 79.

7. Laborit, Huguenard, and Alluaume, "Un nouveau stabilisateur."

8. This is not unlike the U.S. State Department's interest in a specifically Arab psychology in the aftermath of the Six-Day War—see Glidden, "Arab World"—or the current resurgence of interest in Patai, *Arab Mind*, reprinted in 2002 and used at the John F. Kennedy Special Warfare Center at Fort Bragg, North Carolina, for military training purposes; see Starrett, "Culture Never Dies."

9. See, e.g, Pierson, "Chlorpromazine"; Ramée et al., "Effets favorables du Largactil"; and Sutter and Pascalis, "Effets psychologiques de la chlorpromazine"; all presented at Delay's international congress in Paris in 1955.

10. See esp. Estroff, *Making It Crazy*.

11. Healy, *Creation of Psychopharmacology*, 129–77.

12. Macey, *Frantz Fanon*, 24.

Bibliography

Archives

AAP: Archives de l'Assistance Publique, Hôpitaux de Paris, Paris
Ammar Papers: Archives of Sleïm Ammar, Tunis
AN: Archives Nationales, Paris
ANT: Archives Nationales de Tunisie, Tunis
BHRM: Bibliothèque de l'Hôpital Razi-la Manouba, Manouba
BIUM: Bibliothèque Interuniversitaire de Médecine, Paris
BMHE: Bibliothèque Médicale Henry-Ey, Centre Hospitalier Sainte-Anne, Paris
CADN: Centre des Archives Diplomatiques, Nantes
CAOM: Centre des Archives d'Outre-Mer, Aix-en-Provence
CHE: Archives du Centre Henri Ellenberger, Centre Hospitalier Sainte-Anne, Paris
Esch-Chadely Papers: Archives of Salem ben Ahmed Esch-Chadely, Tunis
IBLA: Institut de Belles Lettres Arabes, Tunis
IMT: Institut de Médecine Tropicale, Marseilles
IRMC: Institut de Recherche sur le Maghreb Contemporain, Tunis
ISHMN: Institut Supérieur d'Histoire du Mouvement National, Manouba
MAE: Archives du Ministère des Affaires Etrangères, Paris
SHAT: Service Historique de l'Armée de Terre, Vincennes

Periodicals

L'Algérie médicale
Alger républicain
Annales médico-psychologiques
Bulletin médical de l'Algérie
Bulletin sanitaire de l'Algérie
Congrès des médecins aliénistes et neurologistes de France et de pays de langue française

La dépêche algérienne
La dépêche tunisienne
L'echo d'Alger
L'echo d'Oran
L'echo de Tlemcen
L'etendard tunisien
L'evolution psychiatrique
L'hygiène mentale
Le journal d'Alger
Le journal officiel de l'Algérie
Le journal officiel du Maroc
Le journal officiel Tunisien
Libération
L'information psychiatrique
Maroc médical
Le Monde
Le petit matin (Tunis)
Le phare (Tunis)
La presse (Tunis)
La presse médicale
La Tunisie médicale
Tunis-soir

Government Publications

Gouvernement Général de l'Algérie. *Comptes rendus des Assemblées financières algériennes, Délégations des Colons, des Non Colons et des Indigènes.* Algiers: Société anonyme d'imprimérie rapide, 1920–45.

Gouvernement Général de l'Algérie. Direction de l'Intérieur. "L'assistance et l'hygiène publique en Algérie: Oeuvres et Institutions d'Assistance, Services de Protection de la Santé Publique." Algiers: Carbonel, 1927.

Gouvernement Général de l'Algérie. Direction de la Santé Publique. "Collaboration de la direction de la Santé Publique et du Corps Médical." Algiers: Solal, n. d.

———. "Développement de la Réorganisation Sanitaire en 1934." Algiers: Carbonel, 1935.

———. "L'oeuvre française d'assistance et de protection sanitaire en Algérie." Algiers: Carbonel, 1937.

———. "Organisation des Services de Psychiatrie." Algiers: Carbonel, n. d.

———. "Principes généraux de l'Organisation sanitaire." Algiers: Carbonel, 1935.

———. "Services d'assistance sociale rattachés à la Santé Publique." Algiers: Jules Carbonel, 1935.

Régence de Tunis. Protectorat Français. *Procès-verbaux du Grand Conseil de la Tunisie: Sections françaises et indigènes.* Tunis: Société Anonyme d'Imprimerie Rapide, 1922–39.

Résidence Générale de la République Française à Tunis. *Rapport sur l'activité des services du Protectorat et prévisions budgétaires pour 1928: Grand Conseil de la Tunisie, VIIIe session (Novembre–Décembre 1929).* Tunis: Aloccio, 1929.

Books, Articles, and Films

Abbas, Ferhat. *Guerre et révolution d'Algérie: La nuit coloniale.* Paris: Julliard, 1962.

Abdel-Jaouad, Hédi. "'Too Much in the Sun': Sons, Mothers, and Impossible Alliances in Francophone Maghrebian Writing." *Research in African Literatures* 27, no. 3 (1996): 15–33.

Acker, Caroline Jean. *Creating the American Junkie: Addiction Research in the Classic Era of Narcotic Control.* Baltimore, Md.: Johns Hopkins University Press, 2002.

Adas, Michael. *Machines as the Measure of Men: Science, Technology, and Ideologies of Western Dominance.* Ithaca, N.Y.: Cornell University Press, 1989.

Adohane, Taoufik. "Le nourrisson médusé: Notes de recherche ethnopsychiatrique." *Nouvelle revue d'ethnopsychiatrie* 13 (1989): 183–204.

———. "Un remède pour les pensées: Place et statut de l'objet dans la pratique médicale au Maroc." *Nouvelle revue d'ethnopsychiatrie* 16 (1990): 55–74.

Agamben, Giorgio. *Homo Sacer: Sovereign Power and Bare Life.* Trans. Daniel Heller-Roazen. Stanford, Calif.: Stanford University Press, 1998.

Ageron, Charles-Robert. *Les Algériens musulmans et la France, 1871–1919.* 2 vols. Paris: Presses Universitaires de France, 1968.

———. *Histoire de l'Algérie contemporaine.* Vol. 2, *De l'insurrection de 1871 au déclenchement de la guerre de libération (1954).* Paris: Presses Universitaires de France, 1979.

Alemdjrodo, Kangni. *Rachid Boudjedra: La passion de l'intertexte.* Bordeaux: Presses Universitaires de Bordeaux, 2001.

"Les aliénés en Algérie." *Annales médico-psychologiques* 31, no. 1 (1873): 491–92.

Alleg, Henri, ed. *La guerre d'Algérie.* 3 vols. Paris: Temps Actuels, 1981.

Alliez, J., and H. Descombes. "Réflexions sur le comportement psychopathologique d'une série de nord-africains musulmans immigrés." *Annales médico-psychologiques* 110, no. 2 (1952): 150–56.

Ammar, A. "L'assistance aux aliénés en Tunisie (Quelques étapes)." *L'information psychiatrique* 31, no. 4 (January 1955): 24–27.

Ammar, Sleïm. "Antoine et Maurice Porot à Tunis." *Psychologie médicale* 15 (1983): 1717–18.

———. "L'assistance psychiatrique en Tunisie: Aperçu historique." *L'information psychiatrique* 48, no. 7 (1972): 647–57.

———. "Les désordres psychiques dans la société tunisienne: Leur evolution et fréquence en fonction des transformations socio-économiques et culturelles depuis l'indépendance." Offprint from *La Tunisie médicale* 1 (1964): unpaginated. Ammar Papers.

———. "La folie à travers les âges." *La voix de la santé,* 6–7 (1954). IBLA.

———. *Poème de la folie.* Tunis: L'Art de la composition, 1993.

———. "Les relations de la psychiatrie tunisienne avec la psychiatrie française." In *Annales de thérapeutique psychiatrique,* vol. 4, *La psychiatrie française dans ses rapports avec les autres psychiatries,* ed. Henri Baruk. Paris: Presses Universitaires de France, 1969. 185–93.

———. *Rhazès: Abû Bekr Er-Razi.* Tunis: Imprimerie Principale, 1997.

———. *Trois grands médecins andalous: Ezzahraoui, Ibn Zohr, Ibn Roschd.* Tunis: Congrès International d'Histoire de la Médecine, 1998.

———. "Les troubles mentaux en Tunisie depuis l'indépendance: Aspects psychopathologiques et épidémiologiques centrés sur notre expérience des vingt-cinq dernières années." Offprint from *L'Information psychiatrique* 55, no. 3 (1979): unpaginated. Ammar Papers.

Amir, Mohammed Benaïssa. *Contribution à l'étude de l'histoire de la santé en Algérie autour d'une experience vecue en ALN Wilaya V: Réflexions sur son développement.* Algiers: Office des Publications Universitaires, 1986.

Amrouche, Jean el-Mouhoub. "Aspects psychologiques du problème algérien." In *Un Algérien s'adresse aux Français ou l'histoire d'Algérie par les textes, 1943–1961,* ed. Tassadit Yacine. Paris: L'Harmattan, 1994. 287–92.

Anderson, Warwick. "Immunities of Empire: Race, Disease, and the New Tropical Medicine, 1900–1920." *Bulletin of the History of Medicine* 70 (1996): 94–118.

———. "The Trespass Speaks: White Masculinity and Colonial Breakdown." *American Historical Review* 102 (1997): 1343–70.

———. "Where Is the Postcolonial History of Medicine?" *Bulletin of the History of Medicine* 72, no. 3 (1998): 522–30.

Antheaume, André. "Chronique: L'actualité neuro-psychiatrique." *L'informateur des aliénistes et des neurologistes* 20 (1925): 97–121.

———. "Communiqués: Au Congrès de Tunis." *L'informateur des aliénistes et neurologistes* 7 (1912): 87–106.

———. "L'évolution de l'assistance psychiatrique vers les services ouverts sans internement." *L'informateur des aliénistes et des neurologistes* 20 (1925): 148–62.

Apter, Emily. "Out of Character: Camus's French Algerian Subjects." *Modern Language Notes* 112 (1997): 499–516.

Aresu, Bernard. Introduction to Kateb Yacine, *Nedjma,* trans. Richard Howard. Charlottesville, Va.: CARAF, 1991. xiii–l.

Arnaud, Jacqueline. *Recherches sur la littérature maghrébine de langue française: Le cas de Kateb Yacine.* 2 vols. Paris: L'Harmattan, 1982.

Arnold, David. *Colonizing the Body: State Medicine and Epidemic Disease in Nineteenth-Century India.* Berkeley: University of California Press, 1993.

Arnold, David, ed. *Warm Climates and Western Medicine: The Emergence of Tropical Medicine, 1500–1900.* Amsterdam: Editions Rodopi, 1996.

"Arrêté instituant un contrôle technique permanent des services de psychiâtrie de l'Algérie," 16 August 1934. *L'Algérie médicale* 38, no. 82 (October 1934): 233.

"Arrêté Ministériel portant création d'une Commission d'hygiène mentale au Ministère des Colonies." *Bulletin officiel du Ministère des Colonies* 39 (1925): 1600–1601.

Arrii, Don Côme. "De l'impulsivité criminelle chez l'indigène algérien." Med. thesis, Algiers, 1926.

Artéro, Sylvaine, Isabelle Beluche, Jean-Philippe Boulenger, and Karen Ritchie. "Prévalence des troubles psychiatriques dans une population âgée exposées aux psycho-traumatismes de la guerre d'Algérie: L'étude ESPRIT." Premier Congrés de la Société Franco-Algérienne de Psychiatrie, Paris, 4 October 2003.

Aubin, Henri. "L'assistance psychiatrique indigène aux colonies." *Congrès des médedins aliénistes et neurologistes de France et de pays de langue française,* Algiers (1938): 147–76.

———. "Esquisse d'une ethno-psycho-pathologie." *L'Algérie médicale* 5–6 (1945): 174–79.

———. "Introduction à l'étude de la psychiatrie chez les noirs." Part 1. *Annales médico-psychologiques* 97, no. 1 (1939): 1–29.

———. "Introduction à l'étude de la psychiatrie chez les noirs." Part 2. *Annales médico-psychologiques* 97, no. 2 (1939): 181–213.

Aussaresses, Paul. *Services spéciaux: Algérie, 1955–1957.* Paris: Perrin, 2001.

Bakiri, M. A. "À propos de l'organisation des services de santé mentales dans les pays en voie de developpement." *La Tunisie médicale* 53 (1975): 333–39.

Baldacci, Aimé. *C'était ainsi: Souvenirs d'un Français d'Algérie.* Paris: La Porte de la Rivière, 1983.

Baraket, Hedia. "Pour une psychiatrie ouverte." *Dialogue* (1982) : 45–49.

Barbier. "Les fous et le mal de mer." *Journal de médecine et de pharmacie de l'Algérie* (October 1884): 227–29.

Bardenat, Charles. "Criminalité et délinquance dans l'aliénations mentale chez les indigènes algériens." Part 1. *Annales médico-psychologiques* 106, no. 2 (1948): 317–33.

———. "Criminalité et délinquance dans l'aliénations mentale chez les indigènes algériens." Part 2. *Annales médico-psychologiques* 106, no. 2 (1948): 468–80.

Barthes, Roland. *Critical Essays.* Trans. Richard Howard. Evanston, Ill.: Northwestern University Press, 1972.

Baruk, Henri, David, Racine, Vallancien, and Mlle Owsianik. "Etude expérimentale chez le lapin et le singe des modifications de la circulation cérébrale dans le coma insulinique, l'épilepsie cardiazolique, l'électrochoc et au cours de l'action de la folliculine et du scopochlorase." *Encéphale* 35 (1942–45): 81–89.

Basalla, George. "The Spread of Western Science." *Science* 156, no. 3775 (1967): 611–22.

Bastide, Roger. *Le rêve, la transe, et la folie.* 2nd ed. Paris: Seuil, 2003.

Bates, Robert H., V. Y. Mudimbe, and Jean O'Barr, eds. *Africa and the Disciplines: The Contributions of Research in Africa to the Social Sciences and the Humanities.* Chicago: University of Chicago Press, 1993.

Bedjaoui, Mohammed. "Allocution." http://www.sfapsy.com/Premier-congres/Congres-1.htm, accessed 29 June 2006.

Beers, Clifford. *A Mind That Found Itself: An Autobiography.* Pittsburgh: University of Pittsburgh Press, 1981.

Bégué, Jean-Michel. "Un siècle de psychiatrie française en Algérie, 1830–1939." Mémoire for the Certificat d'Etudes Specialisées, Paris, Universitaire Pierre et Marie Curie, 1989.

Béguin, François. "La machine à guérir." In *Les machines à guérir,* ed. Michel Foucault et al. Paris: Institut de l'Environnement, 1976. 55–69.

Ben Jelloun, Tahar. *French Hospitality: Racism and North African Immigrants.* Trans. Barbara Bray. New York: Columbia University Press, 1999.

———. *Hospitalité française: Racisme et immigration maghrébine.* Paris: Seuil, 1984.

———. *La plus haute des solitudes: Misère affective et sexuelle d'émigrés nord-africains.* Paris: Seuil, 1977.

Bennani, Jalil. *La psychanalyse au pays des saints. Les débuts de la psychanalyse et de la psychiatrie au Maroc.* Casablanca: Le Fennec, 1996.

Bennegadi, Rachid. "Anthropologie médicale clinique et santé mentale des migrants en France." *Médecine tropicale* 56, no. 4 *bis* (1996): 445–52.

Ben Rejeb, Riadh. "À propos de la transe psychothérapeutique de Sidi Da^{cc}âs: Note sur la place du djinn dans les psychothérapies traditionnelles." *Institut de belles lettres arabes* 54, no. 168 (1991): 215–21.

Benslama, Fethi. "À propos de l'*Oumma*: Réponse à Daniel Sibony." *Esprit* (1999): 53–60.

————. "Identity as a Cause." *Research in African Literatures* 30 (1999): 36–50.

————. *La psychanalyse à l'épreuve de l'Islam.* Paris: Flammarion, 2002.

Bensmaïl, Malek, dir. *Aliénations* [film]. Distributed by Paris, Eurozoom. France/Algeria, 2002.

Ben Youssef, Adel. "Le docteur Salem Eschadely." *La revue sadikienne* 19 (2000): 3–10.

Bernard, Stéphane. *Le conflit franco-marocain, 1943–1956.* 3 vols. Brussels: Editions de l'Institut de Sociologie de l'Université Libre de Bruxelles, 1963.

Berque, Jacques. *Le Magrib entre deux guerres.* Paris: Seuil, 1962.

Berthelier, Robert. *L'homme maghrébin dans la littérature psychiatrique.* Paris: L'Harmattan, 1994.

Betts, Raymond. *Assimilation and Association in French Colonial Theory, 1890–1914.* New York: Columbia University Press, 1961.

Bey, Maïssa. *Entendez-vous dans les montagnes.* Paris: Editions de l'Aube, 2002.

————. "Les cicatrices de l'histoire." Paper delivered at the Premier Congrès de la Société Franco-Algérienne de Psychiatrie, Paris, 4 October 2003.

Bhabha, Homi K. *The Location of Culture.* New York: Routledge, 1994.

Bidwell, Robin. *Morocco under Colonial Rule: French Administration of Tribal Areas, 1912–1956.* London: Frank Cass, 1973.

Biehl, João. "Vita: Life in a Zone of Social Abandonment." *Social Text* 68 (2001): 131–49.

Boigey, Maurice. "Étude psychologique sur l'Islam." *Annales médico-psychologiques* 66, no. 2 (1908): 5–14.

Bonn, Charles. "Le roman maghrébin et l'ombre du père, ou: Le désordre de la langue française et Kateb Yacine le fondateur." *Annuaire de l'Afrique du Nord* 27 (1988 [1990]): 449–67.

Bonneuil, Christophe. *Des savants pour l'Empire: La structuration des recherches scientifiques coloniales au temps de "la mise en valeur des colonies françaises," 1917–1945.* Paris: Editions de l'ORSTOM, 1991.

Borel, J. "Nord-Africains malades mentaux condamnés en justice." *Information psychiatrique* 33 (1957): 219–21.

Borreil, Paul. "Considérations sur l'internement des aliénés sénégalais en France." Med. thesis, Montpellier, 1908.

Boucebci, Mahfoud. *Maladie mentale et handicap mental.* Algiers: Ecrits des oliviers, 1984.

Boucebci, Mahfoud, and A. Yaker. "Aspects généraux et tendances évolutives de la psychiatrie en Algérie." *La Tunisie médicale* 53 (1975): 355–65.

Boudjedra, Rachid. *L'insolation.* Paris: Denoël, 1972.

Bourdieu, Pierre, and Abdelmalek Sayad. *Le déracinement: La crise de l'agriculture traditionnelle en Algérie.* Paris: Editions de Minuit, 1964.

Bouquet, Henry. "Les aliénés en Tunisie." Med. thesis, Lyon, 1909.

Boutet de Monvel, Marc. *Boudjedra l'insolé: L'Insolation, racines et greffes.* Paris: L'Harmattan, 1994.

Bouzgarrou, Abdelhamid. "À propos d'une expérience de Transformation Institutionnelle au niveau d'un service de psychiatrie." Med. thesis, Tunis, 1978–79.

Branche, Raphaëlle. *La torture et l'armée pendant la guerre d'Algérie, 1954–1962.* Paris: Gallimard, 2001.

Braslow, Joel. *Mental Ills and Bodily Cures: Psychiatric Treatment in the First Half of the Twentieth Century.* Berkeley: University of California Press, 1997.

Brisset, Charles. "Psychochirurgie." *L'evolution psychiatrique* 14 (1949): 487–516.

Broustra, Jean, and Catherine Simounet. "Maghreb en folie: Aspects structuraux ou sociopolitiques." *Sociologie santé* 9 (1993): 91–110.

Brunner, José. "Psychiatry, Psychoanalysis, and Politics During the First World War." *Journal of the History of the Behavioral Sciences* 27 (October 1991): 352–65.

Bulhan, Hussein A. *Frantz Fanon and the Psychology of Oppression.* New York: Plenum, 1985.

——. "Revolutionary Psychiatry of Fanon." In *Rethinking Fanon: The Continuing Dialogue*, ed. Nigel C. Gibson. Amherst, N.Y.: Humanity Books, 1999. 141–75.

Buono, Clarisse. *Pieds-noirs de père en fils: Voix et regards.* Paris: Belland, 2004.

Burleigh, Michael. *Death and Deliverance.* New York: Cambridge University Press, 1997.

——. *Ethics and Extermination: Reflections on Nazi Genocide.* New York: Cambridge University Press, 1997.

Bursztyn, Pinkus-Jacques. *Schizophrénie et mentalité primitive.* Paris: Faculté de Médicine, 1935.

Carrère, Jean. "Nécessité de l'assistance neuro-psychiatrique en Tunisie." *Information psychiatrique* 24, no. 10 (1948): 278–81.

Castel, Robert. *L'ordre psychiatrique: L'âge d'or de l'aliénisme.* Paris: Minuit, 1976.

Çelik, Zeynep. *Urban Forms and Colonial Confrontations: Algiers under French Rule.* Berkeley: University of California Press, 1997.

Cerletti, Ugo. "Old and New Information about Electroshock." *American Journal of Psychiatry* 107 (1950): 87–94.

Cerletti, Ugo, and Lucio Bini. "L'elettroshock." *Archivio generale di neurologia, psichiatria e psicoanalisi* 19 (1938): 266–68.

Chapman, Herrick, and Laura L. Frader, eds. *Race in France: Interdisciplinary Perspectives on the Politics of Difference.* New York: Berghahn, 2004.

Charpentier, René. Review of Henri Aubin, "Le test évolutif dans l'intoxication par le Kif," *L'Algérie médicale. Annales médico-psychologiques* 103, no. 1 (1945): 487.

——. Review of Henri Aubin, "Epilepsie psychique larvée équivalent d'une ivresse pathologique," *L'Oranie médicale. Annales médico-psychologiques* 103, no. 1 (1945): 488.

——. Review of Antoine Porot, ed., *Manuel alphabétique de psychiatrie clinique, thérapeutique, et médico-légale*, 1st ed.. *Annales médico-psychologiques* 110, no. 1 (1952): 649–50.

——. Review of A. Porot [*sic*], "L'alcoolisme en Algérie," *Bulletin médical de l'Algérie. Annales médico-psychologiques* 99, no. 1 (1941): 73.

——. Review of Maurice Porot, M. Buscail, and Y. Vincent, "La situation familiale des enfants délinquants de la région d'Alger," *L'Algérie médicale. Annales médico-psychologiques* 108, no. 1 (1950): 528.

————. Review of Jean Sutter, "Les indigènes nord-africains au combat (Etude psychopathologique)," *Cahiers médicaux de l'Union française. Annales médico-psychologiques* 107, no. 1 (1949): 196.

Chatinières, Paul. *Dans le Grand Atlas marocain: Extraits du carnet de route d'un médecin d'assistance médicale indigène, 1912–1916.* Paris: Plon-Nourrit, 1919.

Chénieux-Gendron, Jacqueline. *Surrealism.* Trans. Vivian Folkenflik. New York: Columbia University Press, 1988.

Chérif, Ahmed. "Étude psychologique sur l'Islam." *Annales médico-psychologiques* 67, no. 1 (1909): 352–63.

————. "Histoire de la médecine arabe en Tunisie." Med. thesis, Bordeaux, 1907–8.

————. "La médecine arabe en Tunisie: Le neuvième siècle; Ishaq Ibn Amran." *La France médicale* 55 (1908): 146–50.

Cherki, Alice. *Frantz Fanon: Portrait.* Paris: Seuil, 2000.

Cheula, Jeanne. *Hier est proche d'aujourd'hui.* Paris: L'Atlanthrope, 1979.

Chkili, Taieb. "Assistance psychiatrique au Maroc: Problèmes actuels et perspectives d'avenir." *La Tunisie médicale* 53 (1975): 341–53.

Chraïbi, Driss. *Le passé simple.* Paris: Denoël, 1954.

Clancy-Smith, Julia. *Rebel and Saint: Muslim Notables, Populist Protest, Colonial Encounters; Algeria and Tunisia, 1800–1904.* Berkeley: University of California Press, 1994.

Clancy-Smith, Julia, and Frances Gouda, eds. *Domesticating the Empire: Race, Gender, and Family Life in French and Dutch Colonialism.* Charlottesville: University of Virginia Press, 1998.

Clifford, James. *The Predicament of Culture: Twentieth-Century Ethnography, Literature, and Art.* Cambridge, Mass: Harvard University Press, 1988.

Cloarec, Françoise. *Bimaristans, lieux de folie et de sagesse: La folie et ses traitements dans les hôpitaux médiévaux au Moyen-Orient.* Paris: L'Harmattan, 1998.

Code pénal tunisien. Tunis: Imprimerie française, 1913.

Codet, Henri. "Hygiène mentale et évènements sociaux." *L'evolution psychiatrique* 4 (1938): 3–17.

Cohen, William B. "The Colonial Policy of the Popular Front." *French Historical Studies* 7, no. 3 (1972): 368–93.

————. *The French Encounter with Africans: White Response to Blacks, 1530–1880.* Bloomington: Indiana University Press, 1980.

Cohn, Bernard. "The Census, Social Structure, and Objectification in South Asia." In *An Anthropologist among the Historians and Other Essays.* Delhi: Oxford University Press, 1990. 224–54.

————. *Colonialism and Its Forms of Knowledge: The British in India.* Princeton, N.J.: Princeton University Press, 1996.

Collignon, René. "La construction du sujet colonial: le cas particulier des malades mentaux: Difficultés d'une psychiatrie en terre africaine." In *La psychologie des peuples et ses dérives,* ed. Michel Kail and Geneviève Vermès. Paris: Centre national de documentation pédagogique, 1999. 165–81.

Collot, Claude. *Les institutions de l'Algérie durant la période coloniale, 1830–1962.* Paris: Editions du CNRS, 1987.

Colonna, Fanny. *Insituteurs algériens, 1883–1939.* Paris: Presses de la Fondation Nationale des Sciences Politiques, 1975.

Comaroff, Jean. "'The Diseased Heart of Africa': Medicine, Colonialism, and the Black Body." In *Knowledge, Power, and Practice: The Anthropology of Medicine and Everyday Life*, ed. Shirley Lindenbaum and Margaret Lock. Berkeley: University of California Press, 1993. 305–29.

"Commission d'hygiène mentale au ministère des Colonies." *L'hygiène mentale* 21, no. 2 (February 1926): 47–48.

Conklin, Alice. *A Mission to Civilize: The Republican Idea of Empire in France and West Africa, 1895–1930.* Stanford, Calif.: Stanford University Press, 1997.

————. "Redefining 'Frenchness': Citizenship, Race Regeneration, and Imperial Motherhood in France and West Africa, 1914–40." In *Domesticating the Empire: Race, Gender, and Family Life in French and Dutch Colonialism*, ed. Julia Clancy-Smith and Frances Gouda. Charlottesville: University of Virginia Press, 1998. 65–83.

Cooper, Frederick, and Ann Laura Stoler, eds. *Tensions of Empire: Colonial Cultures in a Bourgeois World.* Berkeley: University of California Press, 1997.

Corpet, Olivier, and Albert Dichy, eds. *Kateb Yacine: éclats de mémoire.* Paris: IMEC Editions, 1994.

Costedoat, A.-L.-D. "Les troubles mentaux des militaires indigènes musulmans de l'Afrique du Nord." *Archives de médecine et de pharmacie militaires* 101, no. 2 (1934): 231–52.

Couchard, Françoise. "Psychanalyse du voile." *France Culture.* Radio broadcast, 18 January 2004.

Couderc. "L'assistance psychiatrique dans le Département d'Oran (Algérie)." *Information psychiatrique* 31, no. 4 (January 1955): 19–23.

Courbon, Paul. Review of Antoine Porot and Jean Sutter, "Le primitivisme des indigènes nord-africains," *Sud médical et chirurgical. Annales médico-psychologiques* 97, no. 2 (1939): 440.

Crapanzano, Vincent. *The Hamadsha: A Study in Moroccan Ethnopsychiatry.* Berkeley: University of California Press, 1973.

"Création en France d'une Commission d'hygiène mentale coloniale." *L'informateur des alienistes et neurologistes* 19, no. 6 (June 1924): 143.

Crouzières-Ingenthron, Armelle. *Le double pluriel dans les romans de Rachid Boudjedra.* Paris: L'Harmattan, 2001.

Curtin, Philip. *Disease and Empire: The Health of European Troops in the Conquest of Africa.* New York: Cambridge University Press, 1998.

Dahoun, Zerdalia K. S. "Les us et abus de l'ethnopsychiatrie." *Les temps modernes*, 552–53 (1992): 223–53.

Daoud, Zakya. "Chez les fous." *Lamalif*, 15 May 1966, 21–24.

Das, Veena, Arthur Kleinman, Mamphela Ramphele, and Pamela Reynolds, eds. *Violence and Subjectivity.* Berkeley: University of California Press, 2000.

Daumezon, Georges. "Lecture historique de *L'histoire de la folie*." *Evolution psychiatrique* 36 (1971): 227–41.

Daumezon, G., Y. Champion, and J. Champion-Basset. *L'assistance psychiatrique aux malades mentaux d'origine nord-africaine musulmane en Métropole.* Monographie de l'Institut National d'Hygiène 14. Paris: INH, 1957.

————. "Étude démographique et statistique des entrées masculines nord-africaines à l'Hôpital psychiatrique Sainte-Anne de 1945 à 1954." Part 1. *L'hygiène mentale* 43 (1954): 1–20.

————. "Étude démographique et statistique des entrées masculines nord-africaines à l'Hôpital psychiatrique Sainte-Anne de 1945 à 1954." Part 2. *L'hygiène mentale* 43 (1954): 85–107.

Dean, Carolyn. *The Self and Its Pleasures: Bataille, Lacan, and the History of the Decentered Subject.* Ithaca, N.Y.: Cornell University Press, 1992.

de Grazia, Victoria. *Irresistible Empire: America's Advance through 20th-Century Europe.* Cambridge, Mass.: Harvard University Press, 2005.

Delay, Jean, Pierre Deniker, and Jean-Marie Harl. "Utilisation en thérapeutique psychiatrique d'un phénothiazine d'action centrale elective." *Annales médico-psychologiques* 110 (1952): 112–31.

Delore, P., R. Lambert, and A. Marin. "Enquête sur la pathologie dans la Métropole de l'Algérien musulman." *Concours médical* 77 (1955): 4545–52.

Demassieux, Eliane. "Le service social en psychiatrie: Son application à la Clinique Psychiatrique de l'Université d'Alger." Med. thesis, Algiers, 1941.

Dequeker, J., F. Fanon, R. Lacaton, M. Micucci, and F. Ramée. "Aspects actuels de l'assistance mentale en Algérie." *Information psychiatrique* 31, no. 4 (January 1955): 11–18.

Desruelles, Maurice, and Henri Bersot. "L'assistance aux aliénés chez les Arabes du viiie au xiie siècle: Contribution à l'histoire de l'assistance aux aliénés." *Annales médico-psychologiques* 96, no. 2 (1938): 700.

———. "L'assistance aux aliénés en Algérie depuis le XIXe siècle." *Annales médico-psychologiques* 97, no. 2 (1939): 578–96.

Devereux, Georges. *Basic Problems of Ethnopsychiatry.* Trans. Basia Miller Gulati and George Devereux. Chicago: University of Chicago Press, 1980.

———. "Cultural Factors in Psychoanalytic Therapy." *Journal of the American Psychoanalytic Association* 1 (1953): 629–55.

———. *Essais d'ethnopsychiatrie générale.* Trans. Tinas Jolas and Henri Gobard. Paris: Gallimard, 1970.

———. *From Anxiety to Method in the Behavioral Sciences.* The Hague: Mouton, 1967.

———. "Psychiatry and Anthropology: Some Research Objectives." *Bulletin of the Menninger Clinic* 16 (1952): 167–77.

———. *Psychothérapie d'un Indien des Plaines: Réalité et rêve.* Trans. Françoise de Gruson and Monique Novodorsqui. Paris: Fayard, 1998.

———. *Reality and Dream: Psychotherapy of a Plains Indian.* New York: International Universities Press, 1951.

Devisch, Renaat, and Bart Vervaeck. "Doors and Thresholds: Jeddi's Approach to Psychiatric Disorders." *Social Science and Medicine* 22 (1986): 541–51.

Dine, Philip. *Images of the Algerian War: French Fiction and Film, 1954–1992.* Oxford: Berg, 1994.

Dols, Michael W. *Majnun: The Madman in the Medieval Islamic World.* New York: Oxford University Press, 1992.

Donnadieu, André. "L'alcoolisme mental dans la population indigène du Maroc." *Maroc-médical* 214 (November–December 1940): 163–65.

———. "Psychose de civilisation." *Annales médico-psychologiques* 97, no. 1 (January 1939): 30–37.

———. "Situation actuelle de la syphilis nerveuse indigène à forme mentale." *Maroc-médical* 207 (September 1939): 15–19.

Donzelot, Jacques. *The Policing of Families.* Trans. Robert Hurley. New York: Pantheon, 1979.

Douglas, Mary. *Purity and Danger: An Analysis of the Concepts of Pollution and Taboo.* London: Routledge, 1966.

Douglas, Norman. *Fountains in the Sand*. London: Martin Secker, 1921 [1912].

Doutté, Edmond. *Magie et religion dans l'Afrique du Nord*. Paris: Maisonneuve, 1984 [1909].

Dowbiggin, Ian. *Inheriting Madness: Professionalization and Psychiatric Knowledge in Nineteenth-Century France*. Berkeley: University of California Press, 1991.

Dower, John. *War without Mercy: Race and Power in the Pacific War*. New York: Pantheon, 1986.

du Camp, Maxime. *Le Nil, Egypte, et Nubie*. Paris: Hachette, 1877.

Dumas, Georges. "Mentalité paranoïde et mentalité primitive." *Annales médico-psychologiques* 92, no. 1 (1934): 754–62.

Dumolard. "Au sujet de l'assistance psychiatrique en Algérie: La situation véritable; Mise au point." *L'hygiène mentale* 21, no. 1 (January 1926): 16–18.

———. "Au sujet de l'assistance psychiatrique en Algérie." *L'hygiène mentale* 21, no. 6 (June 1926): 144–45.

Duquesne, Jacques. *L'Algérie ou la guerre des mythes*. Bruges: Desclée de Brouwer, 1958.

Ehlen, Patrick. *Frantz Fanon: A Spiritual Biography*. New York: Crossroads, 2000.

Eisenberg, Leon. "Disease and Illness: Distinctions between Professional and Popular Ideas of Sickness." *Culture, Medicine and Psychiatry* 1 (1977): 9–23.

Elfakir, Abdelhadi. *Oedipe et personnalité au Maghreb: Eléments d'ethnopsychologie clinique*. Paris: L'Harmattan, 1995.

El-Khayat, Ghita. *Une psychiatrie moderne pour le Maghreb*. Paris: L'Harmattan, 1994.

Ellenberger, Henri. "Ethno-psychiatrie." *Encyclopédie médico-chirurgicale*, 37725 A10.

Ernst, Waltraud. "European Madness and Gender in Nineteenth-Century British India." *Social History of Medicine* 9, no. 3 (1996): 357–82.

———. "Idioms of Madness and Colonial Boundaries: The Case of the European and 'Native' Mentally Ill in Early Nineteenth-Century British India." *Comparative Studies in Society and History* (1997): 153–81.

———. *Mad Tales from the Raj: The European Insane in British India, 1800–1858*. New York: Routledge, 1991.

Escande de Messières, Maurice-Émile. *La psychologie des coloniaux: Influence des pays chauds sur l'état mental*. Angoulême: Charentaise, 1905.

Esch-Chadely, Salem ben Ahmed. "Rythme paradoxal de fatigue et équilibre acide-base dans la neurasthenie." Med. thesis, Paris, 1929.

Establet, Colette. *Etre caïd dans l'Algérie Coloniale*. Paris: CNRS, 1991.

Estroff, Sue. *Making It Crazy*. Berkeley: University of California Press, 1978.

Estrosi, Christian. *Insécurité: Sauver la république*. Monaco: Editions du Rocher, 2001.

Ezra, Elizabeth. *The Colonial Unconscious: Race and Culture in Interwar France*. Ithaca, N.Y.: Cornell, 2000.

Fabian, Johannes. *Out of Our Minds: Reason and Madness in the Exploration of Central Africa*. Berkeley: University of California Press, 2000.

Fadiman, Anne. *The Spirit Catches You and You Fall Down: A Hmong Child, Her American Doctors, and the Collision of Two Cultures*. New York: Farrar, Strauss, and Giroux, 1997.

Fall, Mar. "Les marabouts soufis africains: La baraka des saints." *Sociologie santé* 8 (December 1993): 82–87.

Fanon, Frantz. *Black Skin, White Masks*. Trans. Charles Lam Markmann. New York: Grove, 1967.

——. *A Dying Colonialism*. Trans. by Haakon Chevalier. New York: Grove, 1965.

——. *Pour la révolution africaine: Ecrits politiques*. Paris: Maspero, 1964.

——. "Rencontre de la Société et de la psychiatrie (Notes de cours, Tunis, 1959–60)." Oran: CRIDSSH, 1984.

——. *The Wretched of the Earth*. Trans. Constance Farrington. New York: Grove, 1963.

Fanon, Frantz, and Charles Geromini. "Hospitalisation." *La Tunisie médicale* 38 (1959): 689–732.

——. "Le TAT en milieu maghrébin: Sociologie de la perception et de l'imagination." *Annales médico-psychologiques* 114, no. 2 (1956): 495.

Farmer, Paul. *Infections and Inequalities: The Modern Plagues*. Berkeley: University of California Press, 1999.

——. "On Suffering and Structural Violence: A View from Below." *Daedalus* 125, no. 1 (1996): 261–83.

Fassin, Didier. "L'ethnopsychiatrie et ses réseaux: L'influence qui grandit." *Genèses* 35 (1999): 146–71.

——. "Les politiques de l'ethnopsychiatrie: La psyché africaine, des colonies africaines aux banlieues parisiennes." *L'homme* 153 (2000): 231–50.

Feierman, Steven, and John M. Janzen, eds. *The Social Basis of Health and Healing in Africa*. Berkeley: University of California Press, 1992.

Fenech, Georges. *Tolérance zéro: En finir avec la criminalité et les violences urbaines*. Paris: Grasset, 2001.

Féry, Raymond. *L'oeuvre médicale française en Algérie*. Calvisson: Editions Jacques Gandini, 1994.

Flaubert, Gustave. *Première éducation sentimentale*. Paris: Seuil, 1963.

Foster, Hal. "Primitive Scenes." *Critical Inquiry* 20, no. 1 (1993): 69–102.

Foucault, Michel. *The Birth of the Clinic: An Archaeology of Medical Perception*. Trans. A. M. Sheridan-Smith. New York: Vintage, 1973.

——. "Governmentality." In *The Foucault Effect: Studies in Governmentality*, ed. Graham Burchell, Colin Gordon, and Peter Miller. Chicago: University of Chicago Press, 1991. 87–104.

——. *Histoire de la folie à l'âge classique*. Paris: Gallimard, 1972.

——. *The History of Sexuality*, vol. 1, *An Introduction*. Trans. Robert Hurley. New York: Vintage, 1978.

——. *Society Must Be Defended: Lectures at the Collège de France, 1975–1976*. Ed. Arnold Davidson. Trans. David Macey. New York: Picador, 2003.

Freeman, Walter, and James Watts. *Psychosurgery*. Springfield, Ill.: C. C. Thomas, 1942.

Freud, Sigmund. *The Interpretation of Dreams*. Trans. James Strachey. New York: Avon, 1965.

——. "Mourning and Melancholia." In *The Standard Edition of the Complete Psychological Works of Sigmund Freud*, ed. and trans. James Strachey. 24 vols. London: Hogarth, 1952–66. 14:243–58.

——. *Totem and Taboo: Some Points of Agreement between the Mental Lives of Savages and Neurotics*. In *The Standard Edition of the Complete Psychological Works of Sigmund Freud*, ed. and trans. James Strachey. 24 vols. London: Hogarth, 1953–74. 13:xii–162.

Fribourg-Blanc, A. "L'état mental des indigènes de l'Afrique du Nord et leurs réactions psychopathiques." *L'hygiène mentale* 22, no. 9 (November 1927): 135–44.

Friedrichsmeyer, Sara, Sara Lennox, and Susanne Zantop, eds. *The Imperialist Imagination: German Colonialism and Its Legacy.* Ann Arbor: University of Michigan Press, 1998.

Fuller, Alexandra. *Don't Let's Go to the Dogs Tonight.* New York: Random House, 2001.

Gaines, Atwood D., ed. *Ethnopsychiatry: The Cultural Construction of Professional and Folk Psychiatries.* Albany: SUNY Press, 1992.

Gallagher, Nancy Elizabeth. *Medicine and Power in Tunisia, 1780–1900.* New York: Cambridge University Press, 1983.

Garas, Félix. *Bourguiba et la naissance d'une nation.* Paris: René Julliard, 1956.

Gastaut, Yvan. *L'immigration et l'opinion en France sous la Ve République.* Paris: Seuil, 2000.

Gates, Henry Louis, Jr. "Critical Fanonism." *Critical Inquiry* 17 (1991): 457–70.

Geertz, Clifford. "Common Sense as a Cultural System." In *Local Knowledge: Further Essays in Interpretive Anthropology.* New York: Basic Books, 1983. 73–93.

———. *Local Knowledge: Further Essays in Interpretive Anthropology.* New York: Basic Books, 1983.

Geismar, Peter. *Fanon.* New York: Dial, 1971.

Gellner, Ernest, and Charles Micaud, eds. *Arabs and Berbers: From Tribe to Nation in North Africa.* Lexington, Mass.: D. C. Heath, 1972.

Gelman, Sheldon. *Medicating Schizophrenia: A History.* New Brunswick, N.J.: Rutgers University Press, 1999.

Gendzier, Irene. *Frantz Fanon: A Critical Study.* New York: Pantheon, 1973.

Gérente, Paul. "Discussion du budget de l'Algérie (Exercice 1895)." Paris: Imprimerie des Journaux officiels, 1895.

Gérente, Paul, and Henri Colin. *Réforme de la loi du 30 juin 1838 sur les Aliénés: Projet de loi sur le Régime des malades attents d'affectations mentales. Projet de la Commission du Sénat chargée d'examiner la proposition de loi adoptée par la Chambre des Députés (Projet Dubief, 1907).* Paris: Imprimerie Coueslant, 1911.

Gershovich, Moshe. "The Ait Ya'qub Incident and the Crisis of French Military Policy in Morocco." *Journal of Military History* 62, no. 1 (1998): 57–73.

Gervais, Dr. "L'oeuvre sociale de la France en Algérie hier et aujourd'hui." *Bulletin sanitaire de l'Algérie* 508 (1940): 493.

Gilman, Sander L. *Difference and Pathology: Stereotypes of Sexuality, Race, and Madness.* Ithaca, N.Y.: Cornell University Press, 1985.

———. *Picturing Health and Illness: Images of Identity and Difference.* Baltimore, Md.: Johns Hopkins University Press, 1995.

Glidden, Harold W. "The Arab World." *American Journal of Psychiatry* 128, no. 8 (1972): 984–88.

Goffman, Erving. *Asylums: Essays on the Social Situation of Mental Patients and Other Inmates.* Garden City, N.Y.: Anchor, 1961.

———. "Characteristics of Total Institutions." In *Symposium on Preventive and Social Psychiatry, 15–17 April 1957.* Washington, D.C.: Walter Reed Army Institute of Research, 1958. 43–84.

Goldberg, Ann. *Sex, Religion, and the Making of Modern Madness: The Eberbach Asylum and German Society, 1815–1849.* New York: Oxford University Press, 1999.

Goldstein, Jan. *Console and Classify: The French Psychiatric Profession in the Nineteenth Century.* New York: Cambridge, 1987.

Good, Byron J. "Culture and DSM-IV: Diagnosis, Knowledge and Power." *Culture, Medicine and Psychiatry* 20 (1996): 127–32.

Goonatilake, Susantha. "Modern Science and the Periphery: The Characteristics of Dependent Knowledge." In *The "Racial" Economy of Science: Toward a Democratic Future*, ed. Sandra Harding. Bloomington: Indiana University Press, 1993. 259–73.

———. *Toward a Global Science: Mining Civilizational Knowledge.* Bloomington: Indiana University Press, 1999.

Gould, Steven Jay. *The Mismeasure of Man.* New York: Norton, 1981.

Gran, Peter. "Medical Pluralism in Arab and Egyptian History: An Overview of Class Structures and Philosophies of the Main Phases." *Social Science and Medicine* 13 (1979): 339–48.

Greenwood, Bernard. "Cold or Spirits? Choice and Ambiguity in Morocco's Pluralistic Medical System." *Social Science and Medicine* 15 (1981): 219–35.

Guiraud. Response to "Les services hospitaliers de psychiatrie dans l'Afrique du Nord." *Annales médico-psychologiques* 94, no. 1 (1936): 804–5.

Guiraud, A. *Le code de procédure pénale tunisien annoté, suivi d'un Nouveau Commentaire jurisprudentiel du Code pénal tunisien et d'un Répertoire pénal général Tunisien.* Tunis: SAPI, 1947.

Hansen, Emmanuel. "Frantz Fanon: Portrait of a Revolutionary Intellectual." *Transition* 46 (1974): 25–36.

Hargreaves, Alec G. *Immigration and Identity in Beur Fiction: Voices from the North African Community in France.* Oxford: Berg, 1997.

Harrington, Anne. "Unmasking Suffering's Masks: Reflections on Old and New Memories of Nazi Medicine." *Daedalus* 125 (1996): 181–205.

Harrison, Mark. *Climates and Constitutions: Health, Race, Environment and British Imperialism in India, 1600–1850.* New York: Oxford University Press, 1997.

Harrow, Kenneth. "Metaphors for Revolution: Blood and Schizophrenia in Boudjedra's Early Novels." *Présence francophone* 20 (1980): 5–19.

Hartnack, Christiane. "Vishnu on Freud's Desk: Psychoanalysis in Colonial India." *Social Research* 57 (1990): 921–49.

Healy, David. *The Creation of Psychopharmacology.* Cambridge, Mass.: Harvard University Press, 2002.

Herschel, Helena J. "Psychiatric Institutions: Rules and the Accommodation of Structure and Autonomy in France and the United States." In *Ethnopsychiatry: The Cultural Construction of Professional and Folk Psychiatries*, ed. Atwood D. Gaines. Albany: SUNY Press, 1992. 307–26.

Hirsch, Charles-A. "La criminalité des nord-africains en France est-elle une criminalité par défaut d'adaptation?" Paper delivered at the Société Internationale de Prophylaxie Sociale, Paris, 27 March 1959. CHE VI 2, Ethnopsychiatrie III: Criminalité chez certains peuples.

Hoisington, William A. *Lyautey and the French Conquest of Morocco.* New York: St. Martin's Press, 1995.

Hopwood, Derek. *Habib Bourguiba of Tunisia: The Tragedy of Longevity.* New York: St. Martin's Press, 1992.

Horne, Alastair. *A Savage War of Peace: Algeria, 1954–1962.* New York: 1978.

Horne, Janet R. "In Pursuit of Greater France: Visions of Empire among Musée Social Reformers, 1894–1931." In *Domesticating the Empire: Race, Gender, and Family Life in French and Dutch Colonialism*, ed. Julia Clancy-Smith and Frances Gouda. Charlottesville: University of Virginia Press, 1998. 21–42.

Houssin, G. "Un cas de confusion avec onirisme et auto-analyse à la suite d'un électro-choc: Evolution vers la guérison en 24 heures." *Maroc-médical* (April 1949): 228.

Hoyt, David L. "The Reanimation of the Primitive: *Fin-de-siècle* Ethnographic Discourse in Western Europe." *History of Science* 36 (2001): 331–54.

Huot, V. L. "L'aliénation mentale à Madagascar." *Annales de médecine et de pharmacie coloniales* 34 (1936): 5–39.

Jacob, Françoise. "La psychiatrie française face au monde colonial au XIXe siècle." In *Découvertes et explorateurs: Actes du Colloque International, Bordeaux, 12–14 Juin 1992, VIIe Colloque d'Histoire au Présent*. Paris: L'Harmattan, 1994: 365–73.

Jamison, Kay Redfield. *An Unquiet Mind: A Memoir of Moods and Madness*. New York: Vintage, 1995.

Igert, Maurice, and L. Viaud. Bilan d'une année d'électro-chocs." *Maroc-médical* (April 1949): 217–19.

Jacquel, G., and J. Morel. "Sorcellerie et troubles mentaux: Étude faite dans le département de l'Orne." *L'encéphale* 54 (1965): 5–35.

Jayle, F. "La faculté de médecine et l'hôpital de Mustapha." *La presse médicale* (17 January 1934): 97–101.

Jeddi, Essedik, dir. *Al Baab* [film]. Tunisia, 1980.

———. "Aspect sociogène de la morbidité psychiatrique chez l'ouvrier arabe transplanté en France." *Congrès des médedins aliénistes et neurologistes de France et de pays de langue française*, Tunis (1972): 1407–20.

Jeddi, Essedik, ed. *Le corps en psychiatrie: Colloque International Ibn Sina-Collomb*. Paris: Masson, 1982.

Jeddi, Essedik, Abdelhamid Bouzgarrou, C. Mili, and K. Harzallah. "Corps et asile." In *Le corps en psychiatrie: Colloque International Ibn Sina-Collomb*, ed. Essedik Jeddi. Paris: Masson, 1982. 135–55.

Joyaux, Georges. "Driss Chraïbi, Mohammed Dib, Kateb Yacine, and Indigenous North African Literature." *Yale French Studies* 24 (1959): 30–40.

Joyeux, Charles. *Hygiène de l'Européen aux colonies*. Paris: A. Colin, 1928.

Jude, René, and Victor Augagneur. "Utilité de l'étude de la psychologie des indigènes pour les médecins, officiers, administrateurs coloniaux: Necessité d'une collaboration étroite en ce qui concerne les actes administratifs et militaires et pour le dépistage des anomalies mentales." *Congrès des médedins aliénistes et neurologistes de France et de pays de langue française*, Paris (1925): 263–66.

Julien, Isaac, dir. *Frantz Fanon: Black Skin, White Mask* [film]. Produced by Mark Nash for the Arts Coucil of England. United Kingdom, 1996. DVD: California Newsreel, San Francisco.

Kalifa, Dominique. "Les tâcherons de l'information: Petits reporters et faits divers à la Belle Époque." *Revue d'histoire moderne et contemporaine* 40 (1993): 578–604.

Kalinowsky, Lothar B., and Paul H. Hoch. *Shock Treatments, Psychosurgery and Other Somatic Treatments in Psychiatry*. 2nd ed. New York: Grune and Stratton, 1952.

Kateb, Kamel. *Européens, "Indigènes" et Juifs en Algérie, 1830–1962: Représentations et réalités des populations*. Paris: Press Universitaires de France, 2001.

Katz, Jonathan G. "The 1907 Mauchamp Affair and the French Civilising Mission in Morocco." In *North Africa, Islam, and the Mediterranean World: From the Almoravids to the Algerian War*, ed. Julia Clancy-Smith. London: Frank Cass, 2001. 143–66.

Kayanakis, Nicolas. *Algérie 1960: La victoire trahie; Guerre psychologique en Algérie*. Friedberg: Editions Atlantis, 2000.

Kechiche, Abdellatif, dir. *La faute à Voltaire* [film]. France, 2000. DVD: Paris, One Plus One, 2002.

Keller, Richard. "Geographies of Power, Legacies of Mistrust: Colonial Medicine in the Global Present." *Historical Geography* 34 (2006): 26–48.

———. "Madness and Colonization: Psychiatry in the British and French Empires, 1800–1962." *Journal of Social History* 35 (2001): 295–326.

———. "Pinel in the Maghreb: Liberation, Confinement, and Psychiatric Reform in French North Africa." *Bulletin of the History of Medicine* 79 (2005): 459–99.

Khanna, Ranjana. *Dark Continents: Psychoanalysis and Colonialism*. Durham, N.C.: Duke University Press, 2003.

Khélil, Hédi. "Drames à la Manouba." *Le Maghreb* (1981): 28–33.

Khiati, Mostéfa. *Histoire de la médecine en Algérie: De l'antiquité à nos jours*. Rouiba, Algeria: Editions ANEP, 2000.

King, Anthony D. *Colonial Urban Development: Culture, Social Power, and Environment*. London: Routledge, 1976.

———. *Urbanism, Colonialism, and the World Economy: Cultural and Spatial Foundations of the World Urban System*. London: Routledge, 1990.

Kirmayer, Laurence J., and Harry Minas. "The Future of Cultural Psychiatry: An International Perspective." *Canadian Journal of Psychiatry* 45 (2000): 438–46.

Kleinman, Arthur. "Anthropology and Psychiatry: The Role of Culture in Cross-Cultural Psychiatric Research on Illness." *British Journal of Psychiatry* 151 (1987): 447–54.

———. *The Illness Narratives: Suffering, Healing, and the Human Condition*. New York: Basic Books, 1988.

———. *Patients and Healers in the Context of Culture: An Exploration of the Borderland between Anthropology, Medicine, and Psychiatry*. Berkeley: University of California Press, 1980.

———. "What Is Specific to Western Medicine?" In *Companion Encyclopedia of the History of Medicine*, ed. W. F. Bynum and Roy Porter. 2 vols. New York: Routledge, 1993. 1:15–23.

Kleinman, Arthur, and Joan Kleinman. "The Appeal of Experience, the Dismay of Images: Cultural Appropriations of Suffering in Our Times." *Daedalus* 125, no. 1 (1996): 1–23.

Kocher, A. *De la criminalité chez les Arabes au point de vue de la pratique médico-judiciaire en Algérie*. Paris: J. B. Baillière et fils, 1884.

Kohler, Robert E. *Landscapes and Labscapes: Exploring the Lab-Field Border in Biology*. Chicago: University of Chicago Press, 2002.

———. *Lords of the Fly: Drosophila Genetics and the Experimental Life*. Chicago: University of Chicago Press, 1994.

Kortmann, Frank. "Psychiatric Case Finding in Ethiopia: Shortcomings of the Self-Reporting Questionnaire." *Culture, Medicine and Psychiatry* 14 (1990): 381–91.

Kraepelin, Emil. "Vergleichende Psychiatrie." *Centralblatt für Nervenheilkunde und Psychiatrie* 15 (1904): 433–37.

Kraiem, Mustapha. *Mouvement national et front populaire: La Tunisie des années trente.* Tunis: ISHMN, 1996.

Kramer, Jane. "Les pieds-noirs." In *Unsettling Europe.* New York: Random House, 1980. 171–217.

Kuisel, Richard. *Seducing the French: The Dilemma of Americanization.* Berkeley: University of California Press, 1993.

Kuklick, Henrika. *The Savage Within: The Social History of British Anthropology, 1885–1945.* New York: Cambridge University Press, 1991.

Kuklick, Henrika, and Robert E. Kohler, eds. *Science in the Field.* Osiris 11. Chicago: University of Chicago Press, 1996.

Kunzel, Regina G. *Fallen Women, Problem Girls: Unmarried Mothers and the Professionalization of Social Work, 1890–1945.* New Haven, Conn.: Yale University Press, 1993.

Laborit, Henri. "Sur l'utilisation de certains agents pharmacodynamiques à action neuro-végétative en période per-[*sic*; pre-] et postopératoire." *Acta Clinica Belgica* 48, no. 7 (1949): 485–92.

———. "La thérapeutique neuro-végétative du choc et de la maladie posttraumatique." *La presse médicale* (11 February 1950): 138–40.

Laborit, Henri, Pierre Huguenard, and R. Alluaume. "Un nouveau stabilisateur végétatif (le 4560 RP)." *La presse médicale* (13 February 1952): 206–8.

Lacan, Jacques. *De la psychose paranoïaque dans ses rapports avec la personnalité.* Paris: Seuil, 1975 [1932].

———. "Motifs du crime paranoïaque." *Minotaure* 3–4 (1933): 25–28.

———. "Le problème du style et la conception psychiatrique des formes paranoïaques de l'expérience." *Minotaure* 1 (1933): 68.

Lacoste-Dujardin, Camille. *Opération Oiseau Bleu: Des Kabyles, des ethnologues et la guerre d'Algérie.* Paris: L'Harmattan, 1997.

Laing, R. D. *The Divided Self: A Study of Sanity and Madness.* Chicago: Quadrangle, 1960.

Lamartine, Alphonse de. *Voyage en Orient: Éd. critique avec documents inédits.* Ed. Lotfy Fam. Paris: Librairie Nizet, 1959.

Landau, Philippe-E. *Les Juifs de France et la Grande Guerre: Un patriotisme républicain, 1914–1941.* Paris: CNRS, 1999.

Lapipe, M., and J. Rondepierre. "L'électro-choc (2e note): Premières impressions cliniques d'après 250 crises; étude des conditions nécessaires à leur déclenchement." *La presse médicale* (1–4 October 1941) 1069.

———. "Essai d'un appareil français pour l'électrochoc." *La presse médicale* (28–31 May 1941): 582.

Laplantine, François. *Anthropologie de la maladie.* Paris: Payot, 1986.

———. *L'ethnopsychiatrie.* Paris: Seuil, 1988.

Larguèche, Abdelhamid. *Les ombres de la ville: Pauvres, marginaux et minoritaires à Tunis (XVIIIème et XIXème siècles).* Manouba: Centre de Publication Universitaire, Faculté des Lettres, 1999.

Larheribi, Ahmed. "Maladie mentale et acculturation." *Al-Asas* 62 (1984): 35–38.

Lasnet, Alexandre. "Communication sur les mesures de réorganisation des services sanitaires en Algérie." *Bulletin de l'Académie de médecine* 96, no. 35 (1932): 1303–9.

Lasnet, Alexandre, and Antoine Porot. "L'organisation de l'assistance psychiatrique en Algérie." *Congrès des médedins aliénistes et neurologistes de France et de pays de langue française*, Limoges (1932): 385–90.

Latour, Bruno. "Give Me a Laboratory and I Will Raise the World." In *Science Observed: Perspectives on the Social Study of Science*, ed. Karin Knorr-Cetina. London: Sage, 1983. 141–70.

———. *The Pasteurization of France*. Trans. Alan Sheridan and John Law. Cambridge, Mass.: Harvard University Press, 1988.

———. *Petite réflexion sur le culte moderne des dieux faitiches*. Paris: Synthélabo, 1996.

Lauriol, Louis. "Quelques remarques sur les maladies mentales aux colonies." Med. thesis, Paris, 1938.

Le Bon, Gustave. *La psychologie des foules*. Paris: Alcan, 1895.

———. *The Psychology of Peoples*. London: Macmillan, 1899.

Lebovics, Herman. *True France*. Ithaca, N.Y.: Cornell University Press, 1994.

Lefèvre, R. "L'assistance psychiatrique en Indochine." *Congrès des médedins aliénistes et neurologistes de France et de pays de langue française*, Bordeaux (1931): 293–97.

Léger, J. M., A. Péron, and J. N. Vallat. "Aspects actuels de la sorcellerie dans ses rapports avec la psychiatrie. Peut-on parler de délire de sorcellerie?" *Annales médico-psychologiques* 129, no. 2 (1972): 559–75.

Lemanski, Witold. *Hygiène du colon, ou Vade-mecum de l'Européen aux colonies*. Paris: Steinheil, 1902.

Levet. "L'assistance des aliénés algériens dans un asile métropolitain." Part 1. *Annales médico-psychologiques* 67 (1909): 45–67.

———. "L'assistance des aliénés algériens dans un asile métropolitain." Part 2. *Annales médico-psychologiques* 67 (1909): 239–49.

Lévy-Bruhl, Lucien. *Les fonctions mentales dans les sociétés inférieures*. 3rd ed. Paris: Alcan, 1918.

———. *Primitive Mentality*. Trans. Lilian A. Clare. New York: Macmillan, 1923.

Lévy-Valensi, Jean. "Mentalité primitive et psychopathologie." *Annales médico-psychologiques* 92, no. 1 (1934): 676–701.

Lewis, Mary Dewhurst. "The Company of Strangers: Immigration and Citizenship in Interwar Lyon and Marseille." Ph. D. diss., New York University, 2000.

Lheimeur, Majid. "À la croisée d'une rencontre: Parcours et technique d'une thérapeute Gnawia (Maroc)." *Nouvelle revue d'ethnopsychiatrie* 13 (1989): 41–52.

Livet, Louis. "Aliénés algériens et leur hospitalisation." Med. thesis, Algiers, Montégut et Deguili, n. d. [1911].

Longuenesse, Elisabeth, ed. *Santé, médecine et société dans le monde arabe*. Paris: L'Harmattan, 1995.

Lorcin, Patricia. *Imperial Identities: Stereotyping, Prejudice, and Race in Colonial Algeria*. London: Tauris, 1995.

———. "Imperialism, Colonial Identity, and Race in Algeria, 1830–1870: The Role of the French Medical Corps." *Isis* 90 (1999): 653–79.

———. "Rome and France in Africa: Recovering Colonial Algeria's Latin Past." *French Historical Studies* 25, no. 2 (2002): 295–329.

Loussaief, Moncef. "L'assistance psychiatrique en Tunisie et ses problèmes." *La Tunisie médicale* (1970): 77–85.

Lowe, Lisa. *Critical Terrains: French and British Orientalisms*. Ithaca, N.Y.: Cornell University Press, 1991.

Luccioni, J. "Les maristanes du Maroc: Le nouveau maristane de Sidi-Fredj à Fès." *Bulletin economique et sociale du Maroc* 16 (1953): 461–70.

Luhrmann, T. M. *Of Two Minds: An Anthropologist Looks at American Psychiatry.* New York: Knopf, 2000.

Lunbeck, Elizabeth. *The Psychiatric Persuasion: Knowledge, Gender, and Power in Modern America.* Princeton, N.J.: Princeton University Press, 1995.

Lwoff, Solomon, and Paul Sérieux. "Les aliénés au Maroc." *Annales médico-psychologiques* 69, no. 1 (1911): 470–79.

———. "Sur quelques moyens de contrainte appliqués aux aliénés au Maroc." *Bulletin de la Société clinique de médecine mentale* 4 (1911): 168–74.

Ly, Madeleine. "Introduction à une psychanalyse africaine." Med. thesis, Paris, Faculté de Médecine, 1948.

Mabille, Henri. *Notice sur l'asile des aliénés de la Charente Inférieure (Asile de Lafond).* La Rochelle: Martin, 1893.

Macey, David. "The Algerian with the Knife." *Parallax* 4, no. 2 (1998): 159–67.

———. *Frantz Fanon: A Biography.* London: Picador, 2000.

MacLeod, Roy. "On Visiting the 'Moving Metropolis': Reflections on the Architecture of Imperial Science." In *Scientific Colonialism: A Cross-Cultural Comparison,* ed. Nathan Reingold and Marc Rothenberg. Washington, D.C.: Smithsonian, 1987. 217–49.

MacLeod, Roy, ed. *Nature and Empire: Science and the Colonial Enterprise.* Osiris, 2nd ser., 15. Chicago: University of Chicago Press, 2001.

Maier, Charles. *Recasting Bourgeois Europe: Stabilization in France, Germany, and Italy in the Decade after World War I.* Princeton, N.J.: Princeton University Press, 1975.

Mallem, Leïla. "La folie féminine et ses représentations romanesques dans quelques oeuvres algériennes et libanaises." Doctoral thesis, University of Paris XIII, 1999.

Manceaux, A., C. Bardenat, and R. Susini. "L'hystérie chez l'indigène algérien. Quelques aspects de ses manifestations en milieu militaire." *Annales médico-psychologiques* 105, no. 2 (1947): 1–34.

Manderson, Leonore. *Sickness and the State: Health and Illness in Colonial Malaya, 1870–1940.* New York: Cambridge University Press, 1996.

Manue, Georges R. "La guerre psychologique." *France Outremer* 33 (June 1956): 19.

Maran, Rita. *Torture: The Role of Ideology in the French-Algerian War.* New York: Praeger, 1989.

Maréschal, Pierre. "L'héroïnomanie en Tunisie." *Congrès des médedins aliénistes et neurologistes de France et de pays de langue française,* Nancy (1937): 255–59.

———. "Réflexions sur vingt ans de psychiatrie en Tunisie." *La raison* 15 (1956): 69–79.

Maréschal, Pierre, Tahar Ben Soltane, and Victor Corcos. "Résultats du traitement par l'électro-choc appliqué à 340 malades a l'Hôpital psychiatique de La Manouba (Tunisie)." *Congrès des médecins aliénistes et neurologistes de France et de pays de langue française,* Montpellier (1942): 341–46.

Maréschal, Pierre, and Lamarche. "L'assistance médicale aux aliénés en Tunisie." *Congrès des médedins aliénistes et neurologistes de France et de pays de langue française,* Nancy (1937): 393–401.

Margain, L. "L'aliénation mentale aux colonies et pays de protectorat." *Revue indigène* 23 (1908), 7.

Marie, Auguste. "Conférences faite à l'Ecole d'Anthropologie, 16–29 mars 1907." CHE.

———. "Rapport sur la question des Asiles coloniaux (Description de l'Asile d'aliénés d'Abbasieh, Egypte." *Dritter internationaler Kongress für Irrenfürsorge in Wien vom 7.–11. Oktober 1909.* Vienna: Franz Doll, 1909.

Martin, Gustave. "L'influence du climat tropical sur le psychisme de l'Européen." *Les Grandes endémies tropicales* 3 (1932): 101–16.

———. "La mentalité primitive indigène devant nos méthodes de prophylaxie et de thérapeutique modernes." *Les Grandes endémies tropicales* 6 (1934): 93–106.

Martin, Gustave, and Ringenbach. "Troubles psychiques dans la maladie du sommeil." Part 1. *Annales d'hygiène et de médecine coloniales* 13 (1910): 723–56.

———. "Troubles psychiques dans la maladie du sommeil." Part 2. *Annales d'hygiène et de médecine coloniales* 14 (1911): 151–83.

Masson, Agnes. *L'assistance psychiatrique nouvelle.* Paris: Editions Champenoises, 1948.

Mathias, Gregor. *Les Sections Administratives Spécialisées en Algérie: Entre idéal et réalité.* Paris: L'Harmattan, 1998.

Mauss-Copeaux, Claire. *Appelés en Algérie: La parole confisquée.* Paris: Hachette Littératures, 1998.

Maupassant, Guy de. *La vie errante.* Paris: Librairie Paul Ollendorff, n. d. [1900].

Maurin, Armand. *Khenchela.* Paris: La pensée universelle, 1981.

McClintock, Anne. *Imperial Leather: Race, Gender, and Sexuality in the Colonial Contest.* New York: Routledge, 1995.

McCulloch, Jock. *Black Soul, White Artifact: Fanon's Clinical Psychology and Social Theory.* New York: Cambridge University Press, 1983.

———. *Colonial Psychiatry and "the African Mind."* New York: Cambridge University Press, 1995.

Mehta, Uday Singh. *Liberalism and Empire: A Study in Nineteenth-Century British Liberal Thought.* Chicago: University of Chicago Press, 1999.

Meilhon, Abel-Joseph. "L'aliénation mentale chez les Arabes: Étude de nosologie comparée." Part 1. *Annales médico-psychologiques* 54, no. 1 (1896): 17–32, 177–207, 364–77.

———. "L'aliénation mentale chez les Arabes: Étude de nosologie comparée." Part 2. *Annales médico-psychologiques* 54, no. 2 (1896): 26–40, 204–20, 344–63.

Memmi, Albert. *The Colonizer and the Colonized.* Trans. Howard Greenfield. New York: Orion, 1965.

———. *Le statue du sel.* Paris: Gallimard, 1966 [1953].

———. "La vie impossible de Frantz Fanon." *Esprit* (1971): 248–73.

Meriem, Abdelmadjid. "Sociologie et psychiatrie dans l'approche de la maladie mentale des immigrés maghrébins." *Revue sociologie santé* 9 (1993): 111–31.

Meyer, Philippe. "L'antipsychiatrie." *Esprit* (1971): 207–25.

Michaux, Léon. "Professeur Antoine Porot." *Annales médico-psychologiques* 123, no. 2 (1965): 71–72.

Michel, Andrée. "Les Algériens à l'hôtel à Paris: Psychopathologie de la vie quotidienne." *La raison* 15 (1956): 81–87.

Micouleau-Sicault, Marie-Claire. *Les médecins français au Maroc, 1912-1956: Combats en urgence.* Paris: L'Harmattan, 2000.

Mignot, Roger. "Les journées médicales tunisiennes et l'assistance des aliénés en Tunisie." *L'hygiène mentale* 21, no. 6 (June 1926): 159–64.

Miller, Christopher L. *Blank Darkness: Africanist Discourse in French.* Chicago: University of Chicago Press, 1985.

Mills, James. *Madness, Cannabis, and Colonialism: The "Native Only" Lunatic Asylums of British India, 1857–1900.* New York: St. Martin's Press, 2000.

Ministère des Colonies. *Exposition Coloniale Internationale de 1931: Rapport Général présenté par le gouverneur général Olivier (Marcel) Rapporteur Général délégué général à l'exposition.* 9 vols. Paris: Imprimerie nationale, 1933.

Miquel, Pierre. *La guerre d'Algérie: Images inédites des archives militaires.* Paris: Chêne, 1993.

Mitchell, Timothy. *Colonising Egypt.* Berkeley: University of California Press, 1991.

Mohia, Nadia. "Pratiques traditionnelles et psychiatrie dans la société kabyle." *Cahiers de sociologie economique et culturelle* 9 (1988): 47–65.

Mongin, Olivier. "Guerre des cultures ou modernisation avortée?" *Esprit* (1991): 15–18.

Monnais-Rousselot, Laurence. *Médecine et colonisation: L'aventure Indochinoise, 1860–1939.* Paris: CNRS, 1999.

Montgomery, Scott L. *Science in Translation: Movements of Knowledge through Cultures and Time.* Chicago: University of Chicago Press, 2000.

Morel, Pierre, and Claude Quétel. "Les thérapeutiques de l'aliénation mentale au XIXe siècle." In *Nouvelle histoire de la psychiatrie,* ed. Jacques Postel and Claude Quétel. Paris: Dunod, 1994. 314–26

Moreau (de Tours), Joseph. "Recherches sur les aliénés en Orient." *Annales médico-psychologiques* 1, no. 1 (1843): 103–32.

Morton, Patricia. *Hybrid Modernities: Architecture and Representation at the 1931 Colonial Exposition, Paris.* Cambridge, Mass.: MIT Press, 2000.

Nandy, Ashis. *The Intimate Enemy: Loss and Recovery of Self under Colonialism.* Delhi: Oxford University Press, 1983.

——. *The Savage Freud and Other Essays on Possible and Retrievable Selves.* Princeton, N.J.: Princeton University Press, 1995.

Nathan, Tobie. *La folie des autres: Traité d'ethnopsychiatrie clinique.* Paris: Dunod, 1986.

——. *L'influence qui guérit.* Paris: Odile Jacob, 1994.

——. "Psychothérapie et politique: Les enjeux théoriques, institutionnels et politiques de l'ethnopsychiatrie." *Genèses* 38 (2000): 136–59.

Noiriel, Gérard. *Le creuset français: Histoire de l'immigration, XIXe–XXe siècles.* Paris: Seuil, 1988.

Nolan, Mary. *Visions of Modernity: American Business and the Modernization of Germany.* New York: Oxford University Press, 1994.

Nye, Robert. *Crime, Madness, and Politics in Modern France.* Princeton, N.J.: Princeton University Press, 1984.

——. *The Origins of Crowd Psychology: Gustave Le Bon and the Crisis of Mass Democracy in the Third Republic.* Beverly Hills, Calif.: Sage, 1975.

L'oeuvre de la santé publique au Maroc. Paris: Copernic, 1951.

Olivier de Sardan, Jean-Pierre. "Possession, affliction et folie: Les ruses de la thérapisation." *L'homme* 34, no. 131 (1994): 7–28.

Ortigues, Marie-Cécile, and Edmond Ortigues. *Oedipe africain.* Paris: Plon, 1966.

Orwell, George. "Shooting an Elephant." In *Shooting an Elephant and Other Essays.* New York: Harcourt, Brace, 1950.

Osborne, Michael. *Nature, the Exotic, and the Science of French Colonialism.* Bloomington: Indiana University Press, 1993.

Palladino, Paolo, and Michael Worboys. "Science and Imperialism." *Isis* 84 (1993): 91–102.

Pandey, Gyanendra. "In Defense of the Fragment: Writing about Hindu-Muslim Riots in India Today." In *A Subaltern Studies Reader, 1986–1995.* Ed. Ranajit Guha. Minneapolis: University of Minnesota Press, 1997. 1–33.

Pandolfo, Stefania. *Impasse of the Angels: Scenes from a Moroccan Space of Memory.* Chicago: University of Chicago Press, 1997.

Patai, Raphael. *The Arab Mind.* New York: Scribner, 1973.

Paul, Jim. "Medicine and Imperialism in Morocco." *MERIP Reports* 60 (1977): 3–12.

Pelis, Kim. "Prophet for Profit in French North Africa: Charles Nicolle and the Pasteur Institute of Tunis, 1903–1936." *Bulletin of the History of Medicine* 71, no. 4 (1997): 583–622.

Pendola, Marinette. "L'insolation de Rachid Boudjedra ou le refus de la communication." *Présence francophone* 18 (1979): 19–27.

Périale, Marise. "Les formations neuro-psychiatriques du Maroc." *Paris médical,* 25 January 1936, 83–88.

———. *Le Maroc à 60 kms à l'heure.* Casablanca: Imprimerie Réunies, 1936.

Peyre, E.-L. "Les maladies mentales aux colonies." *L'hygiène mentale* 29, no. 8 (September–October 1934): 185–212.

———. "Le suicide et ses aspects dans les troupes coloniales." *Annales de médecine et de pharmacie coloniales* 34 (1936): 939–66.

Philibert, Nicolas, dir. *La moindre des choses* [film]. France, 1996. DVD: Paris, Éditions Montparnasse, 2002.

Pick, Daniel. *Faces of Degeneration: A European Disorder, 1848–1915.* New York: Cambridge University Press, 1989.

Pierson, C. A. "L'assistance psychiatrique au Maroc." *Maroc médical* (April 1949): n. p.

———. "La chlorpromazine et la maitrise de soi dans les angoisses collectives." *L'encéphale* 45, no. 4 (1956): 562–65.

———. "Paléophrénie réactionnelle: Psychopathologie de l'impulsion morbide en milieu nord-africain." *Maroc médical* 360 (1955): 642–47.

Pierson, C. A., R. P. Poitrot, and Rolland. "L'assistance psychiatrique au Maroc." *L'information psychiatrique* 31, no. 1 (January 1955): 30–37.

Pierson, Ruth Roach, and Nupur Chaudhuri, eds. *Nation, Empire, Colony: Historicizing Gender and Race.* Bloomington: Indiana University Press, 1998.

Pinel, Philippe. *The Clinical Training of Doctors: An Essay of 1793.* Ed. and trans. Dora Weiner. Baltimore, Md.: Johns Hopkins University Press, 1980.

———. *Traité médico-philosophique sur l'aliénation mentale, ou la manie.* Paris: Richard, Caille, et Ravier, An IX (1801).

Plichet, André. "L'électro-choc: Le traitement des affections mentales par les crises convulsives électriques." *La presse médicale* (20–23 November 1940) 937–39.

———. Review of Antoine Porot, ed., *Manuel alphabétique de psychiatrie clinique, thérapeutique, et médico-légale,* 1st ed. *La presse médicale* (11 June 1952): 879.

Pontecorvo, Gillo, and Saadi Yacef, dir. *The Battle of Algiers* [film]. Italy/Algeria, 1965. DVD: Criterion Collection, 2004.

Poitrot, R.-P. "Considérations sur le traitement de certaines psychoses par la méthode de la convulsivothérapie électrique et de la pyrétothérapie associée." *Maroc-médical* (April 1949): 220–25.

Porot, Antoine. "L'assistance psychiatrique en Algérie et le futur Hôpital psychiatrique de Blida." *L'Algérie médicale*, no. 65 (May 1933): 86–92.

———. "Au sujet de l'assistance psychiatrique et de l'enseignement en Algérie." *L'hygiène mentale* 21, no. 3 (March 1926): 67–69.

———. "Chronique algérienne." *L'hygiène mentale* 20, no. 9 (November 1925): 269–79.

———. "Dernier mot—en réponse à M. Dumolard—sur l'assistance psychiatrique en Algérie." *L'hygiène mentale* 21, no. 6 (June 1926): 145.

———. "Notes de psychiatrie musulmane." *Annales médico-psychologiques* 76 (May 1918): 377–84.

———. "L'oeuvre psychiatrique de la France aux colonies depuis un siècle." *Annales médico-psychologiques* 101, no. 1 (1943): 356–78.

———. "Résultats d'une expérience de 'Service ouvert' pour psychopathes en Tunisie." *Informateur des aliénistes* 18, no. 5 (May 1923): 111–14.

———. "Les services hospitaliers de psychiatrie dans l'Afrique du Nord (Algérie et Tunisie)." *Annales médico-psychologiques* 94, no. 1 (1936): 793–806.

———. "La situation des aliénés français en Tunisie." *Tunisie médicale* 1, no. 2 (1911): 70–76.

Porot, Antoine, ed. *Manuel alphabétique de psychiatrie clinique, thérapeutique, et médico-légale.* Paris: PUF, 1952–96.

Porot, Antoine, and Don Côme Arrii. "L'impulsivité criminelle chez l'indigène algérien: Ses facteurs." *Annales médico-psychologiques* 90, no. 2 (1932): 588–611.

Porot, Antoine, and Charles Bardenat. *Anormaux et malades mentaux devant la justice pénale.* Paris: Maloine, 1960.

———. *Psychiatrie médico-légale.* Paris: Maloine, 1959.

Porot, Antoine, Charles Bardenat, Jean Sutter, Maurice Porot, Pierre Léonardon, and Th. Kammerer. "Réflexions sur 3.000 électro-chocs pratiqués dans les services psychiatrique de l'Algérie." *Congrès des médedins aliénistes et neurologistes de France et de pays de langue française*, Montpellier (1942): 329–36.

Porot, Antoine, and Angelo Hesnard. *L'expertise mentale militaire.* Paris: Masson, 1918.

———. *Psychiatrie de guerre: Etude clinique.* Paris: Alcan, 1919.

Porot, Antoine, and Jean Sutter. "Le 'primitivisme' des indigènes Nord-Africains: Ses incidences en pathologie mentale." *Sud médical et chirurgical* (15 April 1939): 226–41.

Porot, Antonin [Antoine]. "La question des injections mercurielles dans le traitement de la syphilis nerveuse (étude critique)." Med. thesis, Lyon, 1904.

Porot, Maurice. "Cardiazol." In *Manuel alphabétique de psychiatrie clinique, thérapeutique, et médico-légale*, 3rd ed., ed. Antoine Porot. Paris: PUF, 1964. 104.

———. "Cardiazol-test." In *Manuel alphabétique de psychiatrie clinique, thérapeutique, et médico-légale*, 3rd ed., ed. Antoine Porot. Paris: PUF, 1964. 104.

———. "Electrochoc." In *Manuel alphabétique de psychiatrie clinique, thérapeutique, et médico-légale*, 3rd ed., ed. Antoine Porot. Paris: PUF, 1964. 192–94.

———. "Electrochocs et cardiopathies." *Annales médico-psychologiques* 113, no. 2 (December 1955): 814–21.

————. "Insulinotherapie." In *Manuel alphabétique de psychiatrie clinique, thérapeutique, et médico-légale*, 3rd ed., ed. Antoine Porot. Paris: PUF, 1964. 311.

————. "La leucotomie préfrontale en psychiatrie." *Annales médico-psychologiques* 105, no. 2 (1947): 121–42.

————. "Les intoxications arsenicales par le vin et les produits viticoles." Med. thesis, Algiers, 1938.

————. "Traitements psychiatriques de choc et grossesse." *La presse médicale* (3 December 1949): 118–20.

Porot, Maurice, and E. Bisquerra. "Note préliminaire sur l'utilisation de l'iodure de succinyl-choline dans la curarisation des malades soumis aux électro-chocs." *Annales médico-psychologiques* 112, no. 2 (October 1954): 449.

Porot, Maurice, and A. Cohen-Tenoudji. "Tuberculose et traitements psychiatriques de choc." *Annales médico-psychologiques* 113, no. 1 (March 1955): 376–408.

Porot, Maurice, and Pierre Descuns. "Etat actuel de la psycho-chirurgie." *Afrique française chirurgicale* 13, no. 6 (1955): 525–37.

Porot, Maurice, and G. Duboucher. "La guerison des alcooliques par l'antabus." *La presse médicale* (2 February 1952): 147.

Porot, Maurice, and J. Gentile. "Alcoolisme et troubles mentaux chez l'indigène musulman algérien." *Bulletin sanitaire de l'Algérie* 522 (May 1941): 125–30.

Porter, Roy. *A Social History of Madness: The World through the Eyes of the Insane*. New York: Weidenfield and Nicolson, 1988.

Postel, Jacques. *Génèse de la psychiatrie: Les premiers écrits de Philippe Pinel*. Paris: Institut Synthélabo, 1998.

Postel, Jacques, and Claude Quétel, eds. *Nouvelle histoire de la psychiatrie*. Paris: Dunod, 1994.

Potet. "Au sujet de l'hygiène mentale au Maroc." *Congrès des médedins aliénistes et neurologistes de France et de pays de langue française*, Rabat (1933): 449–51.

Prakash, Gyan. *Another Reason: Science and the Imagination of Modern India*. Princeton, N.J.: Princeton University Press, 1999.

Pressman, Jack D. *Last Resort: Psychosurgery and the Limits of Medicine*. New York: Cambridge University Press, 1997.

Prochaska, David. *Making Algeria French: Colonialism in Bône, 1870–1920*. New York: Cambridge University Press, 1990.

Proctor, Robert. *Racial Hygiene: Medicine under the Nazis*. Cambridge, Mass.: Harvard University Press, 1988.

Pyenson, Lewis. *Civilizing Mission: Exact Sciences and French Overseas Expansion*. Baltimore, Md.: Johns Hopkins University Press, 1993.

————. "Cultural Imperialism and Exact Sciences Revisited." *Isis* 84 (1993): 103–8.

Rabinow, Paul. *French Modern: Norms and Forms of the Social Environment*. Cambridge, Mass.: MIT Press, 1989.

————. *Reflections on Fieldwork in Morocco*. Chicago: University of Chicago Press, 1977.

Ramée, F., R. Lacaton, F. Sanchez, and M. Boulanger. "Effets favorables du Largactil dans la pratique psychiatrique algérienne." *L'encéphale* 45, no. 4 (1956): 821–27.

Raynaud, Lucien. *Etude sur l'hygiène et la médecine au Maroc, suivie d'une notice sur la climatologie des principales villes de l'empire*. Paris: Baillière et fils, 1902.

Régis, Emmanuel. "L'assistance des aliénés aux colonies (note additionnelle)." *L'informateur des aliénistes et neurologistes* 7 (1912): 177–88, 209–16.

―――. "La condition des aliénés dans les colonies néerlandaises (Législation et assistance)." *Journal de médecine légale psychiatrique et d'anthropologie criminelle* 1, no. 3 (25 June 1906): 97–107.

Review of Henri Aubin, "Le Mensonge: Reniement chez les psychopathes." *Congrès des médecins aliénistes et neurologistes de France et de pays de langue française*, Marseille (1948). *Annales médico-psychologiques* 106, no. 2 (1948): 517–18.

Rhodes, Lorna. "The Subject of Power in Medical/Psychiatric Anthropology." In *Ethnopsychiatry: The Cultural Construction of Professional and Folk Psychiatries*, ed. Atwood D. Gaines. Albany: SUNY Press, 1992. 51–66.

Riesman, Paul. "The Person and the Life Cycle in African Social Life and Thought." *African Studies Review* 29, no. 2 (1986): 71–138.

Ritchie, Karen, Sylvaine Artero, Isabelle Beluche, M.-L. Ancelin, A. Mann, A.-M. Dupuy, A. Malafosse, and J.-P. Boulenger. "Prevalence of DSM-IV psychiatric disorder in the French elderly population." *British Journal of Psychiatry* 184 (2004): 147–52.

Roberts, Mary Louise. *Civilization without Sexes: Reconstructing Gender in Postwar France, 1917–1927*. Chicago: University of Chicago Press, 1994.

Robinson, Ronald. "Non-European Foundations of European Imperialism: Sketch for a Theory of Collaboration." In *Studies in the Theory of Imperialism*, ed. Roger Owen and Bob Sutcliffe. London: Longman, 1972. 117–42.

Roheim, Géza. "Psychoanalysis of Primitive Cultural Types." *International Journal of Psychoanalysis* 13 (1932): 1–222.

Rose, Jacqueline. *On Not Being Able to Sleep: Psychoanalysis and the Modern World*. Princeton, N.J.: Princeton University Press, 2003.

Rosenberg, Charles E. "Framing Disease: Illness, Society, and History." In *Framing Disease: Studies in Cultural History*, ed. Charles E. Rosenberg and Janet Golden. New Brunswick, N.J.: Rutgers University Press, 1992. xlii–xxvi.

Rosenberg, Clifford D. "Republican Surveillance: Immigration, Citizenship, and the Police in Interwar Paris." Ph.D. diss., Princeton University, 2000.

Ross, Kristin. *Fast Cars, Clean Bodies: Decolonization and the Reordering of French Culture*. Cambridge, Mass.: MIT Press, 1995.

Rouby. "Un aliéné arabe en liberté." *Bulletin médical de l'Algérie* (30 October 1905): 573–77.

―――. "Les aliénés en liberté." *Bulletin médical de l'Algérie* (15 November 1908): 625–29.

―――. "Les aliénés arabes en liberté: Kabyle inculpé d'homicide volontaire." *Bulletin médical de l'Algérie* (November 1903): 425–32.

Roudinesco, Elisabeth. *La bataille de cent ans: Histoire de la psychanalyse en France.* 2 vols. Paris: Seuil, 1982–85.

―――. *Jacques Lacan*. Trans. Barbara Bray. New York: Columbia University Press, 1997.

Roudinesco, Elisabeth, and Michel Plon. "Paranoïa." In *Dictionnaire de la psychanalyse*. Paris: Fayard, 1998. 764–68.

Rouillon, Frédéric. Introduction, Premier Congrès de la Société Franco-Algérienne de Psychiatrie, 3 October 2003. http://www.sfapsy.com/Premier-congres/Congres-1.htm, accessed 29 June 2006.

Rubenovitch, Pierre. "La notion d'évolution et les rapports de la mentalité primitive avec la psychopathologie." *L'evolution psychiatrique* 11, no. 2 (1935): 77–92.

Rudolph, Luc, and Christophe Soullez. *Insécurité: La vérité.* Saint-Amand-Montrond: Ed. JC Lattès, 2002.

Sadowsky, Jonathan. *Imperial Bedlam: Institutions of Madness in Colonial Southwest Nigeria.* Berkeley: University of California Press, 1999.

Said, Edward W. *Orientalism.* New York: Vintage, 1978.

Sardan, Jean-Pierre Olivier de. "Possession, affliction et folie: Les ruses de la thérapisation." *L'homme* 131 (1994): 7–27.

Sauzay, Paul. "L'assistance aux psychopathes (aliénés et non-aliénés) en Algérie: Etat actuel de la question." Med. thesis, Algiers, 1925.

Savarèse, Eric. *Histoire coloniale et immigration: Une invention de l'étranger.* Paris: Séguier, 2000.

Sayad, Abdelmalek. *La double absence: Des illusions de l'émigré aux souffrances de l'immigré.* Paris: Seuil, 1999.

Schaar, Stuart. "Creation of a Mass Political Culture in Tunisia." *Maghreb Review* 18 (1993): 2–17.

Schaefer, Sylvia. *Children in Moral Danger and the Problem of Government in Third Republic France.* Princeton, N.J.: Princeton University Press, 1997.

Scham, Alan. *Lyautey in Morocco: Protectorate Administration, 1912–1925.* Berkeley: University of California Press, 1970.

Scheper-Hughes, Nancy. *Death without Weeping: The Violence of Everyday Life in Brazil.* Berkeley: University of California Press, 1992.

———. "The Global Traffic in Human Organs." *Current Anthropology* 41, no. 2 (2000): 191–224.

Schiebinger, Londa. *The Mind Has No Sex? Women in the Origins of Modern Science.* Cambridge, Mass.: Harvard University Press, 1993.

———. *Nature's Body: Gender in the Making of Modern Science.* Boston: Beacon Press, 1993.

Schilder, Kees. *Popular Islam in Tunisia.* Leiden: African Studies Centre, 1991.

Schneider, William. "The Scientific Study of Labor in Interwar France." *French Historical Studies* 17, no. 2 (1991): 410–46.

Scott, David. "Colonial Governmentality." *Social Text* 43 (1995): 191–220.

Scott, Joan Wallach. "French Universalism in the Nineties." *Differences* 15, no. 2 (2004): 32–53.

Scull, Andrew. "Somatic Treatments and the Historiography of Psychiatry." *History of Psychiatry* 5 (1994): 1–12.

Secord, James. "The Crisis of Nature." In *Cultures of Natural History,* ed. Nicholas Jardine, James A. Secord, and E. C. Spary. New York: Cambridge University Press, 1996. 447–59.

Shepard, Todd. "Decolonizing France: Reimagining the Nation and Redefining the Republic at the End of the Algerian War." Ph. D. diss., Rutgers University, 2001.

Sherman, Daniel J. "The Arts and Sciences of Colonialism." *French Historical Studies* 23 (2000): 707–29.

Shorter, Edward. *A History of Psychiatry from the Era of the Asylum to the Age of Prozac.* New York: John Wiley and Sons, 1997.

Showalter, Elaine. *The Female Malady: Women, Madness, and English Culture, 1830–1980.* New York: Pantheon, 1985.

Silverstein, Paul A. *Algeria in France: Transpolitics, Race, and Nation.* Bloomington: Indiana University Press, 2004.

Simon, Jacques, ed. *L'immigration algérienne en France: De 1962 à nos jours.* Paris: L'Harmattan, 2002.

Sinha, Mrinalini. *Colonial Masculinity: The "Manly Englishman" and the "Effeminate Bengali" in the Late Nineteenth Century.* New York: Manchester University Press, 1995.

Soubeiga, André. "Syncrétisme et pratiques thérapeutiques des marabouts au Burkina Faso." *Sociologie Santé* 8 (December 1993): 54–64.

Soumeire, Henri. "Meurtre chez les aliénés indigènes algériens." Med. thesis, Marseille, 1932.

Starrett, Gregory. "Culture Never Dies: Anthropology at Abu Ghraib." *Anthropology News* 45, no. 6 (September 2004): 10–11.

Stora, Benjamin. *La gangrène et l'oubli: La mémoire de la guerre d'Algérie.* Paris: Editions la Découverte, 1998.

———. *Histoire de l'Algérie coloniale (1830–1954).* Paris: Editions la Découverte, 1991.

———. *Histoire de l'Algérie depuis l'indépendance,* vol. 1, *1962–1988.* Paris: Editions la Découverte, 2001.

———. *Histoire de la guerre d'Algérie, 1954–1962.* Paris: Editions la Découverte, 2002.

———. "Le Maghreb face à l'Europe." *Esprit* (1999): 215–27.

———. *Le transfert d'une mémoire: De l'"Algérie française" au racisme anti-Arabe.* Paris: Editions la Découverte, 1999.

Stoler, Ann Laura. *Race and the Education of Desire: Foucault's History of Sexuality and the Colonial Order of Things.* Durham, N.C.: Duke University Press, 1995.

———. "Rethinking Colonial Categories: European Communities and the Boundaries of Rule." *Comparative Studies in Society and History* 31 (1989): 134–61.

Sutter, Jean. *L'épilepsie mentale chez l'indigène nord-africain: Étude clinique.* Algiers: Crescenzo, 1937.

———. "Une famille des psychopathes." *Annales médico-psychologiques* 100, no. 1 (1942): 40–50.

———. Review of Suzanne Taïeb, "Les idées d'influence dans la pathologie mentale de l'indigène nord-africain." *Annales médico-psychologiques* 99, no. 1 (1941): 55.

Sutter, Jean, and Maurice Porot. "Hypertension artérielle et électro-choc." *Annales médico-psychologiques* 107, no. 2 (1949): 1–12.

Sutter, Jean, and G. Pascalis. "Effets psychologiques de la chlorpromazine." *L'encéphale* 45, no. 4 (1956): 979–86.

Swain, Gladys. *Le sujet de la folie: Naissance de la psychiatrie.* Toulouse: Privat, 1977.

Swazey, Judith. *Chlorpromazine in Psychiatry: A Study of Therapeutic Innovation.* Cambridge, Mass.: MIT Press, 1973.

Swearingen, Will D. *Moroccan Mirages: Agrarian Dreams and Deceptions, 1912–1986.* Princeton, N.J.: Princeton University Press, 1987.

Taguieff, Pierre-André. "Face à l'immigration: Mixophobie, xénophobie ou sélection: Un débat français dans l'entre-deux-guerres." *Vingtième siècle* 47 (1995): 103–31.

Taïeb, Suzanne. "Les idées d'influence dans la pathologie mentale de l'indigène nord-africain: Le rôle des superstitions." Med. thesis, Algiers, 1939.

Talbott, John. *The War without a Name: France in Algeria, 1954–1962.* New York: Knopf, 1980.

Taleb, Mohamed. Interview in "Souffrances et mémoires Djazaïr 2003." Press release at http://www.sfapsy.com/Premier-congres/Congres-1.htm, accessed 29 June 2006.

Terracini, Jeanne. *Si bleu le ciel, si blanche la ville.* Paris: Albin Michel, 1996.

Thiher, Allen. *Revels in Madness: Insanity in Medicine and Literature.* Michigan: University of Michigan Press, 2000.

Thuillier, Jean. *Ten Years That Changed the Face of Mental Illness.* Trans. Gordon Hickish. London: Martin Dunitz, 1999.

Tillion, Germaine. *L'Algérie en 1957.* Paris: Editions de Minuit, 1957.

Tissot, Sylvie, and Pierre Tévanian. *Stop quelle violence?* Paris: l'Esprit frappeur, 2001.

"Tobie Nathan: L'excision est en quelque sorte un mécanisme de prévention mentale, avec un bénéfice social extraordinaire." *Afrique magazine* 163 (1999): 57.

Torgovnick, Marianna. *Gone Primitive: Savage Intellects, Modern Lives.* Chicago: University of Chicago Press, 1990.

Toulouse, Edouard. "La conduite de la vie." *La prophylaxie mentale* 6, no. 17 (1929): 3–9.

———. "Les hôpitaux et services d'observation et de traitement." *Revue de psychiatrie*, 3rd ser., no. 3 (1899): 165–78; citation at 165.

———. *Le problème de la prophylaxie mentale.* Paris: Imprimerie Chaix, 1929.

Toulouse, Edouard, and Roger Dupouy. "De la transformation des asiles d'aliénés en hôpitaux psychiatriques." *L'hygiène mentale* 22 (1927): 83–89.

Trenga, Victor. *L'âme arabo-berbère: Étude sociologique sur la société musulmane nord-africaine.* Algiers: Homar, 1913.

———. *Sur les psychoses chez les Juifs d'Algérie.* Montpellier: Delord, Boehm et Martial, 1902.

Turin, Yvonne. *Affrontements culturels dans l'Algérie coloniale: Écoles, médecines, religion, 1830–1880.* Paris: Maspero, 1971.

Turner, Patricia. *I Heard It through the Grapevine: Rumor in African-American Culture.* Berkeley: University of California Press, 1993.

Vadon, Raoul. "L'assistance médicale des psychopathes en Tunisie." Med. thesis, Marseille, 1935.

Valensi, Lucette. *Tunisian Peasants in the Eighteenth and Nineteenth Centuries.* Trans. Beth Archer. New York: Cambridge University Press, 1985.

Valenstein, Eliot S. *Great and Desperate Cures: The Rise and Decline of Psychosurgery and Other Radical Treatments for Mental Illness.* New York: Basic Books, 1986.

Variot, G. "Une visite à l'hôpital arabe de Tunis." *La revue scienifique de la France et de l'étranger*, 3rd ser., 1 (23 April 1881): 537–38.

Vaughan, Megan. *CuringTheir Ills: Colonial Power and African Illness.* Stanford, Calif.: Stanford University Press, 1991.

Vergès, Françoise. "Chains of Madness, Chains of Colonialism: Fanon and Freedom." In *The Fact of Blackness: Frantz Fanon and Visual Representation*, ed. Alan Read. Seattle, Wash.: Bay Press, 1996. 46–75.

———. "Creole Skin, Black Mask: Fanon and Disavowal." *Critical Inquiry* 23 (1997): 578–95.

———. *Monsters and Revolutionaries.* Durham, N.C.: Duke University Press, 1999.

Voisin, Auguste. "Souvenirs d'un voyage en Tunisie (1896)." *Annales médico-psychologiques* 54, no. 2 (1896): 89–90.

Wacquant, Loïc. "Sur quelques contes sécuritaires." *Le monde diplomatique* (May 2002): 6–7.

Walker, David. *Outrage and Insight: Modern French Writers and the "Fait Divers."* London: Berg, 1995.

Walkowitz, Judith. *City of Dreadful Delight: Narratives of Sexual Danger in Late Victorian London.* Chicago: University of Chicago Press, 1992.

Wallon, Henri. "L'oeuvre de Lévy-Bruhl et la psychologie comparée." *Revue philosophique* (1939): 254–57.

Weber, Eugen. *France: Fin de siècle.* Cambridge, Mass.: Harvard University Press, 1986.

Weiner, Dora B. *Comprendre et soigner: Philippe Pinel et la médecine de l'esprit.* Paris: Fayard, 1999.

White, Luise. *Speaking with Vampires: Rumor and History in Colonial Africa.* Berkeley: University of California Press, 2000.

Wilder, Gary. *The French Imperial Nation-State: Negritude and Colonial Humanism between the Two World Wars.* Chicago: University of Chicago Press, 2005.

Windholz, G., and L. H. Witherspoon. "Sleep as a Cure for Schizophrenia: A Historical Episode." *History of Psychiatry* 4 (1993): 83–93.

Wojciechowski, Jean-Bernard. *Hygiène mentale et hygiène sociale.* 2 vols. Paris: Harmattan, 1997.

Wright, Gwendolyn. *The Politics of Design in French Colonial Urbanism.* Chicago: University of Chicago Press, 1991.

———. "Tradition in the Service of Modernity: Architecture and Urbanism in French Colonial Policy, 1900–1930." *Journal of Modern History* 59, no. 2 (1987): 291–316.

Wurgaft, Lewis. *The Imperial Imagination: Magic and Myth in Kipling's India.* Middletown, Conn.: Wesleyan University Press, 1983.

Yacine, Kateb. *Le cercle des représailles.* Paris: Seuil, 1959.

———. *Nedjma.* Paris: Seuil, 1956.

———. *L'oeuvre en fragments: Inédits littéraires et textes retrouvés.* Ed. Jacqueline Arnaud. Paris: Sindbad, 1986.

———. "Poésie et vérité de *La femme sauvage.*" In *Kateb Yacine, éclats de mémoire,* ed. Olivier Corpet and Albert Dichy. Paris: IMEC Editions, 1994. 39–41.

———. *Le poète comme un boxeur: Entretiens, 1958–1989.* Paris: Seuil, 1994.

———. *Le polygone étoilé.* Paris: Seuil, 1966.

———. "La rose de Blida." *Les Lettres françaises,* 7–13 February 1963, 4.

Yealland, Lewis. *Hysterical Disorders in Warfare.* London: Macmillan, 1918.

Youssef, Hanafy, and Salah Fadl. "Frantz Fanon and Political Psychiatry." *History of Psychiatry* 7 (1996): 525–32.

Zahar, Renate. *L'oeuvre de Frantz Fanon: Colonialisme et aliénation dans l'oeuvre de Frantz Fanon.* Trans. Roger Dangeville. Paris: Maspéro, 1970.

Zahzah, Abdenour, and Bachir Ridouh, dirs. *Frantz Fanon: Mémoire d'asile* [film]. Algeria, 2002. DVD: Paris: Mille et une Productions, 2002.

Ziou Ziou, A. "Psychiatrie moderne? Psychiatrie traditionnelle?" *Lamalif* 161 (1984): 52–54.

Index

1968, student revolution, 231

Abbas, Ferhat, 159
Abdel-Jaouad, Hédi, 177–78
acclimatization, 41
Action Française, 207
Adas, Michael, 132
Agamben, Giorgio, 179, 249n1
AIDS, 111
Aïssawa, 244n95
Aix-en-Provence, asylum at, 41–43,
  86, 126
Alapetite, Gabriel, 10, 29–30, 150
alcohol, alcoholism, 90–91, 93, 98,
  103, 145, 146, 147, 172
Algeria: civil war, 1990s, 194;
  conquest and settlement of, 3,
  10–11, 24, 40–41, 125, 126;
  elections in, 224, 225; epidemics
  in, 41; governmental organization of, 50; psychiatric reform
  in, 40–45, 47–81; settler community in, 8, 16, 64, 96–97,
  101–2, 128, 138, 140, 152, 164,
  223; urban planning in, 69
Algerian Fiscal Assemblies, 44,
  50–51, 62–79
Algerian war: and end of colonial
  psychiatry, 3, 207, 230; and
  Fanon, 164, 181; and immigration, 148–50, 207; and
  Islamism, 200–201; and Kateb,
  174, 180; and medicine, 110,
  194–96, 198; and memory, 222–
  26; and psychological warfare,

7, 16, 123, 150–59, 250n26; and
  repatriation, 206; and torture,
  105; and violence, 186
Algérie médicale, 144
Algiers: medical faculty, 3, 44, 66,
  137, 194, 196; University of, 99,
  138, 145
Algiers School: and Algerian war,
  152, 154–56, 194, 206, 207,
  230; concern with innovation,
  118, 228, 230; and Esch-
  Chadely, 172–73; and ethnopsychiatry, 3, 16–18, 122–23,
  129–50, 191, 192, 213, 215,
  216, 231, 244n102; and Fanon,
  124, 163, 164–65, 171; and
  Kateb, 184, 187; and Memmi,
  170; A. Porot's direction of,
  57–58
Aliénations (Bensmaïl), 193–94, 200
Alliez, Joseph, 148
Almohad dynasty, Morocco, 34
Ammar, Sleïm, 171–72, 180, 182,
  183, 188, 196, 197–98, 202, 203
Amrouche, Jean el-Mouhoub, 159,
  169–70, 182, 188
Anjanamasina, asylum at, 49
Annales médico-psychologiques,
  42–43, 124, 140, 145, 147, 166
Antabuse (disulfiram), 103
Antheaume, André, 60
antihistamines, 228–29, 230
antipsychiatry, 172, 195, 231,
  252n2
Apter, Emily, 8